D1556461

Menelaus' Orthopaedic Management of
Spina Bifida Cystica

RJ496
S74
m45
1998

Menelaus' Orthopaedic Management of Spina Bifida Cystica

Third Edition

Edited by

Nigel S Broughton FRCS Ed, FRCS, FRACS

Honorary Consultant Orthopaedic Surgeon
Royal Children's Hospital
Melbourne, Australia

and

Malcolm B Menelaus MD, FRCS, FRACS

Senior Orthopaedic Surgeon
Royal Children's Hospital
Melbourne, Australia

WB Saunders Company Limited
London   Philadelphia   Toronto   Sydney   Tokyo

WB Saunders is an imprint of Harcourt Brace and Company Limited

Harcourt Brace and Company Limited 24–28 Oval Road
London NW1 7DX, UK

The Curtis Center
Independence Square West
Philadelphia, PA 19106–3399, USA

Harcourt Brace & Company
55 Horner Avenue
Toronto, Ontario M8Z 4X6, Canada

Harcourt Brace & Company, Australia
30–52 Smidmore Street
Marrickville, NSW 2204, Australia

Harcourt Brace & Company, Japan
Ichibancho Central Building, 22–1 Ichibancho
Chiyoda-ku, Tokyo 102, Japan

© 1998 Harcourt Brace and Company Limited

This book is printed on acid-free paper

All rights reserved. No part of this publication may be reproduced, stored in a retrieval system or transmitted, in any form or by any means electronic, mechanical, photocopying or otherwise, without the prior permission of Harcourt Brace and Company Limited, 24–28 Oval Road, London NW1 7DX, UK

First published 1971
Second edition 1980
Third edition 1998

A catalogue record for this book is available from the British Library

ISBN 0-7020-2149-0

Typeset by Paston Press Ltd, Loddon, Norfolk
Printed and bound at The Bath Press, Avon, UK

Contents

Contributors

Catherine A Abery B App Sci (Phy), Post Grad Dip Phy (Paeds)
Senior Orthopaedic Physiotherapist, Royal Children's Hospital, Melbourne

John S Barnett MB BS, FRACS
Honorary Plastic Surgeon, Royal Children's Hospital, Melbourne
Consultant Plastic Surgeon, Austin Hospital, Melbourne

Shane A Barwood MB BS
Research Fellow, The Hugh Williamson Gait Analysis Laboratory, Royal Children's Hospital, Melbourne

Nigel S Broughton FRCS Ed, FRCS, FRACS
Honorary Consultant Orthopaedic Surgeon, Royal Children's Hospital, Melbourne

Kester Brown MB ChB, MD, FANZCA, FRCA
Director of Anaesthesia, Royal Children's Hospital, Melbourne

Douglas Bryan MB BS, FRACP, FAFRM
Deputy Director, Department of Child Development and Rehabilitation,
Consultant Paediatrician, Spina Bifida Clinic, Royal Children's Hospital, Melbourne

D Robert V Dickens MB BS, FRACS
Director of Orthopaedics, Royal Children's Hospital, Melbourne

Catherine M Duffy MB FRCS(I)
Research Fellow, Mitre Gait Analysis Laboratory, Musgrave Park Hospital, Belfast

Kevin B Dunne MB BS, FRACP
Consultant Paediatrician, Department of Child Development and Rehabilitation, and the Spina Bifida Clinic, Royal Children's Hospital, Melbourne

Jane L Galvin B App Sci (OT)
Senior Occupational Therapist, Royal Children's Hospital, Melbourne

H Kerr Graham MD, FRCS Ed, FRACS
Professor of Orthopaedic Surgery, Director, The Hugh Williamson Gait Analysis Laboratory, Royal Children's Hospital, Melbourne

Jane L Halliday BSc (Hons), PhD
Epidemiology Unit, Murdoch Institute, Melbourne

Geoffrey L Klug MB BS, FRACS
Senior Neurosurgeon, Department of Neurosurgery, Royal Children's Hospital, Melbourne

John O Lavarack MB BS, PhD, FRCPA (Deceased)
Former Reader in Histology and Embryology, University of Melbourne

Malcolm B Menelaus MD, FRCS, FRACS
Senior Orthopaedic Surgeon, Royal Children's Hospital, Melbourne

David Phillips B App Sci (P&O)
Senior Orthotist/Prosthetist, Royal Children's Hospital, Melbourne

John G Rogers MB BS, DCH, FRACP
Senior Medical Geneticist, Murdoch Institute and Victorian Clinical Genetics Service,
Senior Associate, Department of Paediatrics, University of Melbourne

Ian P Torode MB BS, DABOS, FRCS(C), FRACS
Deputy Director of Orthopaedics, Royal Children's Hospital, Melbourne

Preface to the Third Edition

Since the 2nd edition of *Orthopaedic Management of Spina Bifida Cystica* was published in 1980 our knowledge and understanding of the child with spina bifida has progressed considerably. In preparing the 3rd edition of the book, several new sections have been added and most of the chapters have been rewritten, reflecting the advances made in the orthopaedic management of this condition.

We would consider the greatest change that has taken place over the past 16 years has been our understanding of the aetiology of deformity; we now appreciate that muscle imbalance is not the cause of deformity at the hip, knee and foot in most instances, nor is it the cause of dislocation of the hip. Our operative management of the hip in these children has altered with our understanding that dislocation of the hip has little effect on walking ability. We have now abandoned prophylactic muscle-balancing procedures to prevent deformity. Over the years we have refined our indications and type of surgery for the foot and knee and these changes in approach and technique are reflected in the sections on surgery of the lower limb. We have worked on various projects over the years studying the results after surgery, so we now feel that our teaching is based on sound evidence and there have been many alterations in our recommendations since the second edition.

Another area that has developed over the past 16 years has been neurosurgical imaging and the recognition of the harmful effects of cord tethering and syrinx formation producing late deformity in these children.

We are grateful to Geoffrey Klug for a new chapter in this edition appraising the latest developments in this area.

Gait analysis is another area that has developed considerably over the past 16 years. It is already proving a valuable tool to assess these children, but its full potential is still under investigation. We have found that gait analysis can evaluate the effect of surgery more accurately and give some idea of the expectations after surgery much sooner than in the past. We are grateful for an appraisal of the latest developments in this field by our colleague, Professor Kerr Graham, who is a recognized leader in this field.

Spinal surgery in spina bifida has improved, both in the understanding of the mechanics and also the instrumentation used. We are grateful to Ian Torode and Bob Dickens for their contributions to the chapter on spinal surgery conditions.

Orthotic management, the philosophy of physiotherapy and the care of pressure sores in these children have all changed and improved over the years and the text reflects this.

The 3rd edition is therefore an opportunity to document all of the above changes. Many of the recommendations in this edition are at variance with those in previous editions, but we are keen to describe our present management of these children in response to requests by our peers. We hope that at the very least this work will improve management and stimulate further study of this condition.

Acknowledgements

The development of our expertise in the management of children with spina bifida has only been possible with the help of many people throughout the Royal Children's Hospital, Melbourne. We are privileged to work in an institution with excellence throughout its many departments, and the study of and refinement of our techniques is only possible with the support of our many colleagues.

Our studies of the natural history of deformity and the influence of surgery, and similar studies have relied on Professor David Shurtleff of the Children's Hospital, Seattle. He developed the computer database called Patient Data Management System on which all our studies over the past 10 years have been based. David has also improved the study of these children throughout the world by the development of the International Myelodysplasia Study Group.

We are most grateful to Ann Stillwell, Liz Williams, Judy Coates and Cathy Abery in their assessment of these children over the past 20 years. Their contribution and commitment is immeasurable and none of our studies would have been possible without their great care and meticulous collection of data.

The encouragement to develop a specialized service for these children can only come from a well-organized department of orthopaedics and for that we are grateful to Peter Williams and all our present colleagues who give us help and support: Professor Kerr Graham, Bob Dickens, Ian Torode, Roy Carey, Mark O'Sullivan, Gary Nattrass and Bill Doig. We are also grateful to Anne McCoy, Head of Physiotherapy and David Phillips, orthotist, for their continued help and collaboration. The Educational Resource Centre has prepared illustrations to the highest possible standard and Dr S S Tan, Head of Embryology, at the University of Melbourne has helped in preparing the section on embryology.

Nigel Broughton would like to acknowledge Gill Hunt and the late Alan Murley in encouraging his initial interest in the subject and also to document his appreciation to Malcolm Menelaus in being given the opportunity to study these children with him.

Over the past 15 years many Fellows and Registrars at the Royal Children's Hospital have worked on projects studying the natural history of deformity and the effects of treatment. We are grateful to John Mazur, David Brougham, Paul Cooke, Brad Olney, James Wright, John Williams, Geoff Graham, Rob Fraser, Mark Romness, George Godette, P S Sandhu, Phil Frawley, Minne Heeg and Paul Marshall for their hard work in this regard. We also thank Anne Dalby who has worked unstintingly in the preparation of the manuscript.

We are grateful to our wives and families in giving us continued support allowing us to produce this work.

Our greatest acknowledgement must be to the children themselves who put their trust in our management, so we can help them and others similarly affected.

Chapter 1

General Considerations

INTRODUCTION
Nigel S Broughton and Malcolm B Menelaus

Despite increased preventative measures we continue to see significant numbers of children with myelomeningocele, about 65% of whom have normal intelligence. Every doctor who has been involved with this disease has despaired for the future of a baby with myelomeningocele associated with total paralysis of the legs, urinary and faecal incontinence and the likelihood of hydrocephalus; yet with appropriate management, the disability from each of these problems can be considerably reduced.

The management of the orthopaedic disabilities is a challenge to ensure these children fulfil the maximum potential that their neurosegmental deficit imposes on them. Many of the children with high level lesions walk in childhood but later find that they are more mobile in a wheelchair. At an early stage we explain the probability of this to the parents and do what is appropriate to enable walking in childhood. We now know that, although this may often later be abandoned, a period of walking will enhance transfer ability and quality of life in adulthood (Mazur *et al.*, 1989). The development and improvement of reciprocating orthoses since 1980 has greatly improved the ability of children with high level lesions to walk. Many children with spina bifida integrate successfully into normal community life, with the respect and satisfaction that this brings. If we can effect improvement in their ability to lead an independent life then active management is well worthwhile.

The role of the orthopaedic surgeon in spina bifida cystica is to encourage a pattern of development in the child as near normal as possible. There are many factors that influence the pattern of development of each child. These include the neurosegmental level of the lesion, the level of intelligence, the presence of upper motor neurone lesions and upper limb abnormalities and obesity. The orthopaedic surgeon should be aware of these influences and their significance in each child.

In order to establish an appropriate pattern of development it is clearly necessary to provide, by conservative or operative means, stable posture and effective gait. The measures taken to achieve these ends should be aimed to meet not only childhood needs but also be appropriate for the expected pattern of adult life.

To ensure proper management, the orthopaedic surgeon should be aware of the services and expertise offered by a wide range of medical and paramedical specialities. This is necessary in order that the child and his or her family receive co-ordinated support.

The aims of this book are to consider the factors that influence orthopaedic management, to review our own and others' experience, to advocate a particular approach to management and to describe the precise treatment for the individual child.

Definitions

Throughout this book, the following definitions obtain. The terms brace and orthosis are used synonymously and include calipers and splints.

Community walkers

Patients who can walk and live in the community with little or no restriction in walking ability. They may require crutches or braces or both. They can manage ramps, stairs and public transport.

Household walkers

Patients who can walk only indoors or on level outdoor areas. They require apparatus but can transfer themselves in and out of a chair or bed with little or no assistance. They may require a wheelchair for some indoor activities (at home or at school) and for most community activities. They can put on their own braces.

Functional walkers

This includes community and household walkers.

Non-functional walkers

Walking is only carried out during physiotherapy sessions. A wheelchair is used at other times. This is a temporary phase; the patient will either progress to functional walking or become a non-walker.

Non-walkers

Patients who use a wheelchair exclusively but may be able to transfer themselves from the chair to their bed. (These are based on Hoffer *et al.*, 1973.)

Definitions and Incidence of Spinal Lesions

The following terminology has been used throughout.

Spina bifida occulta

An unfused condition of the vertebral arches without any cystic distension of the meninges. This form occurs in approximately 10% of adult spines and most commonly affects the fifth lumbar and first sacral vertebrae. There may or may not be changes in the overlying skin or abnormal neurological signs or pathology in the spinal cord. The latter occurs in a small number of patients and leads to progressive neurological signs, generally between the ages of 8 and 14 years, revealed by progressive deformity of the feet or changes in micturition.

Meningocele

An unfused condition of the vertebral arches with cystic distension of the meninges. The spinal cord is confined to the vertebral canal. It is relatively uncommon, occurring in 6% of cases of spina bifida cystica, but because of the higher death rate in cases of myelomeningocele, it occurs in 11% of survivors. Hydrocephalus is rare, the mental state of the child is generally normal and the overall prognosis is excellent.

Myelomeningocele

An unfused condition of the vertebral arches with cystic distension of the meninges and with cord or roots lying in the sac, resulting in abnormal neurological signs. It occurs in 94% of cases of spina bifida cystica and 89%

of survivors and is the most important, and unfortunately the commonest, variety of the disease.

Spina bifida cystica

Includes meningocele and myelomeningocele.

EMBRYOLOGY
John O Lavarack

The Normal Development of the Spinal Cord and its Coverings

The spinal cord and other parts of the central and peripheral nervous systems develop from the neural plate. Experiments on other vertebrates have shown that the neural plate differentiates, from surface ectoderm, under the inductive influence of the adjacent notochordal process and mesoderm. The chordamesoderm itself differentiates to form the dura and vertebral coverings of the cord.

Formation and development of the neural tube

The neural plate forms neural folds, between which lies the neural groove, by the 20th day. The neural folds begin to close when the embryo has six or seven somites at about the 22nd day. Closure commences in the cervical region and proceeds cranially and caudally.

Closure of the neural tube is completed by closure of the cranial neuropore (at about the 24th day) and of the caudal neuropore (at about the 26th day, when the embryo has about 25 somites).

The segmental level at which the caudal neuropore closes has not been determined. Behind this the caudal extremity of the neural tube is described as forming in the cell mass of the tail but by a process of canalization (Lemire, 1975).

As the neural tube forms, its proliferating cells constitute a neuroepithelium. After closure of the tube these cells begin to differentiate to form neuroblasts, which migrate outwards from the neuroepithelium to become neurones of the spinal cord and their processes. Processes of the motor neurones grow out from the cord as motor axons of the peripheral nerves. The cells at the margins of the neural plate (after folding) form a column on each side, the neural crest, between the dorsal aspect of the neural tube and the ectoderm. The neural crest cells later form the sensory neurones of the posterior root ganglia and their axons, and the peripheral cells and processes of the autonomic nervous system and the pia and arachnoid.

Much of the caudal extremity of the neural tube undergoes regression, and is finally represented by the filum terminale. The spinal cord gradually recedes up the spinal canal as gestation proceeds. The origin of the first sacral nerve from the cord is at the level of the first lumbar vertebra at term. The spinal cord terminates at the level of the third lumbar vertebra at term, and at the first lumbar vertebra in the adult.

Development of coverings of the spinal cord

The arachnoid and pia differentiate from the neural crest cells surrounding the neural tube and the dura from the surrounding mesenchyme. The pia mater differentiates in the mesenchyme surrounding the cord at about the 40th day, at which time chondrification begins from two centres in each vertebral body. Two or three days later the dura mater is recognizable, and chondrification begins in a centre in each vertebral arch. By the 3rd month the cartilagenous vertebral arches are united dorsally and with the centra. Ossification follows.

The Development of Spina Bifida

Spina bifida belongs to a group of disturbances of development of the vertebral arches or cranial vault. These are often associated with disturbances of development of structures derived from the neural tube, and of the meninges, and may give rise to cyst formation. The diversity of the disturbances suggests that causative factors exert their effects at different periods of development.

Spina bifida cystica

Myeloschisis or myelocele (Figure 1.1)
In this, the most severe form of the defect, vertebral arches are deficient and neural plate material is spread out on the surface, sometimes in a shallow depression, more commonly over a cystic swelling of the meninges. It is found most commonly in the lumbosacral region. Although other explanations have been offered (Gardner, 1968; Padget, 1970), it is widely accepted that a defect in closure of the spinal neural tube underlies this condition and that overgrowth of the neural plate is a primary defect (Patten, 1952). Secondarily, the exposed neural plate becomes covered by epithelium (Cameron, 1956).

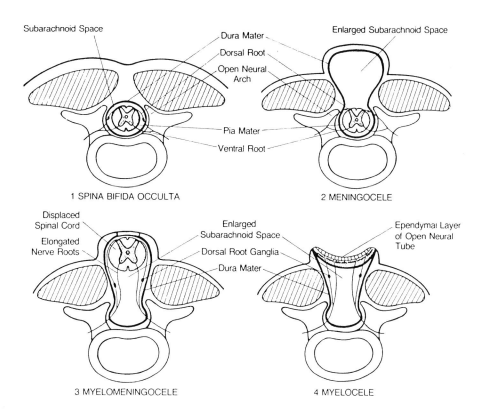

Figure 1.1 Types of spina bifida (based on Patten, 1952).

Myelomeningocele (Figure I.I)

There is a fluid-filled cystic swelling, formed by dura and arachnoid, protruding through a defect in the vertebral arches under the skin, and the spinal cord and nerve roots are carried out into the fundus of the sac. In these cases the neural tube appears to have closed normally, but rarely the central canal is distended to form the whole or part of the cystic swelling – the condition of myelocystocele or myelocele proper.

Meningocele (Figure I.I)

In this relatively uncommon variety of spina bifida cystica, a cystic swelling of dura and arachnoid protrudes through a defect in the vertebral arches under the skin and is filled with fluid. The spinal cord is entirely confined to the vertebral canal, but may exhibit abnormalities.

There is little information on the mode of development of the cystic swelling in myelomeningocele and meningocele, but it may be supposed that the disturbance of development of the meninges manifests itself later than disturbances of neural tube closure. Gardner's theory (1968) is that the development of cysts, whether of the cord or the subarachnoid space, is the result of over-distension with the fluid normally produced by the neuroepithelium after closure of the neural tube. He suggests that over-distension may be of a degree to produce neural tube rupture. On this basis, myeloschises would be the result of secondary reopening of the neural tube after closure. Gardner's suggestion has new relevance as hydrosyringomyelia is a cause of progressive scoliosis in myelomeningocele (Chapter 12).

Spina bifida occulta (*Figure I.I*)

There is a localized defect in one or more of the vertebral arches, presumably developing as a failure of the halves of the vertebral arches to meet and fuse in the 3rd month. The spinal cord and meninges remain within the vertebral canal.

The skin overlying spina bifida occulta may be normal, or there may be a dimple which may connect with the dura mater by a fibrous cord, a patch of hairs, pigmentation, or a lipoma which may connect with an intradural fatty component. All these and the rare intramedullary dermoid are of a theoretical interest as possibly representing abnormalities of separation of presumptive skin from neural tissue during the process of closure of the neural tube.

Associated abnormalities

Abnormalities of the spinal cord which may be associated with spina bifida cystica (or occulta) are duplica-tion of the cord or diastematomyelia, and dilatation of the central canal or hydromyelia. The frequency of occurrence of these associations suggests again that the primary defect in spina bifida is commonly in the neural tube.

The skeletal defect in spina bifida may include any of the wide range of defects in segmentation of vertebral bodies and failure of fusion of two halves of vertebral bodies. This anterior spina bifida is one of a group of malformations thought to be due to persistence of the relationship between the roof of the developing gut and the neural plate, with a bipartite notochord (Feller and Sternberg, 1929).

GENETIC COUNSELLING
John G Rogers and Jane L Halliday

Genetic counselling, prenatal diagnosis, serum screening programmes and folate ingestion can all contribute to the prevention of neural tube disorders.

All parents who have a child with a neural tube defect require genetic counselling. We believe that this counselling is best undertaken in specialist medical genetics clinics because of the reservoir of counselling experience and the freedom to challenge the parents' belief, free of the role of providing medical care. Parents learning that their child has a neural tube defect will experience a grief reaction regardless of whether the child survives or dies. It is important that this is recognized and acknowledged. Families require the opportunity of knowing about and understanding the problems that affect their children. It is thus always important to give the parents a detailed explanation about anencephaly or spina bifida.

Parents who have a child with a neural tube defect that dies require an opportunity to mourn for that child. Studies (Lewis, 1976) have shown it is easier to mourn for a baby that has been seen than for an unseen object. The fantasies of parents about the sort of monsters they have produced are much greater when the baby is unseen. We would thus encourage parents to see and to handle their baby. Babies with spina bifida and anencephaly can be draped in such a way as to make them acceptable. Some parents will wish to look directly at the lesion so they can better understand it.

Neural tube defects have been shown to follow a multifactorial pattern of inheritance (Carter, 1976). In this situation a number of genes are thought to have a small additive effect, together with at present undefined environmental factors. When this compound effect passes a critical threshold there is a liability for the child to have the disorder. Most common malformations such as cleft lip and palate, congenital heart disease, talipes equino-varus and developmental dysplasia of the hip fit this pattern of inheritance.

The birth of a child with spina bifida also predisposes to the birth of a child with anencephaly and vice versa. It has also been shown that having a child with extensive congenital vertebral anomalies (Wynne-Davies, 1975) or with spinal dysraphism (Carter et al., 1976) gives the same predisposition to spina bifida and anencephaly in subsequent children as does the birth of a child with a neural tube defect (NTD).

Aims

Genetic counselling aims to provide a family with sufficient information to make an informed decision about their future and to help them come to terms with the problems that confront them. Counselling is not merely a statistical discussion about risks but an attempt to provide detailed information about the burden of the disease. Parents' knowledge of this burden may be helped if they have already attended a spina bifida clinic and seen and talked to other families with affected children.

Counselling should be done in a quiet, relaxed atmosphere. Both parents should be seen at the same time and the counselling interview usually takes about 1 hour. A detailed family history is obtained and a family tree drawn. The counselling aims to be non-directive but challenges the family to look at their own values to help them with their decision making. It may take more than one interview to assist a family in reaching their decision. It is important that the family know how to put their decision into effect.

After a stillbirth or death of a child, it is important for a family to give themselves some time to come to terms with this experience. Families know when they are ready to embark on another pregnancy. This may take up to 12 months. Sometimes after the death of a baby, the parents are fairly desperate to have another child in their arms. If they pause for a few months, they realize they are not ready to have a child, and, if they wait a little longer, they realize they have reached the point when they are ready to proceed, albeit with anxiety.

Diagnosis

Genetic counselling requires precise diagnosis. Before counselling any parents of a child with NTD, the counsellor must confirm the diagnosis. This point may sound rather trivial in relationship to spina bifida. However, Holmes et al. (1976) showed that amongst 106 stillborn and liveborn infants with anencephaly,

myelomeningocele, meningocele and encephalocele, six different causes were identified. In 12% the problem was due to a chromosome disorder or was part of the Meckel syndrome, an autosomal recessive condition. With the current fall in the rate of post mortems it is easier to mistake a chromosome disorder or syndrome for an isolated NTD.

Once the diagnosis is established, then an estimate of the recurrence risk can be made. The most common situation in counselling is a family with a clear history who have had one affected child. Counselling should be based on local experience; the recurrence risk varies from area to area and population. It has been reported as 3–4% in women in S.E. England (Sellers and Nevin, 1984; Medical Research Council Vitamin Study Research Group, 1991). In Melbourne we talk about 1 in 50 recurrence risk of NTD, 1 in 100 risk of spina bifida and 1 in 100 risk of anencephaly, although actual data are not available. Recently, we have begun to see the adult survivors with spina bifida who are contemplating a family of their own. If either in a couple have spina bifida the approximate risk of recurrence is 1 in 25 (Carter, 1976).

If parents have had two children with an NTD (Carter, 1973a), the risk rises to approximately 10% and after three children to approximately 25%. To help parents comprehend their risk it is useful to compare it to the 1 in 30 (3%) risk of major birth defects (Riley and Halliday, 1996) occurring in the population at large which most people ignore or regard as an acceptable risk. Risks are often better expressed as odds, in other words that there is a 1 in 25 risk of recurrence, as people generally understand this better than percentages.

Burden

The burden varies considerably depending on whether a child has anencephaly or spina bifida. Anencephalics are usually stillborn or die shortly after birth. Although there is the emotional burden for both parents of going through a pregnancy, parents of a baby with anencephaly do not have the ongoing care of a child with severe disability.

Spina bifida is a very variable condition. This range of variability and the treatment necessary, including orthopaedic procedures, shunts and the problems of incontinence should be discussed in detail, as well as problems of intelligence and the chances of future independent living and treatment. When parents already have a child with spina bifida they need to know in detail about future medical plans and prognosis.

Prenatal Diagnosis of Neural Tube Defects

There are now three techniques that can be used to look for anencephaly or spina bifida in a foetus. These may each be used in isolation or combination:

- amniocentesis
- ultrasound
- maternal serum screening

Amniocentesis

Amniocentesis is usually done at 15 or 16 weeks gestation by insertion of a needle into the uterus, under ultrasound guidance, to take a sample of amniotic fluid. The level of an analyte in the fluid, alphafetoprotein (AFP), is measured; elevated levels may indicate the presence of an open neural tube defect in the foetus, which must be confirmed by ultrasound. When an amniocentesis is performed, the cells in the amniotic fluid are usually cultured and the chromosomes are looked at. Parents need to understand that NTDs are not the only diagnoses that can be made by amniocentesis.

Ultrasound

Careful ultrasound by an experienced operator is probably as accurate in detecting anencephaly as amniocentesis. Ultrasound with a vaginal probe at 10–12 weeks pregnancy can detect most foetuses with anencephaly and occasionally one with spina bifida. This is a useful screening procedure for women who are at high risk of an affected child. This should be followed-up by an ultrasound at 18 weeks, the timing of which allows for a detailed assessment of the cranium and spine.

Maternal serum screening

In recent years, in some centres, maternal serum screening has been available routinely for all pregnant women. Between 15 and 18 weeks of pregnancy a small sample of maternal blood is taken and a number of analytes measured in the serum. As with amniotic fluid, an elevated level of maternal serum AFP suggests the presence of a foetus with a NTD. The other analytes measured in the serum are used to detect an increased risk of the foetus having Down syndrome. The mother's age and an accurate gestational age are necessary for these risk estimations.

This is obviously a less invasive procedure than amniocentesis, but has added problems associated with a screening test:

- Some affected foetuses (approximately 10%) will not be detected (false negatives).
- A follow-up diagnostic test must be done to validate the result, to ensure it is not a false positive. Not all elevated AFP levels are due to neural tube defects and this should be checked by amniocentesis with or without ultrasound. A twin pregnancy, any open lesion which puts the foetal circulation in direct contact with amniotic fluid, or one in which there are specific obstetric problems, may result in elevated serum AFP.

General Comments

The logical outcome of prenatal diagnosis is the termination of a pregnancy in which the foetus is affected. This is not acceptable to all parents and doctors. If doctors find because of their personal views, that they are not able to give the parents factual information about these techniques, they are obliged to refer the parents to a doctor who does not feel a similar constraint.

Prenatal diagnostic studies are best performed by experts at centres where a substantial number of tests are done by a few operators. Experience and training with ultrasound improves accuracy of diagnosis and experience with amniocentesis reduces the number of spontaneous miscarriages which can occur as a complication of the procedure.

Ideally, all parents presenting for prenatal diagnosis will previously have had genetic counselling at which they are informed of the methods available to them and the potential outcomes. Parents need to understand that no technique can detect all birth defects. These tests can remove most of the special risk that an individual runs; however, much of the general risk run by the population, of approximately 3% for major birth defects, cannot be removed.

Use of folic acid

It is now recognized that if a woman has adequate levels of folic acid in her diet at least 1 month before conception and for the first 3 months of pregnancy, the chance of having a baby with an NTD is reduced by approximately 70%. This finding was first made in high-risk women who had already had an affected baby, using a multicentre, international randomized controlled trial of folic acid, other vitamins and placebo (MRC Vitamin Study Research Group, 1991). Another randomized trial found a reduction also in women who had never had an affected baby (Czeizel and Dudas, 1992). As a result of these studies the national health authorities in many countries have published recommendations for the use of folic acid for the prevention of NTDs.

To give this important message to all women of child-bearing age, a number of education programmes targeted at the relevant community and health care professionals have been implemented by health authorities. Fortification of some staple foods has occurred in some countries and natural dietary sources of folic acid publicized. In order to increase periconceptional folic acid intake by the recommended additional 0.4 mg per day, supplementation by means of a daily tablet may be offered. In the high-risk category, a dose of folic acid, up to 5 mg daily, is recommended.

There have been no reported adverse effects from folic acid in the vast majority of women of reproductive age. Women on anticonvulsant drugs need special consideration and must seek expert advice. There has been some concern with regard to the possible masking of pernicious anaemia in the elderly if they eat folate-enriched food, but this has not been substantiated.

Folic acid (vitamin folate) is a water-soluble, B group vitamin found naturally in many foods. It has an essential role in the very early development of the human central nervous system and in the healthy growth of cells. The underlying mechanism by which folic acid protects is not yet known.

THE ADOLESCENT
Douglas Bryan

In order to place the orthopaedic treatment of children with spina bifida in perspective, the following pages give a short outline of the disease and its management. Those readers who require more details relating to matters other than orthopaedic management are referred to Smith (1965), Smith (1976), Anderson and Spain (1977), Shurtleff (1986) and Rowley-Kelly and Reigel (1993). The annual proceedings of the Society for Research into Hydrocephalus and Spina Bifida since 1965 provide a wealth of material on all aspects of spina bifida and are published as supplements to the *European Journal of Paediatric Surgery*.

Incidence

Two major developments have emerged since the last edition; first, antenatal diagnosis and termination and second, folic acid supplementation and primary prevention. The incidence of spina bifida (excluding spina bifida occulta, cranial meningocele and anencephaly) in Melbourne was reported by Collman and Stoller (1962) as 0.56 per 1000 hospital births. The overall incidence in Australia has been reported by Simpson (1976) as 0.95 per 1000 births. The incidence in the Australian population is less than that in Western Europe. In this latter region, it is 1.5–3 per 1000 total births (Record and McKeown, 1949; Smithells and Chin, 1965; Carter and Evans, 1973b) although there are certain areas with an even higher incidence (Laurence *et al.*, 1968b; Richards *et al.*, 1972). More recent data from Victoria (see *Figure 1.2*) (Riley and Halliday, 1996) and Seattle (*Figure 1.3*) (Shurtleff and Lemire, 1995) reveal dramatic reductions in live births since 1987 with the Victorian change largely accounted for by termination.

In many parts of Europe, spina bifida has become a rare disease. Antenatal diagnosis and folate are probably influential.

Sex Incidence

Fifty-eight per cent of our myelomeningocele patients are female (see *Table 1.2*). This is statistically significant and corresponds with the experience of other workers. Hayes and Gross (1963) report an incidence of 55.5% of females.

Case Mortality

Our previous studies have shown only 10% of deaths occurred after the age of 2 years. This has implications for orthopaedic treatment: if a child reaches the age of 1 year, death in childhood is unlikely and the orthopaedic surgeon is justified in planning active treatment for the whole of childhood and into adult life.

Vertebral Levels

The lumbar and lumbosacral regions of the spine are predominantly affected by spina bifida cystica. Ninety-two per cent of lesions occur below the second lumbar vertebra and 42% are at the lumbosacral junction (*Table 1.1*). The bony anomalies generally extend over a greater length of the spine than does the soft tissue mass.

Gross neurological abnormalities are less commonly present when the lesion is high; that is, in the cervical or upper thoracic regions. Conversely, most lesions of the lumbar and lumbosacral regions are associated with extensive paralysis. Doran and Guthkelch (1963) reported a 5% incidence of limb paralysis in cervical lesions, a 17% incidence in thoracic lesions and an 87% incidence in lumbosacral lesions.

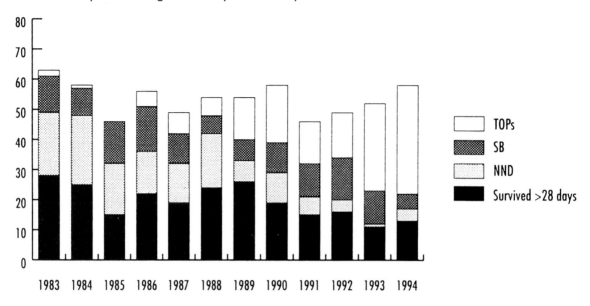

Figure I.2 The incidence of spina bifida in Victoria has remained constant up to 1994. The number of live births has decreased due largely to the number of terminations in those diagnosed *in utero*. TOPs, termination of pregnancy; SB, stillbirth; NND, neonatal death (reproduced from Riley and Halliday, 1996, with permission).

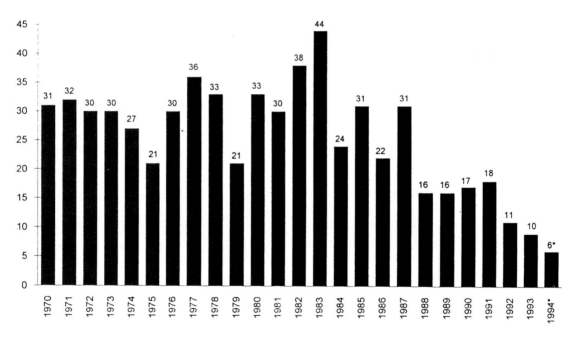

Figure I.3 The number of children with spina bifida in the birth defects clinics in Washington State born 1970–1994. The reduced numbers after 1988 are thought to be due to voluntary termination of pregnancy in those diagnosed before 24 weeks gestation (reproduced from Shurtleff and Lemire, 1995, with permisssion).

Neurological Levels

Table 1.2 indicates the number of patients with varying degrees of neurological deficit and the relationship this has to sex. The basic muscles delineating the levels are psoas and quadriceps muscles. In level 2 the psoas major muscles are paralysed and there is no lower motor neurone muscular activity in the legs; in level 3 psoas muscles are active but the quadriceps muscles paralysed; and in level 4 both psoas and quadriceps

Table 1.1 Vertebral level of spina bifida cystica in 295 patients

Vertebral level of spina bifida cystica	Number of patients	Percentage
Cervical level only	3	1
Thoracic level only	4	1
Lower thoracic plus upper lumbar levels	18	6
Lumbar level only	79	27
Lumbosacral junction	124	42
Sacral level only	62	21
Entire lumbar and sacral levels involved	5	2
Total	295	100

Table 1.2 Sex and level of lesions (1961–1969). Figures in parentheses show percentages

Neurological level	Male	Female	Total
1 Cervical and upper thoracic	1 (1)	1 (1)	2 (1)
2 Lower thoracic	30 (24)	50 (29)	80 (27)
3 Upper lumbar	28 (23)	39 (23)	67 (23)
4 Lower lumbar and upper sacral	60 (49)	74 (43)	134 (45)
5 Lower sacral	4 (3)	8 (4)	12 (4)
	123 (42)	172 (58)	295

muscles are active. In level 5 there is no paralysis of the legs, the paralysis being confined to the bladder, bowel and pelvic floor.

Hydrocephalus

Seventy-two per cent of patients develop significant hydrocephalus. The incidence of hydrocephalus is related to the neurological levels of the lesion; hydrocephalus occurred in 83% of those with high lesions (levels 2 and 3) compared with 60% of those with low lesions (levels 4 and 5).

Hydrocephalus is present at birth in 26% of cases, mostly those with high lesions, and by 1 month of age in 77%. It rarely develops after 6 months of age (4%). Shunts are most commonly inserted for hydrocephalus in the first 2 months of life.

Apart from death in infancy, of which hydrocephalus is a major cause, the main importance of hydrocephalus is its relationship to the intellectual development of the survivors.

Urinary Bladder Management

The innervation of the urinary tract, and in particular of the bladder, is from sacral segments of both the somatic and autonomic (sympathetic and parasympa-

thetic) nervous systems. It would be expected, for practical purposes, that all individuals with spina bifida would have some degree of impairment. Certainly in the newborn period, the possibility of urinary continence problems is discussed with the parents of all infants. However, in an unselected cohort reviewed 25 years after closure, 25% were normally continent (Hunt and Poulton, 1995). Almost all had little or no sensory loss.

The anatomical and pathophysiological manifestations of impairment have been described (Shurtleff, 1986). Ultrasound examination of the kidneys, urodynamics and micturating cystometrographic examinations in the neonatal period and at regular intervals subsequently, define the pathologic anatomy and physiology in any individual. A number of different bladder types have been described (Shurtleff, 1986) which encompass the variation in bladder capacity, bladder pressure, outlet resistance and voiding patterns.

The long-term principles of management continue to be the achievement of continence at a developmentally appropriate time, protection of the upper urinary tract and eventually self-management. There have, however, been massive changes in particular aspects of management since the introduction of the ileal conduit urine diversion device and its incorporation in total care of spina bifida (Smith, 1965) which changed the mortality from up to 90% at the age of 12 years to a situation where survival rates were 50–60%.

Long-term follow up of supravesical diversions of various sorts reveal a continuing morbidity with recurrent urinary tract problems, deterioration in the upper tracts and substantial social stigmatization. Since the early 1970s clean intermittent catheterization has become the mainstay of management of the neurogenic bladder (Lapides *et al.*, 1972). Pharmacological manipulations and a variety of surgical techniques, particularly those devoted to increasing bladder volume and increasing outlet resistance, have supplemented treatment for approximately 20% of children unable to achieve reasonable continence with clean intermittent self-catheterization alone.

Clean intermittent catheterization is most successful in maintaining dryness in the situation where the bladder is hypotonic and holds a good volume and there is some element of outlet resistance. A satisfactory result is the achievement of dryness for a period of 3 or 4 hours. If there is detrusor activity, medications including anticholinergic agents or smooth muscle relaxants such as Imipramine or Oxybutynin either orally or intravesically, can be of assistance.

Increased bladder pressure, particularly in very young children, can cause major upper tract deterioration in the presence of vesico-ureteric reflux. Aggressive management with catheterization and medications may need to be supplemented by surgery in the form of a vesicostomy, particularly if recurrent infections are also present. A small volume bladder, as a result of fibrosis or lowered outlet resistance, will not generally be amenable to management by clean intermittent catheterization alone. A variety of surgical procedures to enlarge the bladder capacity, usually supplemented by an artificial urinary sphincter or a muscle sling, are necessary to achieve continence in this group (Stone, 1995).

Developmental and medical management should proceed side by side so as to ensure successful maintenance of physical health. Appropriate responsibility for self-care from early childhood is promoted so as to ensure that by adolescence there exists knowledge and motivation for independent self-care.

As large numbers of individuals with spina bifida are now reaching adult life, end-stage renal disease is becoming evident in significant numbers of patients. In a recent study, haemodialysis was the most common form of treatment with satisfactory results in up to 70% of patients. Of those individuals who come to renal transplantation, up to 80% survive at 5 years following surgery (Patrick *et al.*, 1994).

Bowel Management

Bowel control is of major concern to the majority of individuals with spina bifida. However, by adult life about a quarter are fully continent (Hunt, 1995). This group is largely comprised of people with at least a degree of sensation, either bilateral or unilateral. For the majority where sensation is lacking, bowel incontinence is a substantial social difficulty at home, with peers at school and at work. In addition to, and complicating, the social implications of incontinence there are some medical concerns with bowel function in this group.

The pathophysiology has been described in detail (Shurtleff, 1986) with constipation being a major issue for people with neurological or functional increased lower bowel outlet resistance. This group is also prone to spurious diarrhoea. The second major group is patients with lowered outlet resistance who have frequent small stools throughout the day. In any of these situations lowered self-esteem and social interaction are major issues in childhood (Younoszai, 1992).

The basics of management of these situations revolve around three premises; that is, commitment to:

- Dietary and fluid intake.
- Regular evacuation of the bowel (on a daily basis) at a time that suits the person.
- Behavioural management to ensure compliance with recommended management procedures.

Early in their child's life, most families find foods which ensure the child's stool consistency is appropriate and which result in a bowel motion. Fibre-containing foods either in their natural state or processed in some way are usually a major part. There is strong evidence that active measures early in life are necessary to subsequent attainment of continence in the important school years (Rudeberg *et al.*, 1995). Adequate fluid intake throughout the course of the day is important so as to allow fibre-containing foods to be effective. Evacuation is achieved by regular sitting, often in combination with oral laxatives or more direct intervention with enemas and bowel washouts. Whilst children with outlet resistance problems can usually be managed well with bowel washouts, children with weak sphincters often pose a problem. Recently, balloon-tipped enema catheters have played a part in assisting this group (King *et al.*, 1994). Biofeedback training has been demonstrated to be useful particularly for those who can or have the potential to recognize their sensory function (Younoszai, 1992).

Early intervention has been demonstrated to have a substantial impact on continence by school age (Rudeberg *et al.*, 1995). Chronic constipation on the other hand has substantial deleterious effects on social functioning at school.

Finally, it is important to recognize that not all bowel disturbances in children with spina bifida have a neurological or mechanical basis. These children are at risk of other conditions associated with diarrhoea, for example giardiasis, and should always be investigated appropriately should any suggestion of a non-spina-bifida cause be evident.

Skeletal Growth

Skeletal growth is significantly affected in individuals with spina bifida with or without hydrocephalus (Rotenstern et al., 1995) and in individuals with hydrocephalus alone (Lopponen et al., 1995).

Short stature has been reported in children and those with the greatest degree of paralysis are most at risk. Spinal curvature, associated vertebral anomalies and contractures contribute to the short stature. The presence of a ventriculoperitoneal shunt further contributes, suggesting the possibility of hypothalamic dysfunction. In addition, chronic ill health particularly with infection, swallowing disorders with the Chiari malformation, and precocious puberty observed particularly in those with hydrocephalus, may be factors.

Recently, anthropomorphic data have become available describing the large number of young adults with myelomeningocele. Here, too, short stature relates to the level of the lesion and the presence of hydrocephalus (Rotenstern et al., 1995).

Children with hydrocephalus alone experience slow linear growth prior to puberty but an earlier than expected adolescent growth spurt (Rotenstern et al., 1995).

Obesity develops in later prepubertal childhood in up to 60% of children with spina bifida with increasing risk in those with higher lesions (Mita et al., 1993). However, obesity is also more prevalent in those with hydrocephalus alone, suggesting a metabolic aetiology in addition to the potential impact of decreased physical activity.

Measurement of growth parameters in this population is difficult particularly because of mechanical factors and the presence of aids and appliances that interfere with easy measurement. Arm span has been suggested as a method of measuring length but this has recently been questioned as not being interchangeable with length (Rotenstern et al., 1995); however, it may be useful to monitor growth rates to screen for growth failure as well as monitoring the results of treatment (Satin-Smith et al., 1996).

Young people with spina bifida often have low self-esteem and disabled girls in particular place very high importance on physical appearance (Appleton et al., 1994). In addition, adults of very short stature have difficulty with the physical environment at work, in motor vehicles and the like.

A recent report from the National Co-operative Growth Study Group reveals that 106 prepubertal children were treated with growth hormone (71% had maximal stimulated growth hormone levels less than 10 μg per litre). The treatment had a significant effect on growth, obesity and muscle strength over a 4-year period (Rotenstern et al., 1995). Any effect on adult stature has not yet been demonstrated.

Latex Sensitivity

The first reports of sensitivity to latex in children with spina bifida appeared in 1989 (Slater, 1989). Children with this condition are at risk of exposure to latex, particularly from rubber gloves and catheters in everyday life and to a variety of rubber-based products in hospital and operative settings.

Since those early reports, many other case studies have demonstrated this significant possible complication of therapeutic intervention. The allergic response is a type 1 Ige-mediated response to residual free protein found in latex products. Subsequent studies of at-risk populations have demonstrated a serological prevalence (RAST) of 38% but a clinical prevalence of 10% (Tosi et al., 1993) False-negative RAST testing has been reported (Shaer et al., 1992).

With present knowledge, a detailed history is the most sensitive way to detect individuals at risk for a latex reaction. Prophylactic measures include a latex-free environment at home and in the hospital and the education of health care workers, families and individuals with spina bifida.

Up to 40% of sero-positive patients may ultimately become clinically reactive. It would seem sensible to limit the exposure of patients to this material.

Prophylactic medication in the form of corticosteroids, Diphenhydramine and H_2-agonists has been recommended. The treatment for an established allergic reaction includes epinephrine, beta-agonists and intravenous fluids (Banta et al., 1992).

Adolescence – Psycho-social Adjustment, Independence, Sexuality and Transitional Issues

Advances in the last 15–20 years have seen increased survival in individuals with spina bifida occurring in parallel with decreased incidence at birth in many countries. The majority of individuals with spina bifida in any given community will increasingly be adolescents or young adults. The issues affecting adolescents with chronic illness and disability have been of increasing interest and importance to clinicians. They include the development of independence, particularly self-care, relationships with the family and peer groups, a range of behavioural and educational issues, sexuality and human relationships, occupational opportunities, recreation and transition to adult health care.

Much research on psycho-social adjustment to disability and chronic illness suggests a similarity across conditions with some degree of variation of severity according to the burden of the illness. However, there is some recent evidence that adolescents with spina bifida and other brain-based conditions have more problems with behaviour, independence and school achievement (Howe *et al.*, 1993).

Independence is the acquisition of developmentally appropriate self-care skills and attitudes. Many studies demonstrate that individuals with spina bifida across the age spectrum have a high level of dependence on personal carers, usually parents and mostly mothers, for a range of personal care, in particular bowel programmes, skin care, social relationships and the organization of general medical and developmental care (Blum *et al.*, 1991). This phenomenon exists in spite of the fact that the risks of such difficulties developing were identified in the disability literature in the mid-1970s (Anderson, 1976) and subsequently in the adolescent medicine literature (Blum, 1983). Increasingly, the focus on developing independence is moving into early childhood and infancy. Early intervention groups are being used to study the impact on such diverse facets of functioning as urological management, schooling and independent locomotion (Rudeberg *et al.*, 1995).

Policies of integration of children with disabilities into mainstream schooling offer the opportunity for appropriate peer relationships to develop. Indeed, in a recent study more than 50% of children with spina bifida indicated they had a best friend who was not disabled (Blum *et al.*, 1991). However, only 15% had been on a date as part of a heterosexual relationship. Seventy-five per cent of individuals indicated that they hoped to marry. For these aspirations to be achieved, strenuous and urgent efforts will need to be made to ensure opportunity of access of social interaction, for otherwise socially isolated, young people.

Physical sexual development can be significantly affected in spina bifida. Girls with myelomeningocele menstruated (along with other aspects of secondary sexual development) significantly earlier than the mean (Furman and Mortimer, 1994). Boys have similarly an increased risk of early physical sexual maturation. The complex neurological processes involved in male erection and ejaculation are theoretically very much at risk in almost all individuals with spina bifida. Objective measures of impotence measuring the number and duration of erections in sleep indicate that only a minority (mostly those with sacral lesions) will have normal functioning (Sandler *et al.*, 1996). More young men report an ability to obtain and sustain an erection with stimulation than is evident from the nocturnal studies. Frequency of sexual intercourse in published studies is very low, usually under 5%. On the other hand, an interest in sexual relationships has been reported repeatedly since Dorner's landmark work in 1976–1977 (Dorner, 1977). More recent work indicates that three-quarters have aspirations of marriage.

Many of these issues are more comfortably and appropriately the province of adolescent and adult health care than conventional paediatric practice. They are also issues that confront young people and their families well beyond the usual time of formal departure from paediatric care. The development of transition programmes, which provide the opportunity for adult and adolescent physicians to meet, interact and work with young people with spina bifida from early- to mid-teens to develop partnerships with their paediatric colleagues, would seem to offer the best opportunity for young people to explore their predicament with experienced and informed health care professions in a developmentally appropriate way. The subsequent transfer into the adult health care service can be achieved in a way that best meets the continuity of care needs of this group of patients. Unfortunately, many young people with spina bifida continue to be involved with paediatric health care services into their late teens, 20s and even 30s. More recently, a number of reports of the establishment of adult spina bifida service clinics offering multidisciplinary and appropriate developmental services have appeared (Morgan *et al.*, 1995).

Education

Most individuals with spina bifida have some degree of learning problems with the greater degree being in those with hydrocephalus. Formal psychological assessment in this group is difficult and assessments should always be done by a neuropsychologist with considerable experience with this population and their other physical difficulties. In addition, it is critically important to examine not just the results of tests, but quality of the approach taken to the task by the child. For example, it may be difficult to differentiate between an ability to perform a task because of physical limitations, such as fine motor control problems, or whether disorganization and confusion is the issue rather than a motor problem. Assessments also need to be conducted in a serial fashion over a period of time, prior to and in the early stages of primary and secondary school, to be reliable and valuable to the student.

Difficulties in many areas of cognitive functioning

have been described. They include problems with short-term memory, visuo-spatial perceptual skills, difficulties with numerical skills, particularly abstract mathematics in secondary school, motor planning difficulties and, in a small minority, frank intellectual disability. There is often statistically significant difference between the verbal and performance scales in IQ testing, particularly in those with hydrocephalus (for any cause, not just that associated with spina bifida) who show evidence of the 'cocktail party syndrome'. In this condition, hyperverbal but inappropriate language use may seduce casual or inexperienced observers into believing that the individual has a greater degree of understanding of situations and concepts than is really the case. A deeper analysis of understanding of the level of words used and the lack of insight with which they are used, reveals a qualitative difficulty even if on quantitative estimation verbal performance seems satisfactory. Additional cognitive/behavioural phenomena often occur in instances of hydrocephalus (with or without spina bifida) in which inappropriate behaviours, particularly those associated with short concentration span, limited ability to control one's attention and impulsivity occur. This attention deficit hyperactivity disorder-like syndrome may pose substantial difficulties in a classroom situation.

In spite of this extensive and complex array of potential difficulties, in most countries children with spina bifida attend mainstream schooling, a change which has taken place progressively over 20 years. Most require substantial education resourcing, however, for the educational implications of the learning difficulties as well as assistance with mobility, continence, seizure control, and assistance with integrating into the psycho-social culture and context of the school situation.

Case Management, Rehabilitation and Early Intervention

Developmental programmes focusing on early intervention have been progressively introduced to the health and behavioural programmes for children with spina bifida and their families since the first large numbers of such children emerged following the development of successful ventriculo-atrial shunting procedures for hydrocephalus in the early 1960s. Initially, programmes very much focused on the deficits experienced by the children. Great efforts were devoted by medical, allied health and nursing professionals towards remediation of specific physical difficulties. More recently, the focus on early intervention has shifted towards supporting families in their efforts to assist their children to develop social competencies in parallel with the attainment of physical skills.

There is some evidence (Rudeberg et al., 1995) that early intervention provided in a structured setting improve a number of functional outcomes for children. They include increased likelihood of independent mobility with a reduction in the number of orthopaedic procedures, increased likelihood of social continence with a reduction of the urological procedures and an increased likelihood of involvement in regular school. Decreased stress on families and increased quality of life were also reported. These changes in developmental outcomes occurred at a time of substantial change in medical and surgical practice which may have also affected outcome.

The development of multidisciplinary spina bifida clinics with co-ordinated care has been a feature in many areas, which is a reflection of the needs of patients for co-ordinated yet specialized care, and the very complex organizational problems imposed upon hospital systems to provide appropriate support for individuals with multisystem disorders. Continuity of care is a critical issue for these children and their transition from early intervention into school age and subsequently adolescent and adult programmes is of major importance to them.

Self-esteem and Quality of Life

Children, adolescents and young people with spina bifida are at risk of experiencing difficulties in self-esteem. Adolescents, in particular, are at risk of isolation at a time when peer support is crucial. Poor self-esteem is likely to mean poor motivation for the development of self-care skills, so critical to maturation of all young people. A number of factors appear to have an influence. Parents who take an age-appropriate approach to their young people and are permissive in social participation can provide positive support for their children (Wolman and Basco, 1994) whereas difficulties at school and negative perceptions by their peers of their disability can have a negative impact on self-esteem. The degree of disability can have a direct relationship with the level of self-esteem. Increasing levels of disability may be associated with increasing levels of self-esteem and vice versa. Presence or absence of continence or hydrocephalus appears to have little effect (Minchom et al., 1995). It is not clear why reducing levels of disability often lead to markedly impaired self-esteem. The relationship is likely to be complex but may be associated with a feeling of having just missed out.

Appearance may play a role, with disabled girls appearing to be particularly susceptible to the role of appearance on self-esteem (Appleton *et al.*, 1994). Generally, physical appearance is strongly associated with self-esteem.

Families

Spina bifida is a condition which almost always is apparent at the time of birth. Parental reaction to the news that their child has been born with a problem of substantial significance with the potential for an impact on life-long health and functioning, is usually intense and characterized by the various stages of reaction to bad news that have been described for many human circumstances. These encompass shock, anger, grief and varying degrees of adjustment to the change in circumstances over time. Whilst there are some evolutionary developments to the diagnosis, particularly as it affects intellectual functioning and to some degree continence, a good deal of reliable information can be given to families at an early stage and there is evidence that people deal rather better with their feelings if they have reasonably accurate information about what it is they will have to manage. The development of supportive relationships at an early time with health care givers and others, particularly family members (Kronenberger and Thompson, 1992), is the beginning of early intervention programmes that have as their basis the twin goals of supporting the child and the family.

In spite of the potentially very considerable stresses experienced by these families at the birth and care of severely impaired children, there is increasing evidence that parents of children in this situation cope remarkably well and are not dissimilar to parents of non-disabled children matched for age and sex in similar circumstances (Capelli *et al.*, 1994). Certainly there were more similarities than differences between families in these circumstances (Lie *et al.*, 1994).

The mother's role is critical in these circumstances. There is evidence that most of the responsibility for the care of the disabled child lies with her (Lie *et al.*, 1994) and that her positive adjustment to the situation has a positive impact on the child (Barakat and Linney, 1992). The mother's own adjustment seems to be little affected by the severity but more related, in a positive way, to support from her own family and her spouse (Kronenberger and Thompson, 1992). These mothers provide the principal physical and psychosocial support and with increasing survival, even of significantly impaired individuals, continued support into adult life (Hunt, 1995). Support for the mother is of immense importance and seems to have huge potential for positive outcomes.

Inevitably in families where the child with severe impairment and high health care needs requires extra support from the family, siblings will, at least potentially, have less than equal parental support. Nevertheless, there is good evidence for believing that siblings have empathic relationships with their disabled brothers and sisters (Kiburz, 1994).

The negative side to establishing supportive relationships with families at an early time can be the development of dependencies (which are sometimes mutual) between paediatric health care providers and families. This has, on occasions, impeded the development of transition programmes and effective transfer to adult health care systems (Rosen, 1994). Great care needs to be taken in the development of such relationships so they are supportive but empowering rather than tending to create dependency.

THE ADULT
Kevin B Dunne

Surgical advances beginning in the mid-1950s, resulted in dramatically improved survival rates for children born with spina bifida. Forty years later, we are now seeing large numbers of adults with spina bifida. However, there is little information on the health problems that these adults face. It is becoming clear that there is potential for ongoing deterioration and problems more specific to the adult years are emerging (Shurtleff and Dunne, 1986). Bax *et al.* (1988) found a sharp decline in the use of health services by a group of young disabled adults once they left the paediatric setting and noticed a deterioration in their health. The reasons are unclear but adults with spina bifida are at risk of receiving suboptimal care. This may be because they fail to attend appointments, possibly because of their cognitive difficulties, or because there is no suitable facility available to continue their management.

Background – Historical Perspective

Population studies from England suggest that without surgical treatment available 12.8% of children born with spina bifida survived until their 11th birthday (Lawrence and Tew, 1971). Death was commonly due to infection, uncontrolled hydrocephalus or renal failure. Survival rates have dramatically improved since the mid-1950s. As survival rates increased with the introduction of cerebrospinal fluid (CSF) shunts and better surgical techniques to preserve the kidneys, so did the number of children surviving with severe intellectual and physical disabilities; however, such aggressive treatment was not recommended for all (Lorber, 1971).

When evaluating adults, one must keep in mind both the medical treatment available to them when they were children plus the society's attitudes at the time. Historically, medical treatment can be broadly broken up into three phases: first, the period prior to the mid-1950s when there was no adequate treatment for hydrocephalus. Survivors generally had no hydrocephalus and low level lesions (Evans *et al.*, 1974; Shurtleff *et al.*, 1975; Laurence and Beresford, 1975).

The period from the mid-1950s to the mid-1970s was characterized by the introduction of CSF shunts and surgical techniques to protect the kidney, such as ileal diversion. As with any new technology or procedure, there were teething problems with infection, shunt failure and the need for frequent shunt lengthening with ventriculo atrial shunts. Infection rates and frequent shunt revisions have been shown to affect cognitive outcome (McClone, 1989). Additionally, there were difficulties managing patients urologically and ileal diversions were developed in an attempt to improve social continence and to protect upper renal tracts from infection, hydronephrosis and subsequent renal impairment. The social thinking of those times was for specific schools for the physically disabled and it was common for patients to live in institutions. There were community-based organizations that provided birth-to-death care.

Since 1975, there have been further medical and social advances that should improve outcome. There is better neonatal intensive care and better antibiotics. Shunt technology has improved with the development of ventriculo peritoneal shunts, which do not require frequent replacement. Non-invasive neurodiagnostic techniques such as CT (computerized tomography) scans and MRI (magnetic resonance imaging) enable better monitoring of shunt dysfunction as well as better imaging of the brain and spinal cord. Clean intermittent catheterization has resulted in better urological management with reduced infections and better protection of the upper renal tracts as well as improved social continence. There have been major social changes. The concept of normalization and general awareness of the rights of the disabled have resulted in persons with physical or intellectual disabilities living and being supported in their communities, rather than being segregated in special schools or living in institutions.

In summary, today's adults were born before 1975 and would have received treatments such as ventriculo atrial shunts and ileal diversions that have been superseded. Additionally, they grew up in an environment where children with disabilities were frequently segregated and were not often expected to achieve within a competitive society.

Medical Status

Increasing information is becoming available about the medical problems adults face. There are few population-based studies reported and much of the medical information is anecdotal. Hunt and Poulton (1995) reported a 25-year follow-up with 100% ascertainment of 117 children born between 1963 and 1970. Of the 61 still alive in this cohort, the major medical problems included seizures (23%), visual defect (44%), recurrent pressure sores (31%), hypertension requiring treatment (15%), depression on treatment (7%), and obesity (26%). Kinsman and Doehring (1996), when analysing all 353 admissions to a tertiary hospital over an 11-year period judged 166 (47%) preventable. Common preventable admissions were mainly urological problems such as pyleonephritis, urinary tract infection and renal calculus or pressure sores.

Our own population of adults was surveyed by a questionnaire and physical examination as part of a research project conducted during 1989–1992 (Dunne *et al.*, 1992). Broadly, this is a follow-up of the group reported by Smith and Smith (1973). The medical problems of adults will be discussed with reference to information contained from this cohort (*Tables 1.3, 1.4*).

Between 1951 and 1970, 648 children were treated at the Royal Children's Hospital, 352 survived and 114 (32%) agreed to be assessed. The whereabouts of 107 of the remaining 238 is unknown. The purpose of the study was to obtain medical status, access to health services and social status.

Neurosurgical

Ongoing neurosurgical problems associated with spina bifida include review and revision of CSF shunts, and monitoring for any deterioration (Tomlinson and Sugarman, 1995). Tethered cord syndrome occurs during childhood, adolescence and in adults (Filler *et al.*, 1995) but its prevalence in the adult is unknown. There is evidence, particularly in pregnancy, of progressive disc degeneration causing sciatica and permanent motor loss (Shurtleff and Dunne, 1986). Other problems include seizures and syringomyelia. In 4% of our patients (*Table 1.4*) the shunt was clinically malfunctioning. Fourteen per cent had recent onset of symptoms such as reduced muscle power or increasing spasticity, indicative of neurological deterioration requiring a neurosurgical review. Many of the group had weaker upper limb power than expected and some had evidence of wasting which may indicate a syrinx. In total, 25% of the group were felt to be in need of a neurosurgical review.

Table 1.3   Characteristics of 114 adults with spina bifida (figures shown as percentages)

Sex	
Females	57
Age	
18–24 years	71
25–29 years	18
>30 years	11
Diagnosis	
Myelomeningocele	83
Meningocele	9
Lipomeningocele	8
Cerebrospinal fluid shunts	49
Motor level	
Thoracic	26
L1–L2	10
L3	15
L4–L5	23
Sacral	17
No loss	9
Ambulation	
Community ambulation	72
Urine collection	
Ileal diversion	74
Normal	15
Clean intermittent catheterization	7
Bowel programme	
Accidents	52

Table 1.4   Medical status: 114 adults with spina bifida (figures shown as percentages)

Urological	
Recurrent urinary tract infection	38
Hypertension	11
Stoma stenosis, ulcers	58
No imaging within 2 years	39
Review recommended	36
Orthopaedic	
Backache	25
Knee pain or instability	15
Hip pain	14
Contractures	14
Shoulder pain	10
Arthritis	6
Review recommended	26
Neurosurgical	
Symptoms of cord tethering	14
Shunt review	4
Seizures	2
Review recommended	25
Skin	
Decubiti present	20
Chronic decubiti	9
Psychological	
Depression	5
Severe anxiety	3
Psychosis	2
Suicide attempts	7
Substance abuse	7
Review recommended	11

Urology

The issues are preservation of renal function and minimizing urinary incontinence. Many adults have had a variety of operative procedures to achieve the above aims. Some older persons had indwelling catheters. From the mid-1950s, ileal diversions were common but were found to have a limited lifespan before needing revision. Clean intermittent catherization (CIC) was introduced in the mid-1970s (Diokno *et al.*, 1976).

Ileal diversions are common in adults. In our adult group 74% have diversions (*Table 1.3*) and 29% of the adult members of the Spina Bifida Association of America have diversions (Dunne *et al.*, 1986). Stomal complications such as ulceration and stenosis are common. Recently, dysplastic changes were noted in ileal conduits raising concerns that carcinoma may develop. Many adults were aware of the undiversion procedures with a view to CIC but are either technically unsuitable for undiversion or do not want further operations with no guarantee of improved continence.

CIC is the main technique used since the mid-1970s. There are complications such as prostatitis in the male but otherwise no major long-term complications are reported to date. Currently, bladder augmentations are performed to enlarge the bladder using segments of bowel and the long-term complications are unknown. The main problems reported by our adults were recurrent urinary tract infection, hypertension, renal stones and, in those with diversions, bleeding and ulceration of the stoma (*Table 1.4*).

The need for regular ongoing surveillance is emphasized. Rickwood *et al.* (1984) demonstrated that renal tract deterioration may occur at any time, even in urologically stable adults, and stressed the need for ongoing regular urological review to prevent needless deterioration.

Other ongoing problems include recurrent urinary tract infection, pyelonephritis, calculi, hypertension and renal impairment. All may result or contribute to renal impairment. Some adults have had renal transplants (Little *et al.*, 1994).

Orthopaedic

Adults with spina bifida have ongoing problems with their musculoskeletal system, but this has not been studied in any systematic way. Ambulation is decided by adolescence and whether further deterioration in walking ability occurs is unknown. Musculoskeletal complications, such as fractures, symptomatic contractures and osteomyelitis, are reported. Many have had extensive spinal surgery and complications from the procedures may occur. Degenerative joint disease is an emerging problem. Twenty-four per cent of 72 ambulating adults with spina bifida had significant knee symptoms and had both clinical and radiological evidence of degenerative change (Williams *et al.*, 1993). Many adults complain of joint pain affecting the spine and hips (*Table 1.4*). Many also complained of upper limb joint pain and weakness, but it was not clear whether it was neurological or whether it was due to abnormal stresses (e.g. using crutches, or a tenosynovitis due to repetitive movements such as pushing a wheelchair).

Pressure sores

Pressure sores remain a persistent problem mainly due to ill-fitting braces, inappropriate wheelchair seating, poor pressure care or incontinence. The prevalence in our population was 20% (*Table 1.4*) with 9% having a chronic problem. Pressure sores are a common cause for prolonged hospitalization in adults (Kinsman and Doehring, 1996).

Obesity

Many adults become obese and are at risk of obesity-related diseases, such as heart disease and diabetes. Obesity also interferes with walking, transfers and self-esteem, and may result in reduced quality of life. The exact prevalence is unclear due to difficulties in measurement. Obesity is most likely to be related to reduced energy consumption due to wheelchair use.

Urinary continence

Social continence requires a combination of good urological management and a consistent urinary continence programme. Only 15% of our group reported no problem, with 26% recording frequent wetness and

18% significant odour. There have been improvements in continence aids and ongoing contact with a continence nurse is essential.

Bowel management

Considerable time and energy goes into developing a bowel management programme. A variety of approaches is used including going normally, timed toileting, digital stimulation, enemas and bowel washouts. Antegrade enemas through a stoma are currently being evaluated and are promising. The adults in our programme used a number of methods, the main one being timed sitting. In 52%, intermittent bowel accidents were reported. Twenty-seven per cent felt that they had a significant problem with faecal odour or staining. Intermittent diarrhoea is a problem for 26% and is often diet related.

Pregnancy and fertility

Many women with spina bifida have babies. Reported problems include disc herniation resulting in permanent motor loss (Shurtleff and Dunne, 1986), recurrent urinary tract infection, obstruction of ileal diversions, obstruction of ventriculo-peritoneal shunts and premature labour. The best mode of delivery is unknown.

We recently reported on 17 women having 23 pregnancies (Dunne *et al.*, 1996). Antenatal complications requiring hospital admission included pyelonephritis, recurrent urinary tract infection, back pain and pressure sores. Two women had temporary deterioration in their mobility but none had permanent loss. Of the 23 pregnancies, 11 were vaginal deliveries and 12 were by Caesarean section. Those women who delivered by Caesarean section had more postnatal complications resulting in longer than expected postnatal admissions.

Psycho-social Considerations

Psychology

There have been a number of studies which indicate that many adolescents have feelings of misery, low self-esteem, poor body image, sexuality concerns and concerns about their health (Dorner, 1976; McAndrew, 1979). However, it is important to remember that many able-bodied adolescents have feelings of misery and suicidal thoughts. Hayden *et al.* (1979) in a controlled study found that adolescents had lower self-esteem compared to controls but there was no difference in the level of depression or sadness between the groups.

In our adult follow-up study, a few were found to

suffer from significant anxiety or depression (*Table 1.4*), although 60% reported intermittent depression. Twenty-seven per cent reported suicidal thoughts, and 7% reported suicide attempts. The number with completed suicides is unknown. Substance abuse occurs. Psychological follow-up was recommended in 11%.

Education

Educational outcomes need to be compared to a control group as over the past 40 years there have been large increases in those completing secondary and tertiary studies. In a controlled study, Tew and Laurence (1984) found that in a group of 16 year olds, 42% of those with spina bifida completed high school compared to 75% of the controls. In our adult group, 16% had completed high school, of whom 8% were undertaking or had completed tertiary studies. Twenty-eight per cent attended a special school.

Regarding employment, 33% were in competitive employment, and a further 13% were students. Fifty-four per cent were not working. Sixty-two per cent were still living with their parents, with the remainder living independently or married. Proportionately more of the over 30 year olds were employed and living independently.

Health Maintenance

Many centres around the world have been grappling with the issue of transition of care to an adult facility and the best way to achieve a successful transition of care. Often no suitable facility is available in the community. The literature is clear that there is an ongoing need for regular health checks to prevent or investigate any deterioration. There are orthopaedic, urological and neurosurgical acute problems requiring hospital admission for treatment. Further corrective surgery may be necessary. As in childhood, the primary and tertiary carers should be familiar with the natural history of spina bifida as there are pitfalls for the inexperienced.

We attempted to ascertain what care adults who had previously attended our clinic were receiving. In the 2 years before assessment, 58% had seen a urologist, 38% a neurosurgeon and 30% an orthopaedic surgeon. Only 45% have been involved with a stomal therapist, 24% an orthotist and 18% had seen a physiotherapist. (Dunne *et al.*, 1992). The physiotherapist assessed 28% of the group as requiring a major intervention, such as a new orthosis, equipment, wheelchair or gait retraining.

There is an increasing consensus that we need to develop services similar to the multidisciplinary paediatric clinics where physicians with knowledge about the natural history of the condition and their specialist colleagues provide continuity of care. Rehabilitation physicians with their expertise in managing traumatic spinal cord injury are the obvious group to manage adults with spina bifida. Additionally, there is the need for ongoing allied health follow-up to maximize health, quality of life and access to the community.

Chapter 2

Causes of Deformity, Examination and Assessment

Malcolm B Menelaus

The factors responsible for deformity and gait and postural abnormalities are less certain than formerly believed.

Sharrard (1964b) related limb deformity and dislocation of the hip to the muscle imbalance produced by the particular neurological level of the lesion; his description provided a tidy explanation for the causes of these conditions. However, we had observed (Menelaus, 1980) that many patients did not fit nicely into Sharrard's groupings, sometimes due to the presence of spasticity. A study carried out at the Royal Children's Hospital, Melbourne and at the Children's Orthopaedic Hospital, Seattle (Shurtleff *et al.*, 1986) demonstrated, from a study of 966 children, that hip flexion contracture is not merely due to muscle imbalance; indeed the most significant and progressive forms of hip flexion contracture were found in patients in whom there was no muscle imbalance. Beeker and Scheers (1986) also found that hip deformity and dislocation were not as common as the muscle imbalance theory would predict and that the presence of deformity and dislocation could not be predicted on the basis of the level of the lesion. Broughton *et al.* (1993a) studied 1061 children with myelomeningocele and reviewed 3184 pelvic radiographs from 802 patients. It was found that hip dislocation was not inevitable even when there was maximal muscle imbalance about the hip. The average hip flexion contracture in children aged 9–11 years was significantly greater in those with thoracic-level lesions than those with L4, L5 or sacral

levels. It was thus established that muscle imbalance is not a significant factor in the production of flexion deformity or dislocation of the hip. These findings carried the implication that restoration of muscle imbalance should no longer be considered an aim of management at the hip (see Chapter 11). Studies of the incidence of foot deformity in high-level spina bifida patients (Broughton *et al.*, 1994) and in low-level spina bifida patients (Frawley *et al.*, 1997) demonstrate that the development of foot deformity cannot be explained on the basis of muscle imbalance related to specific levels of lesions (see Chapter 9). Furthermore, a study of the natural history of knee contractures in myelomeningocele (Wright *et al.*, 1991) demonstrated that muscle imbalance and spasticity play a minimal role in the development of knee contractures.

Thus we cannot implicate muscle imbalance as the predictable cause of specific deformities in spina bifida. Nevertheless, some patients do have deformities that are secondary to neurological abnormality.

Although the cause of deformity in the individual circumstance is unproven and there are unknown influences we here endeavour to untangle the web to a degree by discussing the following influences:

- muscle imbalance secondary to the neurological abnormality;
- habitually assumed intrauterine posture;
- habitually assumed posture after birth;
- coexistent congenital malformations;

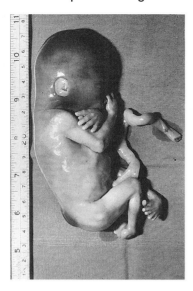

Figure 2.1 A 16-week foetus with a lumbosacral myelomeningocele and rigid equinovarus deformity of both feet at this early stage of development (photographs kindly provided by Dr Gordon Stark of Edinburgh).

- arthrogryposis;
- tethering of neural tissue;
- sensory, cerebral, cerebellar and upper limb abnormalities;
- leg-length discrepancy in association with unilateral paralysis.

Frequently, several of these factors are responsible for the production of a single deformity; for example, muscle imbalance may lead to a particular *in utero* position which has a tendency to become fixed (*Figure 2.1*). Commonly, there are several factors responsible for the various deformities found in a single limb; for example, some deformities will be due to muscle imbalance demonstrably caused by a lower motor neurone paralysis of the lumbar nerve roots, yet other deformities of the same leg may be due to an upper motor neurone lesion of the sacral roots. Added to these causes of deformity there may be deformity of the same limb due to the effects of habitually assumed posture before and after birth.

MUSCLE IMBALANCE SECONDARY TO THE NEUROLOGICAL ABNORMALITY

The nature of the basic spinal cord lesion in myelomeningocele is still not fully understood. For a long time it was believed that the basic defect was a failure of development of anterior horn cells or myelo-dysplasia,

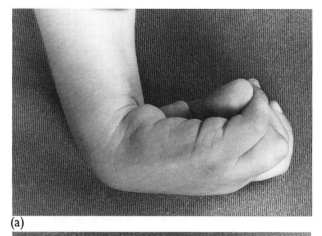

(a)

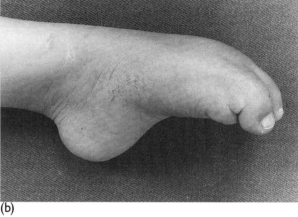

(b)

Figure 2.2(a,b) The left hand and left foot of a boy aged 5 years with a thoracic myelomeningocele and no voluntary function in either leg nor in the left hand. There is marked spasm of the flexors of wrist, ankles and toes.

and that the patient was suffering from a typical lower motor neurone lesion. However, it has become increasingly apparent that upper motor neurone lesions are frequently present (*Figure 2.2a,b*) with preservation of isolated cord segments distally. Attention has been drawn to this by Carr (1956), Doran and Guthkelch (1963), Guthkelch (1964), Stark and Baker (1967) and by Stark and Drummond (1971). Stark and Baker had found clinical evidence of upper motor neurone activity in two-thirds of children with myelomeningoceles.

Stark and Drummond (1971) clarified the relationship between the myelomeningocele plaque and the neurological disorder in the lower limbs. Clinical examination and plaque stimulation was performed on 75 infants. On plaque stimulation almost all the distal muscles responded. Clinical assessment showed that approximately one-third of the muscles responding were under voluntary control and two-thirds had either no activity or reflex activity; yet innervation of these muscles by the lower motor neurone was intact as judged by plaque stimulation. The amplitude of the response was normal so that there must have been a normal number of motor units; a deficiency of anterior horn cells can therefore be discounted as a cause of paralysis. Stark and Drummond also deduced that, in high lesions, the upper motor neurone lesion is probably immediately above the plaque and in low lesions the upper motor neurone lesion is probably within the plaque itself. No muscle, paralysis of which could explain a fixed deformity present, failed to respond to plaque stimulation with a high amplitude action potential; therefore the condition cannot be explained as being due to a lower motor neurone paralysis. Stark and Baker (1967) and Stark (1971) have typed the varying patterns of neurological abnormality in myelomeningocele into two types and have subdivided the second type into three subtypes. These are considered in some detail.

Type I Lesions

Infants in this group have normal function down to a particular level below which there is flaccid paralysis, loss of sensation and loss of reflexes. The pattern of weakness and deformity depends on the upper level of spinal cord involvement in the circumstances. This is the situation described by Sharrard (1964b); though this simple explanation is less commonly applicable than was formerly believed.

This neurological situation is probably due to spinal shock from birth trauma rather than to failure of development of the cord. A proportion of these patients later develop distal reflex activity.

The following description of the effects of paralysis below various levels (*Table 2.1*) is largely based on the work of Sharrard (1964b), somewhat modified by McDonald *et al.* (1991).

The mechanism by which paralysis of muscle produces deformity is variable. The unopposed muscle may not grow in length as rapidly as the other elements of the limb lengthen with resultant fixed deformity. The paralysed muscles may lengthen or shorten depending on their relationship to the axis about which the fixed deformity is occurring, for example if the tibialis anterior acting alone produces a calcaneovarus deformity then the paralysed peroneal muscles become lengthened and the paralysed tibialis posterior will become shortened.

Ralis and Duckworth (1974), in their discussion of feet with congenital vertical talus deformity, found that the most severely atrophied and contracted muscles were on the lateral or tight side of the deformity (as if their contracture had been a factor in producing the deformity) rather than on the elongated side.

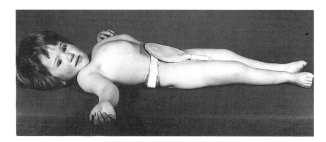

Figure 2.3 Paralysis below the 12th thoracic roots. This child is aged 6 years and the legs lie, as they did at birth, in a position dictated by the effect of gravity.

Paralysis below the twelfth thoracic root (*Figure 2.3*)

There is no muscle activity in the leg. At birth the limb lies in an externally rotated position. There may be twitching muscles distally but no voluntary activity. There may also be continuous uninterrupted activity in certain muscle groups and features seen in type II lesions.

Paralysis below the first lumbar root (*Figure 2.4*)

There is typically weak flexor power at the hip due to the activity in sartorius and some weak action in iliacus and psoas.

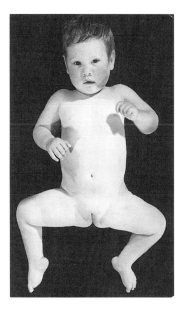

Figure 2.4 Paralysis below the first lumbar roots. There is flexion and external rotation of the hips which leads to an abducted posture and a fixed abduction contracture may result.

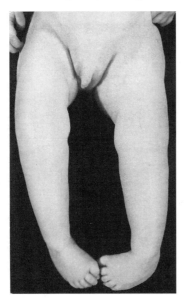

Figure 2.5   Paralysis below the second lumbar root on the right: the right hip is adducted and flexed. On the left there is paralysis below the fourth lumbar segment (see *Figure 2.7* for a better example of paralysis at this level).

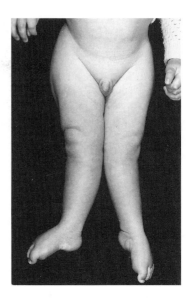

Figure 2.6   Paralysis below the third lumbar roots. The hips lie in flexion and adduction and the knees in extension or hyperextension. There is no muscle power in the feet.

Paralysis below the second lumbar root (*Figure 2.5*)

There is characteristically strong hip flexion and moderately strong adduction. The muscles typically acting are sartorius, iliacus, psoas, pectineus, gracilis and the adductors and rectus femoris. McDonald *et al.* (1991) indicate modifications to the traditional description of the segmental innervation of the lower limb muscles in children with myelomeningocele. They found that the medial hamstring strength more frequently correlated with the ilio psoas and quadriceps and the gluteii with tibialis anterior. They suggested that children with myelomeningocele should be grouped by specific muscle strength in preference to neurosegmental level.

Paralysis below the third lumbar root (*Figure 2.6*)

The power of the flexors and adductors of the hip is normal and quadriceps power only slightly diminished. There is some medial hamstring activity.

Paralysis below the fourth lumbar root (*Figure 2.7*)

In addition to the muscles that are acting in higher lesions, the quadriceps is at full strength. Tibialis anterior can be felt to produce dorsiflexion and inver-

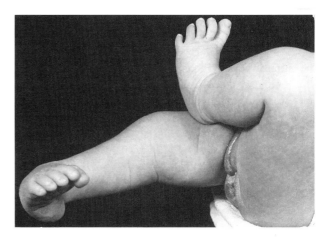

Figure 2.7   Paralysis below the fourth lumbar root in the right lower limb. There is flexion, adduction and external rotation of the hip, extension of the knee and equinovarus of the foot.

sion of the foot, there is some gluteal function and there may be some activity in tibialis posterior. There is good power in the semitendinosus and semimembranosus.

Paralysis below the fifth lumbar root (*Figure 2.8*)

In addition to those muscles that are spared by higher lesions, the tensor fascia lata, gluteus medius and gluteus minimus are functioning strongly and there is strong knee flexion due to semitendinosus and semi-

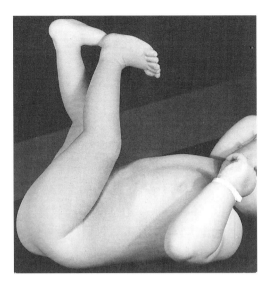

Figure 2.8 Paralysis below the fifth lumbar roots. There is flexion at the hip, some flexion of the knee and a calcaneus posture of the feet.

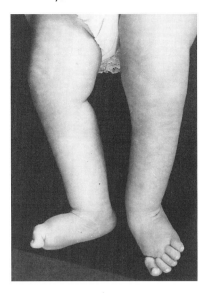

Figure 2.9 Paralysis below the first sacral root in the right lower limb. There is flattening of the sole of the foot and clawing of the toes. Unless the strongly acting toe and ankle extensors are divided, such a foot has a tendency to develop the deformity of paralytic convex pes planus. The left foot demonstrates spasm of the peroneus tertius which is one of the commonest manifestations of an upper motor neurone lesion.

membranosus. Tibialis posterior is strongly acting and there may be power in the peroneal muscles. There is normal power of the long toe extensors and peroneus tertius. Modifications to this pattern, as suggested by McDonald *et al.* (1991) are to be noted.

Paralysis below the first sacral root (*Figure 2.9*)

In addition to those muscles spared by higher lesions there is moderate power in gluteus maximus, biceps femoris, gastrocnemius soleus and flexor digitorum longus. Flexor hallucis longus and brevis are functioning.

Paralysis below the second sacral segment

The only weakness lies in the intrinsic muscles of the foot which may, with growth, produce clawing of the toes. The grading of muscle power that we employ to indicate the neurosegmental level of the lesion is specified in *Table 2.1*.

The extent of the paralysis is commonly different in either leg due to asymmetry of cord involvement.

Type II (a) Lesions

This group of infants has a 'gap' in cord function (with loss of motor, sensory and reflex activity) and, distal to this, intact but isolated cord segments (*Figure 2.10*).

In the isolated territory, spasticity and stretch

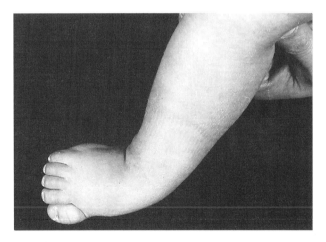

Figure 2.10 Spasticity in the peroneal muscles. This is a common manifestation of spasticity in spina bifida (as is spasm of the hamstrings, *Figures 8.1b, 8.2*, and spasm of extensor hallucis longus). In this child there was paralysis of the quadriceps muscles indicating a 'gap' in cord function and distal intact but isolated cord segments. This is a type II (a) lesion (as categorized by Stark (1971)).

reflexes may be striking but more often are mild. Exteroceptive tonic reflexes can be elicited, for example stroking of the dorsum of the foot evokes toe

Table 2.1 The assessment of neurosegmental level in children with myelomeningocele modified from Sharrard (1964b)

Level	
Thoracic	No active movement at the hip
L1	Iliopsoas grade 2 or better
L2	Iliopsoas, sartorius and adductors all grade 3 or better
L3	Quadriceps grade 3 or better, also meet criteria for L2
L4	Medial hamstrings or tibialis anterior grade 3 or better; also meet criteria for L3
L5	Lateral hamstrings grade 3 or better; also meet criteria for L4 plus one of the following three: gluteus medius grade 2 or better, peroneus tertius grade 4 or better, tibialis posterior grade 3 or better
S1	Two of the following three: gastrocnemius/soleus grade 2 or better, gluteus medius grade 3 or better, gluteus maximus grade 2 or better; also meet criteria for L5
S2	Gastrocnemius/soleus grade 3 or better and gluteus medius and gluteus maximus grade 4 or better, also meet criteria for S1
No loss	All leg muscles have normal strength

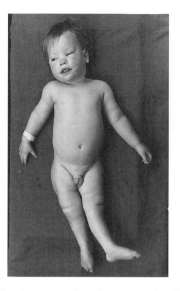

Figure 2.11 Spasm in hip flexors and adductors and knee extensors. Both hips were dislocating and there was a 30° fixed flexion deformity. This was treated by bilateral adductor tenotomy and psoas excision followed by 6 weeks in a broomstick cast.

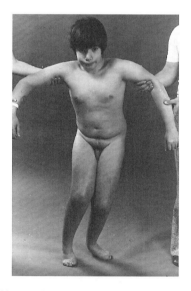

Figure 2.12 A 12-year-old boy as he presented at this age for treatment. A myelomeningocele had been repaired at birth and he had undergone lengthening of the left tendo Achillis at the age of 5 years. He had increased tone in the hip adductors, in the hamstrings and calves bilaterally with increased ankle jerks and the posture and gait of cerebral diplegia. He has since undergone hamstring and calf releases with improved function. This is a type II (c) lesion with voluntary activity in the quadriceps muscles and thus a mixture of spasticity and voluntary activity below the level of incomplete cord transection.

extension. Those infants who have spasticity of the pelvic floor have a deep natal cleft.

Type II (b) Lesions

Members of the group have a narrow 'gap' in cord function and resemble patients with spinal cord transection (*Figure 2.11*). Though there is no movement of the legs on vigorous crying and no central response to pin-prick, the slightest stimulation at any point of the leg generally evokes a flexion withdrawal reflex.

Type II (c) Lesions

There is incomplete transection so that the infant has spastic paraplegia but incomplete loss of voluntary movements and sensation (*Figure 2.12*).

Stark (1971) found the following neurosegmental patterns in a series of 100 consecutive infants with myelo-meningocele examined under the age of 24 hours:

Normal	8%
Type I lesion	28%
Type II (a)	37%
Type II (b)	18%
Type II (c)	9%

Thus, a majority of patients had upper motor neurone lesions and Stark believes that some of the normal and type I lesions will later develop spasticity.

In hemimyelomeningocele the cord is split and only half is involved in the myelomeningocele; one leg is normal or near normal and the other may have any pattern of lesions. The better leg has sometimes later developed neurological signs due to tethering.

The sensory loss in the trunk and lower limbs in myelomeningocele usually follows, within one or two segments, the motor loss. Vasomotor control is frequently disturbed with coldness and discoloration of the skin.

That spasticity is common was indicated by Stark and Drummond (1971) and the incidence was more precisely defined by Mazur *et al.* (1986b). These workers indicate the persistance of spasticity into adolescence and its significance.

HABITUALLY ASSUMED INTRAUTERINE POSTURE

It would seem that intrauterine posture is a factor affecting the degree and rigidity of the deformity initiated by muscle imbalance and perpetuated by lack of foetal movement. Those spina bifida children born with equinovarus feet commonly have rigidity whereas the calcaneus feet in spina bifida are seldom rigid. The rigidity parallels that of the ordinary form of congenital talipes equinovarus and the pliancy that of congenital talipes calcaneovalgus. Thus, if an equinovarus posture is assumed *in utero* it takes on rigid and treatment-resisting characteristics (*Figure 2.1*).

HABITUALLY ASSUMED POSTURE AFTER BIRTH

Flail legs will fall into a position of external rotation and abduction at the hips, flexion at the knees and equinus at the ankles and these may become fixed deformities. Mazur *et al.* (1989) found that patients with high-level lesions who had habitually been seated and never walked had significantly greater hip flexion contracture than those who had walked for a period.

The influence of habitually assumed posture at other sites is conjectural.

COEXISTENT CONGENITAL MALFORMATIONS

Some authors have considered that limb deformities in spina bifida are largely due to coexistent congenital anomalies. In particular, club feet (Smith, 1965) have been regarded as congenital anomalies in association with spina bifida.

Some congenital anomalies not due to muscle imbalance do occur in the limbs of spina bifida children. These include hemihypertrophy, absent fibula and absent foot. Other congenital abnormalities occurring in association with spina bifida are hemivertebra, sacral agenesis (*Figures 2.13, 2.14*), fused vertebrae, diastematomyelia, spondylolisthesis, double ureter, renal anomalies, imperforate rectum and congenital cardiac lesions (Smith, 1965).

ARTHROGRYPOSIS

Deformities are encountered in spina bifida similar to those that occur in children with arthrogryposis multiplex congenita who have no evidence of anterior horn cell or of anterior spinal root abnormality (*Figures 2.15–2.17*). The hips and knees may be just as rigid and have the same featureless appearance and the club feet have the same rigidity, short big toe and treatment-resisting qualities in both circumstances. Muscle imbalance *in utero* would seem to produce occasional arthrogrypotic deformities, but it is not known why this occurs in some cases only. Even when there are no arthrogrypotic features the flail limbs in spina bifida seldom have the same joint mobility as have the floppy flail limbs seen in poliomyelitis. It would seem that muscle imbalance *in utero* leads to degrees of rigidity of which the arthrogrypotic type limb represents the extreme degree. Moreover, muscle imbalance *in utero* may be a factor in all cases of arthrogryposis multiplex congenita which is not a disease entity but may result from one of the following causes (Adams *et al.*, 1962; Pena *et al.*, 1968):

- a degeneration and loss in number of anterior horn cells;
- a focal collagenous proliferation in the anterior spinal nerve roots;
- infantile muscular dystrophy.

All these causes would produce *in utero* muscle denervation in arthrogryposis as in spina bifida.

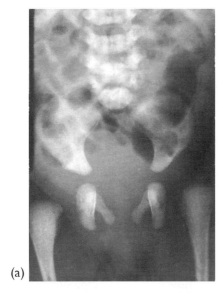

(a)

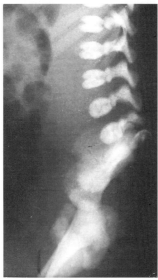

(b)

Figure 2.13(a,b) Antero-posterior and lateral radiographs of the pelvis of a child with congenital absence of the sacrum. There was paralysis of the gluteal muscles on the left with dislocation of this hip (see also *Figure 2.14*).

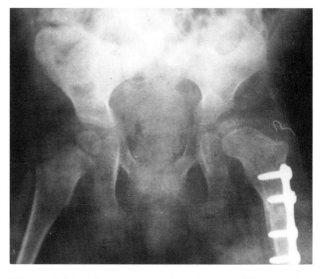

Figure 2.14 The same child at the age of 3 years following left iliopsoas transfer and femoral derotation osteotomy.

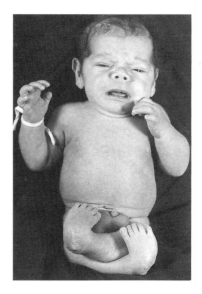

Figure 2.15 Rigid deformities, similar to those seen in arthrogryposis multiplex congenita, in a baby with spina bifida with extensive paralysis of the lower limbs. There is bilateral dislocation of the hip, genu recurvatum and bilateral talipes equinovarus (see also *Figures 2.16, 2.17*).

SENSORY, CEREBRAL, CEREBELLAR AND UPPER LIMB ABNORMALITIES

It is frequently forgotten that, apart from the obvious spinal plaque and the enlarged cerebral ventricles, many other cerebral and spinal malformations occur in children with spina bifida (*Table 2.2*). These malformations provide the basis for the deficits described below, although definite clinicopathological correlations cannot often be made for each individual pathological entity.

Variend and Emery (1973) found a uniform reduction in the weight of the cerebellum in all patients with myelomeningoceles. This is in contrast to their findings that the cerebral hemispheres in these patients are generally larger than in the normal individual. The residual cerebellum shows areas of necrosis, approximately a 50% fallout of Purkinje cells, dysplastic areas in the central lobes of the cerebellum and cystic

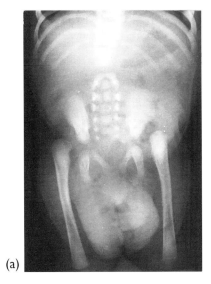

(a)

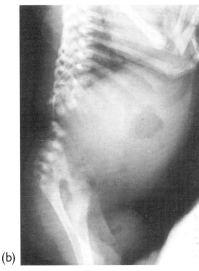

(b)

Figure 2.16(a,b)   Antero-posterior and lateral radiographs of the child illustrated in *Figure 2.15* show the unusual anomaly of absence of the third lumbar vertebra; in addition there is spina bifida distal to this level. Both hips are dislocated and have the rigidity of arthrogrypotic hips; this rigidity led to the decision not to treat the hip dislocation (see also *Figure 2.17*).

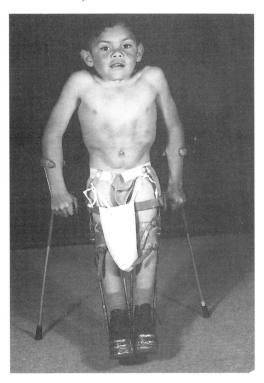

Figure 2.17   The same child at the age of 8 years. He walks with a swing-through gait and has a 5 cm raise on his boots to compensate for his very short stature. He wears a Chiron bag as he has undergone an ileal conduit urinary diversion procedure. This boy's condition at maturity is seen in *Figures 11.3, 11.4*.

degeneration of the white matter. With the added affect of crossed cerebellar atrophy due to hydrocephalic frontal lobe damage, it is not surprising that ataxia is conspicuous in the upper limbs of patients with spina bifida. The cerebellar disturbances are presumably responsible for nystagmus, which is commonly seen in these patients.

The other conspicuous abnormality in upper limb function is that of pyramidal tract disturbance resulting in mild weakness, hyper-reflexia and clumsiness of fine movements. The neuropathological basis for this is presumably a condition of white matter disruption due

to hydrocephalus, pressure on, and distortion of, the pyramidal tracts due to the Arnold–Chiari malformation and the direct effect of the cervical cord anomalies so frequently present in these patients. MacKenzie and Emery (1971) found hydromyelia at the eighth cervical level in 40% of autopsy cases and 20% showed syringomyelia. A smaller percentage had diplomyelia in the cervical region, mid-line arachnoid cysts and central canal anomalies, such as obliteration and forking. Hydromyelia, syringomyelia and hydrosyringomyelia have special significance as causes of scoliosis (see Chapter 12).

In a study of hand function in children with myelomeningocele, Sand *et al.* (1974) showed poor hand functioning, as judged by a series of timed manual activities, in all patients with hydrocephalus and in the majority of patients judged to be free of hydrocephalus. Wallace (1973) found that 69% of a group of 225 children with myelomeningocele had neurologically abnormal arms; only 38% of these had the ability to get about adequately without a wheelchair whereas 77% of those with normal arms were not disabled in this way. The upper limb abnormalities were classified as follows: bilateral pyramidal tract

Table 2.2   The pathology of spina bifida

Pathology	References
Cerebral	
Arnold-Chiari malformation	
Hydrocephalus	Milhorat, 1972
Aqueduct stenosis	
Communicating	
Outlet obstruction of the fourth ventricle	
Cerebellar hypoplasia and anomalies	Variend & Emery, 1973
Cerebral micropolygyria	Peach, 1965
Megalencephaly	Emery, 1974
Subependymal cortical heterotopias	Emery, 1974
Enlargement of the interthalamic body	Emery, 1974
Fusion of the corpora quadrigemina	Emery, 1974
Partial obliteration of the great longitudinal fissure	
Agenesis of the corpus callosum	Milhorat, 1972
Hydrobulbia	Milhorat, 1972
Spinal	
Meningocele	
Myelocele	
Diastematomyelia	Doran & Guthkelch, 1961
Flattening of the cervical cord	Mackenzie & Emery, 1971
Winged cord	Mackenzie & Emery, 1971
Hydromyelia and syringomyelia	Mackenzie & Emery, 1971
Central canal anomalies	Mackenzie & Emery, 1971

dysfunction, unilateral pyramidal deficits, cerebellar dysfunction and other mixed disorders (*Table 2.3*). There was a higher incidence of upper limb abnormalities in patients with hydrocephalus and in those with lumbar, as opposed to sacral, deficits. Minns *et al.*

(1977) found no correlation with the vertebral or neurological level; they demonstrated considerable functional difficulties in these children which might not be detected by formal neurological testing.

Children with hydrocephalus commonly have problems in visuospatial perception. Miller and Sethi (1971) suggest that in children who have had hydrocephalus (even those with an intelligence quotient as high as 105) there are two areas of difficulties: (i) an inability to perceive a presented shape in its totality and to appreciate its particular spacial configuration; and (ii) inability to ignore irrelevant aspects of a total stimulus display.

The difficulties in learning to stand and walk can be better understood if we appreciate these difficulties in perception and if we recall that children with these perceptual defects commonly have upper limb abnormalities and poor tactile discrimination. Furthermore, those children with poor upper limb function also commonly have complex disorders in the lower limbs including ataxia and pyramidal tract dysfunction.

Lack of sensory information from skin, muscles and joints affects posture and gait as does impaired intelligence.

Table 2.3   Upper limb abnormalities in 225 patients with spina bifida (reproduced from Wallace, 1973, with permission)

	Patients
Bilateral pyramidal tract dysfunction	25
Unilateral pyramidal tract dysfunction	21
Cerebellar ataxia	40
Chorea	8
Dyspraxia	5
Mixed pyramidal tract and cerebellar dysfunction	51
Other mixed disorders	6
Total with upper limb abnormalities	156

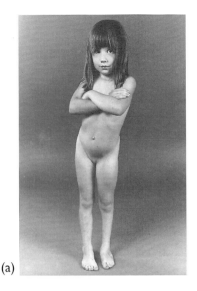

(a)

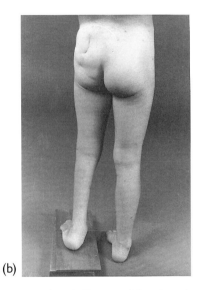

(b)

Figure 2.18(a,b)   A 5-year-old girl with a left hemi-myelomeningocele. There is a leg length discrepancy of 2 cm. The left foot has undergone a postero-medial release for equinovarus deformity at the age of 5 months. At the age of 5 years cavovarus deformity of the right foot was noted. Spinal surgery disclosed tethering of the nerve roots to the right leg.

Leg Length Discrepancy Secondary to Unilateral Paralysis (*Figure 2.18*)

This is seldom a major factor. Its management is considered in Chapter 9.

PHYSICAL EXAMINATION, ASSESSMENT AND SPECIAL INVESTIGATIONS

The first physical examination is made immediately after the baby is admitted to hospital (see Neonatal Assessment below). A thorough examination is then carried out to assess the child's general condition and the state of the spinal lesion; careful note is made of the neurological state and the presence of deformity in the legs and dislocation of the hips. Further assessments of the power of the leg muscles are made while the baby remains in hospital and during the first 2 years of life. Muscle power and joint deformity and range of movement are recorded on a Patient Data Management System, 6-monthly for the first 2 years of life and then annually.

The orthopaedic surgeon will compare his or her findings with those of the neurologist and the physiotherapist. Sharrard (1973) frequently refers to the value of faradic stimulation; we have not found this investigation to be useful.

The following are special considerations in the assessment of muscle power in spina bifida patients:

- Accurate grading of muscle power is frequently impossible and simple statements are then preferable – 0; weak; full strength.
- Whilst an endeavour is made to record the strength of individual muscles, this also may be impossible when examining a baby; if so, the power of a group of several muscles, such as the hip adductors, knee extensors and knee flexors is recorded.
- The resting posture of a child may indicate the muscles that are likely to be functioning and the level of the lesion (as indicated in *Figures 2.3–2.9*).
- Special care must be taken in assessing flexor power at the hip as a strong sartorius may mask a weak psoas. When testing for hip flexion there may be no apparent flexor power until the examiner takes the lying child by both hands and assists him or her to flex the head and trunk whilst observing the hips. If there is flexor power, the hips will flex during this manoeuvre.
- Note that if there is an area of anaesthesia in the feet and legs then a sensory stimulus to this area will not produce voluntary muscular activity. It may produce involuntary activity, such as the withdrawal reflex, if there is an upper motor neurone lesion.
- Care must be taken to note the continuous and uninterrupted activity of muscles that suggests an upper motor neurone lesion.

During the first 2 years of a child's life, discussion with all those involved in management is particularly necessary as all aspects of the child's health and emotional development must be taken into consideration in planning the orthopaedic programme. Information from the neurologist and physiotherapist should be noted.

As the child grows older and attends a special school where one physiotherapist gets to know him or her well then it is desirable for the surgeon to visit that school and see the child in school surroundings in the presence of the usual physiotherapist. If this is impossible then the physiotherapist should occasionally attend the orthopaedic outpatient clinic with the child. Only in these ways can one find out how the child spends their school days, how much walking they do, how much they tire as the day progresses and what problems exist.

NEONATAL ASSESSMENT

Stark (1971) provides much useful information which has been incorporated in the following account.

History

Details of the family and social history are obtained from the father and grandparents. These are later supplemented at the time of genetic counselling. The obstetrician will have provided details of the obstetrical history, which is frequently complicated; only 66% of myelomeningocele patients are born by spontaneous or low forcep delivery and there is a high incidence of breech births and frequent birth injury. Those babies delivered by Caesarean section at 36 weeks gestation are less prone to be severely paralysed than those delivered vaginally (Shurtleff, 1986).

Neurological Examination

The early examination will usually have been carried out by someone other than the orthopaedic surgeon but he or she must be aware how a full examination should be carried out so that they can carry out such examination themselves when difficult decisions have to be made.

Infants who are cold and apathetic (one-third have rectal temperatures below 35.5°C) or who are in poor condition, are warmed. The general condition of the child is assessed and the spinal lesion examined.

The child's alertness and the presence of any cranial nerve lesions are noted. The latter are a common complication, the most common being an abducens nerve palsy.

Spinal cord function

Upper limbs

This examination is difficult at birth and rarely are abnormalities found then, except in the rare cervical myelomeningocele. The upper limb abnormalities found at a later age are described earlier in this chapter.

Lower limbs

Sensory testing is best carried out with the child quiet but not too apathetic. The aim is to obtain the lowest level of normal sensation. Starting in the lowest sacral territory, the perianal region, the skin is stimulated. The examiner then passes to the posterior aspects of the buttocks, thighs and legs; then upwards over successive dermatomes of the anterior surface of the legs and thighs and on to the abdomen. Sensation is indicated by a cry, a grimace or a Moro response. The level is noted as is the presence of any purely reflex response, such as withdrawal reflex. In general, determination of the sensory deficit provides less valuable information than does testing of muscle power.

Motor testing should be carried out with the infant warm, hungry and active and showing vigorous arm movements. If the neural plate is inadvertently pressed upon there may be brisk leg movements which may be mistaken for voluntary movement. Initially voluntary or rather spontaneous movement is assessed by stimulating the arms and tickling the trunk. Each muscle can be tested with gravity eliminated. Whilst Stark is able to grade muscle power according to the Medical Research Council grading, we cannot be as accurate as this, and grade the muscles as – no activity; weak; strong. The lowest segmental level of voluntary function can be assigned to each leg. Palpation of the limb enables some assessment of muscle bulk and this may aid in the delineation of the neurosegmental level.

After this examination has been carried out then purely reflex activity is assessed by stimulating the lower limbs and perineum with a straightened paperclip. Difficulty in distinguishing voluntary from reflex activity may be encountered. Stark states that these difficulties can generally be dispelled by observation of the limb responses to the Moro reflex, the asymmetrical tonic reflexes and stepping reflexes.

Bladder and bowel

Frequent, small volume dribbling of urine increased by crying or movement or by suprapubic pressure suggests that the child is likely to be incontinent.

A patulous anus or a continuous leak of meconium suggests incontinence of the bowel. If one leg is normal or normal apart from a mild upper neurone lesion then the bladder function can be expected to be normal. Infants who have neither voluntary nor reflex

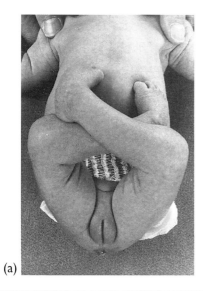

(a)

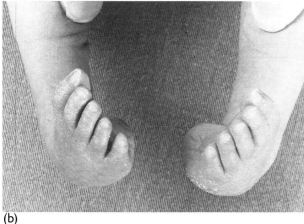

(b)

Figure 2.19(a,b) Baby aged 4 days with a lumbar myelomeningocele that has been repaired. Note the lack of a natal cleft which bespeaks paralysis of the pelvic floor. The legs lie rigidly in the posture shown here and in these circumstances it is impossible to assess the voluntary function which will persist into childhood.

function in muscles innervated from the second, third or fourth sacral segments tend to have complete paralysis of the bladder.

Examination for deformity

Lower limb deformities are noted and recorded and the pattern of deformity may indicate the probable level of the lesion. It must be remembered that the deformity may be a residue of intrauterine muscle imbalance no longer present or to upper motor neurone imbalance.

The presence of rigid deformity in the neonatal period may preclude an assessment of voluntary function (*Figure 2.19a,b*).

The child shown in *Figure 9.1* has deformity typical of paralysis below the fourth lumbar segment but there was no muscle power in the legs at birth. Stark (1971) illustrates a foetus (*Figure 2.1*) with foot deformities consistent with a L4 segmental level in a 16-week foetus with a lumbosacral myelomeningocele. He comments that 'in such cases, the prenatal neurological disorder is, as it were, "fossilised" in the deformity it has produced'.

Special Investigations

- Radiological examination is made of skull, spine and hips. Vertebral anomalies are frequently found (see Chapter 12).
- Concentric needle electrode electromyography may reveal activity in muscles that are difficult to assess clinically. We do not use this technique.
- Faradic stimulation may be used instead of electromyography but is less precise and subject to greater technical limitations in the newborn. We do not use this technique.
- Photographs of the whole child and of leg and foot posture are taken routinely as they provide a useful record of deformity as can be seen from the figures in this chapter, all of which are included in the hospital case records of each child.

Other special investigations of a non-orthopaedic nature will be carried out on the newborn – bacteriological swab from the myelomeningocele and umbilicus, urinary tract investigations and ventriculography.

The neurological assessment outlined above is a description of what may be discovered by careful examination. Not always can the relevant physical signs be elicited at a single examination; repeated examinations may be rewarding. Examination in our hands sometimes gives rise to expectations which are not fulfilled; we may mistake reflex activity for voluntary activity. In type II (c) lesions the degree of voluntary activity is frequently difficult to assess. However, neurological examination in the first few months of life indicates the minimum disability that can be expected. Greater disability may occur due to the error mentioned above or to ventriculitis or to serious valve complications. Late-developing spasticity or tethering of the cord will alter the pattern of neurological disturbance.

Chapter 3
Neurological Deterioration

Geoffrey L Klug

INTRODUCTION

Children born with spina bifida cystica have a markedly abnormal structure of the central nervous system (CNS) which from the outset is associated with impairment of neurologic function of variable degree. Such impairment of neurologic function results in multi-system dysfunction including the musculo-skeletal system.

It is not possible to correct the primary structural anomalies leading to these defects of function but it may be possible in certain situations to prevent deterioration of function arising from secondary structural changes occurring after the time of birth. The most obvious example of such in the neonatal period is the insertion of a shunt to control hydrocephalus. Such a procedure does not alter the structural anomalies leading to defective CNS dynamics but prevents deterioration of brain function if such treatment is not undertaken.

It is important to stress that early repair of the myelomeningocoele sac does not improve function but should not be responsible for deterioration if surgery is undertaken with the required degree of skill. Delayed repair, if infection has occurred in the interim, may be followed by a worse outcome.

Following primary repair of the sac and, if required treatment of hydrocephalus, the anatomic anomalies of the CNS are such that further structural changes can occur which in turn lead to deterioration of function. The aim of this chapter is to discuss the nature of these changes, the clinical manifestations of such changes, the investigations required and finally give a brief indication as to the forms of appropriate treatment and their outcomes.

DELAYED STRUCTURAL CHANGES LEADING TO A DETERIORATION OF NEUROLOGICAL FUNCTION

It is important to detect changes early when they may be more easily correctable and, in particular, correct such changes before the secondary effects are obvious and to a greater or lesser extent irreversible.

Hydrocephalus

The late onset of progressive hydrocephalus is most uncommon in children with a myelomeningocoele. In general, the disorder becomes apparent in the neonatal period. Full evaluation is required at that time to decide whether or not treatment, such as a ventriculo-peritoneal shunt or third ventriculostomy, is deemed necessary. The majority of infants fulfil such criteria and are so treated within the first 4 weeks of life. The remaining patients commonly exhibit some degree of ventricular dilatation which remains stable and is not thought to be responsible for any lessening of neurological function. Such children do not require a cerebrospinal fluid (CSF) diversion procedure but it is essential that they be regularly reviewed clinically and with imaging to ensure this stable condition is maintained.

The cause of late-onset progressive hydrocephalus is unclear in the small number of patients who develop such a condition. In some, it may reflect a very slowly, yet undiagnosed, developing disorder and as such is not strictly an example of progression following a period of stability. In others, such factors as an intercurrent infection or head trauma, often minimal, appear to be related to the onset of progressive ventricular dilatation.

The most common cause of late neurological deterioration due to hydrocephalus is related to a malfunction of an existing shunt system. The mechanical obstruction of the shunt system, commonly but not invariably, leads to a recurrence of hydrocephalus which in turn is responsible for neurological deterioration. The rate of change following such an obstruction varies greatly and depends on such factors as the extent of shunt dependence and the degree of mechanical obstruction. At one extreme, obstruction can be followed by rapid ventricular enlargement and extreme elevation of intracranial pressure. Under these circumstances neurological deterioration is rapid and life may be threatened. At the other extreme, the rate of change following obstruction may be extremely slow and mimic the pattern of change seen in late-onset hydrocephalus. The symptoms and signs of this type of obstruction are subtle and diagnosis of shunt malfunction may be delayed. It is this group who may present with some deterioration of motor function, particularly in the lower limbs, together with other signs such as a lessening of cognitive function, visual deterioration and a general decline in the level of activity. It is believed that deterioration of motor functions, such as increasing spasticity and weakness, is a direct result of a disturbance of the motor pathways associated with the alteration in ventricle size.

It is important to stress that in the majority of children with a shunt obstruction the symptoms fall between these two extremes. Symptoms of raised intracranial pressure, such as headache and vomiting, are dominant and diagnosis is generally readily established and the disorder rectified before the more subtle changes described above eventuate.

In general, it may be stated that deterioration in orthopaedic function may result from late-onset hydrocephalus of slow progression or from chronic shunt obstruction which leads to a slow recurrence of the disorder in which the usual symptoms of raised intracranial pressure are absent or not readily ascertained.

A rare form of hydrocephalus, which may be associated with deterioration of motor function, is the so-called isolated or encysted fourth ventricle. In this condition the fourth ventricle is isolated from the remainder of the ventricular system and the subarachnoid space. The distal obstruction appears to be related to the hind brain anomalies while the aqueduct becomes secondarily obstructed. The fourth ventricle therefore becomes dilated whereas the more proximal ventricles remain collapsed due to the presence of a functioning lateral ventricular shunt. This rare disorder may present with increasing ataxia, gait deterioration and other signs of disturbed brain stem function. Characteristically, signs and symptoms of raised intracranial pressure are absent.

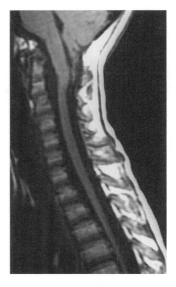

Figure 3.1   MRI image of Chiari type 2 malformation showing the typical findings. Note the inferior displacement of the medulla, fourth ventricle and cerebellar vermis and the kink at the cervico-medullary junction.

Untreated hydrocephalus may adversely effect other structural anomalies, which are subsequently discussed.

Hind Brain Anomalies: The Chiari Type 2 Malformation

All patients with spina bifida cystica have a hind brain anomaly. The complex anatomic changes in this area are encompassed by the term Chiari type 2 malformation. There is no doubt that these changes may be responsible for late neurological deterioration (*Figure 3.1*).

In the neonatal period such changes may be associated with considerable morbidity and may result in death. There is considerable controversy as to whether or not such deterioration results from the primary anomaly or secondarily as a result of distortion and compression of the abnormal structures at the level of the foramen magnum and upper cervical spine. There appears to be evidence supporting both theories. Post-mortem studies have shown changes in the brain stem which appear likely to be congenital in origin (Gilbert *et al.*, 1986) and also changes which could be described as secondary resulting from distortion or compression of that area (Park *et al.*, 1983). In the neonatal group symptoms of brain stem dysfunction usually develop some weeks after birth and may be progressive and thus support the concept of a progressive structural change being responsible rather than a static anomaly.

It is more difficult to precisely define the role of the Chiari type 2 malformation in late orthopaedic deterioration other than via the mechanism of hydromyelia, which will be subsequently discussed. It is conceivable and likely that compression of the neural structures at the level of the foramen magnum and upper cervical spine could lead to impairment of motor function resulting in quadriparesis and increased spasticity. In older patients such symptoms appear to predominate and may be relieved by a decompressive procedure. In neonates and infants a disturbance in this area is more frequently associated with direct signs of brain stem dysfunction, such as stridor, dysphasia and cranial nerve signs. Unfortunately, in this group an adequate decompressive procedure is frequently associated with a poor outcome although Pollack *et al.* (1996) described far better results following early surgical evaluation and intervention. The unsatisfactory outcomes have been attributed to the presence of congenital structural changes in the brain stem or to irreversible changes that have occurred after birth prior to the performance of a decompressive procedure.

Hydromyelia

With the widespread use of magnetic resonance imaging (MRI) this disorder has become increasingly recognized as a common component of the late structural changes that develop in children with spina bifida cystica. The mechanism of development is much debated but there is general agreement that the hind brain anomalies in the region of the foramen magnum are responsible for the progressive dilatation of the central canal of the spinal cord. The hind brain herniation and impaction at the foramen magnum alter CSF dynamics in such a way that CSF accumulates within and dilates the central canal. It is only rarely possible to define a communication between the fourth ventricle and the central canal and it appears most likely that the fluid within the syrinx originates in the spinal subarachnoid space and passes across the cord itself. The driving mechanisms for such a flow pattern are obscure (*Figure 3.2*).

The hydromyelic cavity may extend through the entire cord or be confined to one or two segments. Often the dilatation may be quite extreme. Lesser degrees of this finding appear to be associated with unaltered function, whereas more extreme examples are almost certainly associated with various changes.

In this group of patients the manifestations of this disorder are related largely to disturbances of motor function. The classic motor signs of a lower motor

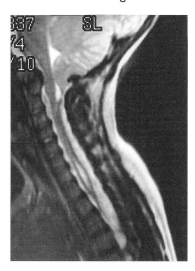

Figure 3.2 This T2 MRI image demonstrates a Chiari type 2 malformation together with hydromyelia which in this projection is most obvious at the cervico-thoracic region.

neurone disturbance in the upper limbs and increasing spasticity in the lower limbs may occur but usually only when the disorder is far advanced. Sensory signs, such as disassociated sensory loss in the upper limbs, are again inconspicuous in the majority of patients in this group.

The principal disorder related to hydromyelia is scoliosis. Spinal curvature has other causes, such as structural vertebral anomalies and terminal tethering (McLone *et al.*, 1990–91) but there does appear to be a firm relationship between hydromyelia and progressive paralytic scoliosis. The exact mechanism producing the deformity is unclear but considered most likely to be a result of paraspinal muscle imbalance.

Tethering

In almost all patients tethering occurs at the site of repair of the myelomeningocoele sac. This is a consequence of the original operative procedure. The original placode attaches to the dorsal aspect of the dural sac while additional intradural adhesions may extend to a higher level (*Figure 3.3*). Rarely, other disorders such as diastematomyelia or a dermoid cyst may contribute to such fixation of the elongated cord.

There appears to be no doubt that under certain poorly defined circumstances tethering of this type may be associated with a deterioration of neurological function. The manifestations of such deterioration include increasing muscle weakness frequently with spasticity, increasing sensory loss, an alteration in bladder and less

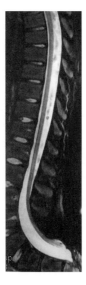

Figure 3.3 This T2 MRI image shows tethering in a 6-year-old child who presented with typical symptoms of a tethered cord syndrome (TCS). The elongated cord is tethered to the dorsal dural sac at the site of the original repair.

commonly bowel function, pain in the back with or without lower limb radiation and scoliosis. These manifestations have been reported in up to one in four children with spina bifida (Tamaki *et al.*, 1988; McLone 1992) and when present constitute the so called tethered cord syndrome (TCS).

Experimental evidence suggests that the deterioration is in the cord itself rather than the nerve roots. Yamada *et al.* (1981) showed evidence of altered metabolic function in the terminal cord in the presence of intermittent and constant stretching and postulated that such altered metabolism could contribute to structural damage at the cellular level. These authors further demonstrated that detethering had a favourable influence on this disturbed metabolism. Earlier experimental evidence seemed to suggest that the mechanical effects of tethering extended no more than four or five segments above the point of tethering (Goldstein, 1966).

The TCS in general is of slow onset. The early manifestations in a child with an already existing neurologic impairment are often not readily apparent. Increasing deformity and complaints of altered gait may be a consequence of growth factors, including increasing obesity, and not be a result of altered neurological function. The diagnosis of lower limb deterioration due to a tethered cord requires a precise analysis of the clinical symptoms and, if possible, the finding of a specific neurologic change, such as increased spasticity, an alteration in reflex activity and altered areas of sensory perception. Repeated muscle charting is of considerable assistance in detecting an altered pattern of muscle strength. If scoliosis is to be attributed solely to tethering it is essential to exclude such causes as structural vertebral anomalies and hydromyelia. Often, however, in this group more than one cause of scoliosis may be present and it may be difficult to define the dominant aetiology.

In a small but important group of children the presence of a tethered cord may be responsible for a sudden and dramatic deterioration in function. The author has seen two teenage children in whom a sudden flexion extension force applied to the spine had produced an immediate profound deterioration of lower limb function. In both patients the deterioration was permanent and presumed due to acute traction and distortion of the already tethered cord. In a further example a 4-year-old child with a past history of a repaired cervical myelomeningocoele developed, after a fall, extensive paralysis of both upper limbs which only partially recovered.

The other situation where presumed acute traction and distortion occur, leading to deterioration, is in the performance of spinal procedures which involve a technique which will of necessity stretch and distort the tethered cord. Procedures of this type have been followed immediately by a marked and permanent deterioration of function. It is essential, before undertaking such operations, to define any such risk. If present it may be necessary to correct an anomaly, such as tethering, prior to the undertaking of the spinal operation.

Other Structural Causes of Deterioration

Diastematomyelia and an intraspinal epidermoid or dermoid cyst have already been indicated as possible, but infrequent, causes of progressive deterioration. In general, the diagnosis of such causes may be identified by currently utilized imaging techniques. Intraspinal arachnoid cysts may be a cause of cord compression leading to deterioration and even with current MRI evaluation a diagnosis may be missed. Such cysts may lie dorsal to the cord and extend over a large segment, such as the entire thoracic component. In many patients with spina bifida cystica the thoracic cord appears to be thinned and lies close to the anterior dural sac. This is usually in the context of a gentle kyphosis and there is a very widened subarachnoid space posteriorly. A long intraspinal arachnoid cyst may be mistaken for this frequent anatomic finding and direct compression of the thoracic cord from the cyst may not be appreciated (*Figures 3.4, 3.5*). Careful

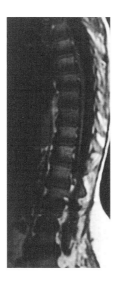

Figure 3.4 This TI image indicates the findings in a child who presented with a progressive and profound deterioration in gait during a 12-month period. The thoracic cord appears thin with a wide space behind this structure.

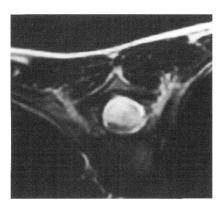

Figure 3.5 The T2 axial image confirms marked anterior displacement of the cord which appears compressed. The cerebrospinal fluid (CSF) containing space behind the cord was a loculated collection of this fluid, which was causing cord compression over the entire thoracic segment. Fenestration resulted in a complete recovery of function.

evaluation of the pattern on good-quality MRI scans may enable the true situation to be ascertained but on occasions it may be necessary to perform additional procedures which involve the insertion of a radio-opaque material into the thecal sac. Such an investigation would allow the area of loculated CSF in the cyst to be defined.

Diagnosis of Neurological Deterioration

As already indicated, neurological deterioration has multiple causes. In any one patient there may be more than a single factor and diagnosis of the precise mechanism may be difficult. Imaging has the ability to define the abnormal anatomy but may not necessarily enable one to define the aetiology of neurological deterioration. The diagnosis relies on analysis of the pattern of change in conjunction with the results of various investigations.

Investigations

MRI

This investigation is the most elegant way of defining the abnormal anatomy of the CNS in patients with spina bifida cystica. Hydrocephalus is readily defined but it is analysis of the changes in the hind brain and within the spinal canal where this investigation is superior to all other modalities of imaging.

There is much to commend the undertaking of MRI studies of the entire spine in all children with spina bifida cystica even in the absence of any evidence of deterioration. Such an investigation will provide baseline information which will alert the clinician to the possibility of late deterioration and result in increased surveillance of that particular patient.

In the presence of suspected deterioration such an investigation is mandatory and rarely needs to be complimented by other imaging techniques.

CT scan

In the older child when the fontanelle is closed a CT scan, together with clinical assessment is useful in defining whether or not there is normal function of a shunt system.

It is possible to define abnormalities at the foramen magnum and within the spinal canal but definition is far less precise than with MRI. A tight foramen magnum, hydromyelia and terminal tethering may be defined.

In the presence of prior spinal instrumentation it may not be possible to interpret MRI or CT scans.

Myelography

This investigation is now rarely if ever required in this group of patients and if undertaken is usually combined with CT (CT/myelogram). The low conus in these patients makes a lumbar puncture a potentially hazardous procedure although in practice such a technique appears to have a low rate of complication.

The main indication for this type of investigation is to define a loculated CSF collection which may be causing cord compression and which is not clearly defined by MRI. If prior spinal instrumentation precludes the use of MRI or CT such imaging may be necessary.

Other investigations

Assessment of spinal cord and nerve root function using electrophysiology is not routinely employed in this group of patients other than in the group undertaking spinal surgery, including orthopaedic instrumentation. There is no doubt that this investigation undertaken at the time of such surgery may alert the surgeon to the possibility of neurological deterioration associated with the procedure.

In the case of suspected deterioration of function of the bladder and bowel, appropriate investigations will be required to confirm or deny such deterioration. Similarly deterioration in spinal function may require plain radiographs with accurate measurements of an increase in curvature to define progression of scoliosis.

PRINCIPLES OF NEUROSURGICAL TREATMENT

If a deteriorating patient has a shunt system or who in the past has had a procedure such as a third ventriculostomy it is imperative to ensure that such a patient has a correctly functioning drainage system. Altered CSF dynamics due to a malfunctioning shunt may not only alter higher brain level function but may also adversely effect the function of the brain stem and the spinal cord. There appears to be evidence that unstable hydrocephalus may induce brain stem signs, particularly in the neonate, and also contribute to the progression of hydromyelia in the older patient. Malfunction of drainage systems can usually be deduced by an analysis of clinical signs and appropriate imaging.

If an orthopaedic surgeon or neurosurgeon contemplates spinal surgery it is essential to ensure that CSF dynamics are satisfactory. The sudden escape of CSF during such a procedure may cause an acute deterioration while persistent elevation of CSF pressure may increase the likelihood of complications such as a CSF fistula or pseudo-meningocoele in the early and late postoperative period.

It is thus essential in the patient with neurological deterioration to first ensure that CSF dynamics are normal. Correction of an anomaly such as would occur with shunt revision may in its own right alleviate the deterioration but it is also essential to perform such a procedure prior to embarking on other forms of spinal surgery, whether they be to correct a disorder such as scoliosis or a procedure designed to reverse deterioration such as a detethering procedure. The rare symptomatic isolated fourth ventricle will require separate drainage either by incorporation into an existing shunt or via an alternate system.

In deteriorating patients there is invariably terminal tethering, changes in the region of the hind brain, and in a sizeable number, hydromyelia. If the symptoms and signs of deterioration relate to the lower limbs and/or the bladder and bowel and there is no associated hydromyelia, then the appropriate procedure after ensuring that hydrocephalus is controlled is to detether the terminal cord. Pain in the back with or without radiation to the lower limbs is also an indication for such an operative procedure as is the isolated development of progressive scoliosis when no other cause for this disorder can be found.

When hydromyelia coexists with tethering a decision regarding the appropriate treatment is less clear. It is the author's opinion that when both conditions exist the primary procedure should be detethering and only be followed by treatment of hydromyelia if the condition for which treatment was undertaken does not stabilize or improve. The author recalls a 16-year-old child with gait deterioration and progressive scoliosis who initially had a posterior fossa and upper cervical decompressive procedure. Preoperative shunt function was considered normal while imaging had demonstrated the Chiari malformation, substantial hydromyelia and terminal tethering. Following what appeared to be a complication-free procedure there was a dramatic deterioration in brain stem function which was only reversed by the undertaking of a detethering procedure 5 days later.

The aim of a detethering procedure is to overcome traction and distortion of the terminal nervous tissue, avoid any additional damage to such tissue and finally endeavour to prevent retethering at some time in the future. In general, the first two aims can be met although a meticulous technique involving magnification is required. Intraoperative electrophysiological monitoring is helpful in deciding which tethered tissue can be safely divided and which must be preserved. Prevention of retethering usually requires the insertion of a substantial dural graft, which enables the thecal sac to be significantly expanded (*Figures 3.6, 3.7*). Even with such techniques, retethering can still occur and may be responsible for the recurrence of a TCS.

Hydromyelia is initially treated by a posterior fossa and upper cervical decompressive procedure. This

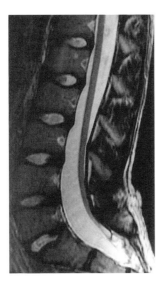

Figure 3.6 This T2 MRI image shows terminal tethering in a 10-year-old child with a tethered cord syndrome (TCS).

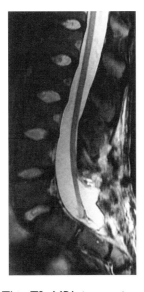

Figure 3.7 This T2 MRI image in the same child shows the findings 3 months after a detethering procedure. In addition to detethering, the dural sac was significantly expanded by the insertion of a dural graft.

is a major undertaking in such patients and is designed to stabilize intracranial and intraspinal CSF dynamics. In these patients it is not necessary or advisable to remove more than just the posterior rim of the foramen magnum but it may be necessary to undertake a multi-segment cervical laminectomy for decompression of the upper cervical cord. As in the lumbar region, a dural graft may be required and the author favours the insertion of a stent to promote flow of CSF from the fourth ventricle to the expanded subarachnoid space.

The extensive laminectomy, particularly performed in a small child, may be followed by late cervical spine deformity (Aronson *et al.*, 1991).

If this procedure is not followed by reduction in size of the hydromyelic cavity then consideration may be given to a direct shunt procedure. Syringo pleural or peritoneal shunts have on occasions been utilized but have a significant complication rate. The fine catheter tends to become occluded in the collapsed hydromyelic cavity.

On occasions an hydromyelic cavity extends into the terminal cord tissue at the site of tethering and may be opened either intentionally or unintentionally during a detethering operation. The term 'terminal ventriculostomy' has been coined to describe such a procedure and has been followed by improvement in the patient's presenting symptoms. Whether or not such improvement is due to such drainage or the detethering is unclear but current concepts regarding the aetiology of hydromyelia would seem to suggest the latter as being the dominant factor leading to improvement.

The rare causes of late deterioration require an appropriate neurosurgical procedure. If diastematomyelia is present the procedure involves the removal of the bone or cartilaginous spur, excision of the dural sleeve around the spur and any intradural adhesions, and finally the reconstitution in a water-tight manner of a single dural tube. An intraspinal dermoid or epidermoid cyst require a complete excision to prevent recurrence while an arachnoid cyst generally requires wide fenestration to prevent late recurrence.

If spasticity persists after an adequate detethering procedure and is responsible for interference with function and increasing deformity then consideration should be given to the undertaking of a selective dorsal rhizotomy. A decision to proceed with such treatment must be very carefully evaluated as in some children such spasticity in the presence of muscle weakness may be providing some benefit. Loss of spasticity under such circumstances may lead to deterioration in ambulatory function and postural abilities.

RESULTS OF SURGICAL TREATMENT

All the above described procedures carry the risk of causing further deterioration. A shunt revision can be associated with problems such as intraventricular or intracerebral haemorrhage while a detethering procedure has a small but not insignificant risk of causing further damage leading to deterioration in function. It is therefore imperative to balance the risks of such procedures against the potential gain. In the correctly selected patient and with the utilization of meticulous technique, deterioration of a progressive nature can be arrested and in many children improvement of function will follow. There is no doubt that the progression of scoliosis may be arrested and there are numerous examples where a detethering procedure or operation for hydromyelia have led to lessening of the scoliotic curve. If pain is the indication for a detethering procedure there is invariably a very satisfactory resolution of the complaint. Improvement in muscle strength and a lessening of spasticity occur in a majority of patients while in the remainder the procedure leads to no clearly defined improvement but rather a cessation of the previous progressive neurological deterioration. Less frequently, deteriorating bladder function may be improved or stabilized by this technique.

The question arises as to whether or not it is justified to undertake prophylactic procedures such as detethering in a child who appears to be neurologically stable. It is the author's opinion that such should not be performed. As previously indicated, TCS only occurs in a minority of patients with demonstrated tethering and as further indicated there is always some risk that such a procedure may in its own right be associated with some deterioration. It is concluded that procedures should only be undertaken if there is well-documented evidence of deterioration, a reasonably clear indication as to the site of the cause of that deterioration and facilities enabling such procedures to be undertaken with the utmost care.

Chapter 4
General Principles in Orthopaedic Management

Malcolm B Menelaus

AIMS OF MANAGEMENT

The aim of management in spina bifida is to establish a pattern of development for the child that is as near normal as the level of paralysis allows. Orthopaedic management should enhance and not interfere with physical and psychological development.

Orthopaedic management should be designed to meet not only the childhood needs but also the expected pattern of adult life for that child. It must be accepted that frequently the child's adult life will be spent seated and orthopaedic management for these children should involve simple limb surgery but maintain high standards in the prevention of pelvic obliquity and the correction of spinal deformity. It is not considered a failure of management if a paraplegic child who walks in childhood does not continue walking in adult life.

Orthopaedic management should place as little strain as possible on the child and the family; they must receive co-ordinated support from the members of an organized spina bifida clinic.

The aim of orthopaedic management of the spine and lower limbs in spina bifida is to establish stable posture (*Figures 4.1, 4.2*). If affected children are to stand for long periods and to remain on their feet in adult life, they must have their centre of gravity over the feet, with minimal flexion deformity at the hips and knees (*Figure 4.3*). Indeed, it is desirable that there be some hyperextension at both hips and knees. It is the posture of these children, when seen from the side, that will largely decide their abilities. They must have extension posture if they are to remain on their feet for long periods and not to tire in the arms, to balance when using one hand for support, and to be able to stand and at the same time have both hands free. This is impor-

tant, since 60% of spina bifida children have neurological abnormalities in their arms and need to use both hands for some activities which unaffected children can perform with one hand.

Figure 4.4 demonstrates flexion posture or flexion deformity. Flexion posture at the hips imposes a flexion posture at the knees; flexion deformity or flexion posture at the knees imposes a flexion posture at the hip. An extension posture at the hip and knee can be maintained with a minimum of support from leg and arm muscles, whereas a flexion posture tends to be a collapsing posture and is commonly associated with lumbar lordosis.

It is important not to be distracted from the principle of producing an extension posture at the hip by the lure of producing a pleasing radiograph of the hips. This is particularly true of those children who require long braces and crutches. Frequently, those children with this severe degree of disability who have the most mobile hips, the greatest ability to remain on their feet all day, and a history of the fewest admissions to hospital and the fewest pathological fractures have radiological appearances which one would hide from one's colleagues. Seldom in spina bifida should we aim at the same excellence of containment of the femoral head within the acetabulum that we aspire to in the management of congenital dislocation of the hip without paralysis.

The chief aim in the management of scoliosis in spina bifida is also the maintenance of stable posture for sitting and standing. In the management of kyphosis and foot deformity, our aim is stability of posture and stability of skin.

To achieve the aim of stable posture, the orthopaedic surgeon must not merely be concerned with

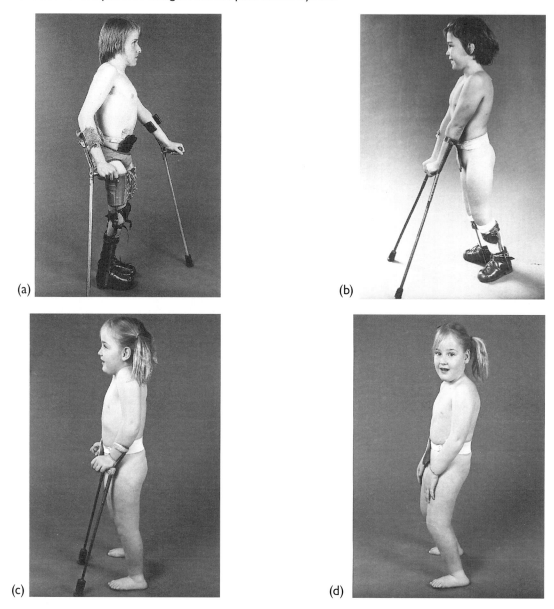

Figure 4.1   Extension posture. These children have varying levels of paralysis and will remain community walkers if they retain this posture and do not develop obesity. The boy illustrated in (a) has bilateral untreated hip dislocation and continues as a community walker at the age of 17 years. He has had hip, knee and foot releases and bilateral triple arthrodeses. The girl illustrated in (c) can walk about the house with crutches, but has to aid her quadriceps muscles by placing her hands on her thighs (d). The children in (b) and (c) have undergone bilateral anterior hip releases and iliopsoas transplantation and soft-tissue surgery to the feet.

surgery and bracing. His or her responsibility includes the continuing care of motor development in order to establish a pattern of development which is as near to normal as the level of paralysis allows. Children who cannot sit by the age of 6–8 months should be provided with a simple sitting aid. Standing with appropriate support usually commences between the 1st and 2nd years, and before the age of 4 years we endeavour to perform all the limb surgery necessary, frequently under one anaesthetic.

PRINCIPLES OF ORTHOPAEDIC SURGERY

Selection of Orthopaedic Surgery

Smith and Smith (1973) drew attention to the fact that spina bifida children had a very much better quality of life if they had strong quadriceps muscles. The quality of life they described included walking ability, need for

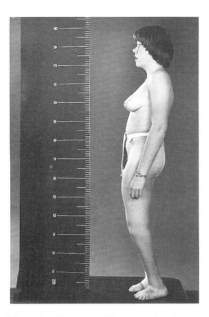

Figure 4.2 A 15-year-old girl who has undergone bilateral iliopsoas transfer, acetabuloplasty of the left hip, posterior knee releases and surgery to the left foot. She has good urinary function and strong quadriceps muscles and benefits considerably from these multiple procedures; if they had been denied her she would have assumed a flexion posture.

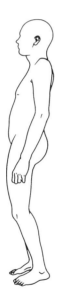

Figure 4.3 Extension posture. Hips and knees extended, feet plantigrade; the posture aimed for regardless of what bracing is necessary.

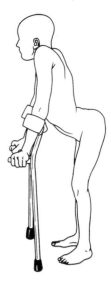

Figure 4.4 Flexion posture. If there is flexion posture at the hips this imposes lumbar lordosis and the patient must use both arms as weightbearing limbs and thus loses their other, more valuable functions.

bracing and wheelchairs, bowel and urinary care, and intelligence and the ability to be educated and later to be employed. Those with strong quadriceps muscles have the most to gain from surgery at the hips. Children with low lesions deserve and benefit from much more complex surgery at the knees and feet, although often this is at the expense of a longer period in casts and a higher complication rate than would be acceptable for those with high lesions. As examples of the application of more complicated surgery, some of the low-lesion group who had an in-toed gait have had the medial hamstrings transferred laterally (Golski and Menelaus, 1976), supramalleolar tibial osteotomies and lateral inlay fusions rid them of short braces, and a small but important group of patients benefit from acetabuloplasty in combination with other hip surgery.

On the other hand, children who do not have adequate bilateral quadriceps power have little to gain from complex surgery. More appropriate are simple soft-tissue releases for fixed deformity, and tendon division or excision to render the joints flail. This prevents recurrence of deformity, a complication which plagued us in the past. The necessity to perform simple procedures for children with high lesions runs contrary to the course of development of surgery, indeed of any science; this is why we have been slow to admit its desirability in these circumstances.

Because the surgery necessary in children with high lesions is relatively minor, it can be performed at several levels and in both limbs under one anaesthetic.

Performing a Minimum of Orthopaedic Surgery

This is merely the restatement of two well-recognized principles: that deformity should be completely corrected and permanently corrected. It is restated in this form – that surgery must be minimized – because there continues to be a widespread need that this requirement be stressed. There has been a high rate of recurrence of deformity, and this must not be accepted as inevitable.

The need is demonstrated by the high failure rate of surgery, a rate which we are in danger of accepting as inevitable. Our incidence of further surgery for recurrent deformity was over 30% for equinovarus deformity and for flexion deformity at the hip and knee. Nor is this unhappy experience confined to the southern hemisphere; Carroll and Sharrard (1972) reported on 149 operations performed on 58 hips.

Deformity must be completely and permanently corrected. Any operation performed on the varus foot must result in a foot that can be placed in some degree of the calcaneovalgus position. Any procedure designed to correct flexion deformity of the hip and knee should enable the joint to be placed in some hyperextension. When we fall short of these aims we have either been insufficiently radical or we have selected the incorrect procedure.

To prevent recurrent deformity it is frequently necessary to divide the tendons of normally acting muscles, even to divide the only functioning motors at hip, knee or foot. It is necessary to overcome our natural reluctance to sacrifice motor function, as there are few reliable tendon transfers for spina bifida children. Associated and sometimes unrecognized spasticity is a potent cause of failure of tendon transfers in this condition.

It must be our aim to perform a single operation on each hip. Many surgeons are reluctant to weaken the psoas which may be the only strong hip motor; we know of no alternative.

Surgery should not be performed as a prophylactic measure. The development of hip deformity or dislocation cannot be predicted on the basis of neurosegmental level. However, it has been advocated, as recently as 1996, that tendon transfers be performed at the hips of patients when there is less than a 50% risk of deformity or dislocation.

Condensed Management

This concept involves the performance of as much surgery as possible under one anaesthetic. When it is not possible to perform all the surgery under one anaesthetic, then operations should be performed a short time apart so that only one period of plaster immobilization is necessary for the total limb surgery. Early weight-bearing in plaster is encouraged.

Correction of Muscle Imbalance

Muscle imbalance plays a part in the production of deformity and should be corrected. Many studies carried out by the authors of this work and referred to in the chapters on limb surgery, show that muscle imbalance is not as potent a cause of deformity as has formerly been believed. Flexion contracture at the hip and knee is more common in the absence of any motor power at these levels and foot deformity is as common in the flail foot as in the foot with active motors. Nevertheless, there are some situations where muscle imbalance is clearly significant, such as the common circumstance where there is a strong tibialis anterior and weak calf leading to calcaneus deformity. Although imbalance between the flexors and extensors of the hip is not the major cause of deformity or dislocation it may be relevant and should be dealt with by lengthening or division of the psoas tendon.

Absence of Sensation Dictates Specific Techniques in the Treatment of Deformity (see Chapter 5)

Fixed deformity in spina bifida must be corrected by means that will not result in pressure on anaesthetic skin. For this and other reasons operative correction of deformity is preferable to the use of conservative measures.

Risk of Pathological Fractures

All management in spina bifida must involve immobilization of the child, and of the individual limbs, for as short a period as possible so that localized osteoporosis and pathological fractures can be avoided. This is a further reason for operative correction of deformity.

Integration with Other Specialist Treatment

The orthopaedic management must be carried out in a centre where there is a specific organization of specialists planned to co-ordinate the various aspects of treatment and to ease the social problems of the child and family. It is preferable to travel 1000 km to such a clinic rather than to receive treatment, in isolation, from a nearby orthopaedic surgeon. Ideally, there should be a clinic where several specialists and ancillary workers can be consulted at one visit to the hospital.

Orthopaedic management cannot be properly carried out in isolation from other specialist management.

The Age of Orthopaedic Treatment

Whereas we normally treat congenital dislocation of the hip as soon as possible after birth, in spina bifida it is generally best to manage the congenital paralytic dislocation of the hip, if at all, at a later age when the spinal defect has healed and the child is thriving.

Wound Infection

Children requiring major surgery should have pre-operative urinary culture. A course of appropriate antibiotics should be commenced 24 hours before operation. This is particularly necessary in relationship to spinal surgery.

THE EFFECTS OF CHANGES IN THE PATTERN OF ORTHOPAEDIC MANAGEMENT

That the persuance of the principles listed above (and notably the first three principles) is effective from some view points, is demonstrated by the following study (Menelaus, 1976a).

Figure 4.5 shows the average number of hospital bed-days per child, and the proportion of these bed-

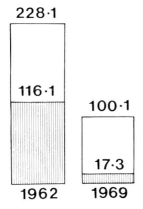

Figure 4.5 Average number of hospital bed-days per child during the first 5 years of life. Shaded areas indicate number of bed-days for orthopaedic management, white areas those for other than orthopaedic management. The 1962 column represents 30 consecutive children born in 1962 and early 1963, the 1969 column represents the same number born in 1969 and early 1970.

days spent in hospital for orthopaedic reasons in a consecutive series of children, born in 1962, who survived for a minimum of 5.5 years. More than half the bed-days spent in hospital during that period were for orthopaedic reasons. Too many operations were performed during these years, often with unrealistic aims. With distressingly high failure rates, operations frequently succeeded in restoring a localized portion of the anatomy to normal but did nothing to enhance walking. Operations were sometimes necessary to treat the complications of previous procedures, and post-immobilization pathological fractures were common. That this problem is not peculiar to one hospital is demonstrated by the world literature; in one series (Lorber, 1971) 41 children, subsequently adjudged to be permanently chairbound, had a total of 333 ortho-paedic operations. It is quite justified to perform orthopaedic procedures to enable walking in childhood in the knowledge that the child will later elect to use a wheelchair, but it is not justifiable to perform an average of more than eight operations on such children.

Over the years we have slowly changed our aims, our principles and our techniques. As a result, the number of bed-days spent in hospital for orthopaedic reasons in a second series (born in 1969) reduced to about one-seventh that for the group born in 1962 (*Figure 4.5*). This reduction was not brought about by orthopaedic lassitude; indeed, the reduction in the number of operations in the two series was merely in a ratio of 4:3; that is, far less than the reduction in the duration of stay in hospital for each child. We did operate on fewer children with high lesions, but the major reduction of time spent in hospital was brought about by performing effective surgery and by condensing the management so that only a single period of plaster immobilization was necessary, despite multiple operations.

Figure 4.6 shows the reduction in the average number of bed-days in hospital for orthopaedic reasons per child per year of life. Unfortunately, the measures taken to bring about this reduction have not been widely adopted and, at some centres, there is still a tendency for major surgery to be performed on the hips when the surgery is unlikely to benefit the patient.

There have been reductions in the average number of operations on each hip from 2.2 to 1.2, and in the incidence of pathological fractures following surgery from 12% to 7%.

REALISTIC AIMS RELATED TO EXTENT OF DISABILITY

Orthopaedic management is directed towards the goal appropriate to the neurosegmental level for that child

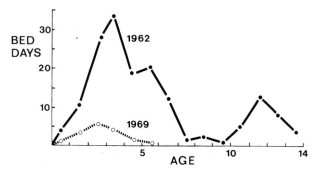

Figure 4.6 Average numbers of hospital bed-days per child per year (same two groups as in *Figure 4.5*). The rise in admissions in the 1962 group between 11 and 12 years is largely because of admissions for foot stabilization and surgery for scoliosis. The earlier peak in the 1969 series reflects earlier soft-tissue surgery for muscle imbalance and deformity of hip, knee and foot.

(Kupka *et al.*, 1978). Whilst these levels are not always clear cut and cannot always be determined early, they can generally be discerned in the 1st year of life. Children do not always fulfil the potential for their neurosegmental level; the potential outlined below represents the maximal potential that can be expected for a given child. These levels are approximations of the lowest group level of active muscle innervation; the situation is complicated by the presence of spasticity and other factors.

Hoffer *et al.* (1973) found that of children with sacral lesions, all became community walkers and of those with thoracic lesions all became non-walkers. Those with lumbar lesions were much more diverse in their walking ability but none with significant deformity at the hips remained walking (though two patients with dislocated hips and up to 25° of fixed flexion remained community walkers).

Barden *et al.* (1975), in a review of the fate of 63 patients with myelodysplasia who had survived 20 years or more, found that 19 of 20 patients with a deficity at the third lumbar level were functional walkers.

Swank and Dias (1992) reported that children with spina bifida walk later than normal. Hoffer *et al.* (1973) also found that those who were ultimately to progress from non-functional to functional walking invariably did so by the age of 9 years; physiotherapy to make children functional walkers is not indicated beyond this age. Generally, it is apparent whether functional walking will be achieved by the age of 6 years.

Upper Thoracic Lesions

These children have poor, long spinal and abdominal muscles and are unable to sit without support. They frequently have evidence of upper motor neurone lesions in their arms and their functional ability is largely determined by the degree of disability in their arms.

These children require spinal support to enable them to sit without supporting themselves with their hands. Approximately 85% develop scoliosis which generally will be of a severe degree and will require surgical correction and fusion.

The goals for children with upper thoracic lesions are good sitting balance, walking ability in a reciprocating orthoses until somewhere between the age of 8 and 14 years if they have good upper limb function, ability to transfer from a chair, wheelchair propulsion and social acceptability. They will always need assistance with activities of daily living and with activities of community living.

Surgery at the hip should be aimed at reducing a fixed flexion deformity so a Reciprocating Gait Orthosis (RGO) can be used in childhood. Surgery at the foot should enable the ability to transfer and so the foot looks normal when placed on the footrest of a wheelchair in later life.

Lower Thoracic Lesions

These children have sufficient innervation of their trunk musculature to be good sitters. They usually have enough upper limb strength to transfer independently and are good wheelchair users. They usually ambulate during the first 10–14 years of life but are largely wheelchair users as adults. As for the upper thoracic lesions, a high percentage will require surgery for flexion deformity at hip and knee and many require surgery for foot deformity. There is a high risk of trophic ulceration. Good skin care, parent and child education and prophylactic skin assessments are necessary to prevent the social, educational, vocational and psychological setbacks that can occur as a result of skin breakdown.

Upper Lumbar Lesions

These children have activity in the flexors and adductors of the hips and weak power in the quadriceps muscles. Hip and knee flexion deformities, both of which require surgical management, are frequent. They should become household ambulators in long leg braces for a period. They will always require crutches and from the second decade will frequently use wheelchairs for increasing periods of the day.

Lower Lumbar Lesions

These children are usually community ambulators although they usually require below-knee orthotics. Strong quadriceps muscles gives them a better quality of life as previously explained. If the hip abductors are weak they may require one or two crutches. A lower percentage will require surgery for hip deformity, than for higher lesions; some will require surgery for, usually unilateral, hip dislocation. Foot deformity will commonly require surgical management to enable them to meet the heavy demands of which they are capable.

Sacral Lesions

Here the aim is brace-free community ambulation. Surgery is necessary for foot deformities only. About 95% become community ambulators in adulthood and a significant number, by adulthood, have complications such as osteomyelitis which may necessitate amputation (Brinker *et al.*, 1994).

FAILURE TO ACHIEVE WALKING POTENTIAL

Children who fail to achieve their walking potential may do so because of a variety of factors: inadequately corrected deformity, poor orthotic care, obesity, low intelligence, development of tethering or syrinx, defective eyesight and lack of motivation in the parents and hence in the child. Trophic ulceration and difficulties with bowel and bladder control may lead to social, educational, vocational and psychological setbacks which prevent children from achieving the potential outlined in the preceding paragraphs. It is not clear why some children fail to achieve the abilities described above or achieve them in the second decade only to deteriorate later; but unfortunately this is common.

If cerebellar, cerebral, high spinal and upper limb pathology is considerable (see Chapter 2) then these features may not be discerned early, in which case the neonatal assessment of potential will have been too optimistic (*Figure 4.7*).

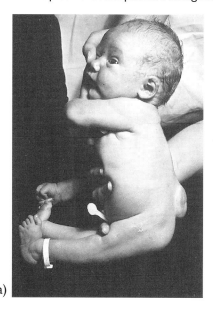

(a)

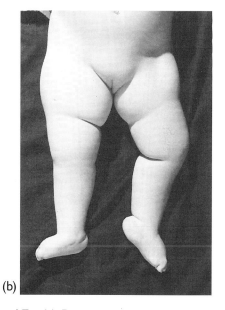

(b)

Figure 4.7 (a) Demonstrates the posture of a baby at presentation on day I. There is strong continuous and uninterrupted activity in the hip flexors, knee extensors and foot dorsiflexors. The neurosegmental level was considered to be such that the fifth lumbar roots were spared. The sac was closed the same day; there was then a gradual reduction in muscle activity in the legs so that by the age of I year (b) there was only a flick of activity in the previously functioning muscles. The possibility that this phenomenon may occur should lead the clinician to caution in making a prognosis for walking potential.

SHOULD ALL CHILDREN BE ENCOURAGED TO STAND AND WALK?

Many children achieve such a poor gait that they use a wheelchair almost exclusively once they are in a position to make their own decision. The question therefore arises as to whether this short period of ambulation in childhood is worth the stresses of hospitalization, surgery and physical therapy.

It is best to assume that all children who are not severely mentally retarded or who do not have gross spasticity will walk and to encourage them to this end. All children, except those who have multiple factors suggesting that they will not walk, should be taught to stand and walk as soon as this becomes feasible.

Mental functions are, in part, derived from motor actions – there must be a continuous interaction between the organism and the environment for normal mental functioning. Unless the child can achieve an upright posture and progress there will be abnormal interaction between the child and his or her surroundings and abnormal mental development. Hostler (1976) also points out that the normal child of 10 months has innumerable experiences of crawling into trouble and has heard 'No, no' innumerable times and consequently understands 'No, no'. However, the infant with spina bifida hears this less often because of his motor problem and thus misses a major language milestone. Similarly at 18 months the child who is handicapped has not been asked to fetch familiar objects or to put toys away and consequently he or she does not understand such instructions. Hostler points out that walking is not only necessary for other gross motor activities but also for socialization, language, self-help, fine motor and cognitive experiences. In addition, prolonged sitting

Table 4.1   Orthopaedic management related to stage of development and age

Developmental stage	Management
Birth ↓ Head control	Assessment commences with view to determining realistic aims; posturing to correct deformity; correction of equinovarus deformity Developmental stimulation
Head control ↓ Sitting	Encourage sitting balance Encourage hand skills and co-ordination
Sitting ↓ Prone mobility	Encourage upper limb strength and co-ordination hand function Provide sitting aids
Prone mobility ↓ Upright stance	Continued assessment; increased social stimulation Provide standing orthosis
Upright stance ↓ Upright mobility	Physiotherapy and orthoses appropriate to the neurosegmental level Soft-tissue releases for hip deformity; open tenotomy of psoas and adductors; reduction of hip dislocation (in combination with appropriate soft-tissue procedure); Pemberton osteotomy ± femoral osteotomy
2.5 years ↓ 6 years	Tendon excision of deforming foot tendons Kyphosis surgery; Grice procedure; correction of fixed flexion at knees; quadriceps release
6 years ↓ 10 years	Surgery for recurrent hip and foot deformity Correction of the early developing spinal deformity
10 years ↓ 16 years	Scoliosis and lordosis surgery; osteotomy for fixed hip and knee deformity Foot stabilization

leads to decubitus, ulcers, urinary stasis and flexion deformities; it is desirable to get these children into the standing position as early an age as is feasible, which will usually be between the ages of 1 and 2 years. Mazur *et al.* (1989) demonstrated the late advantages or earlier walking in patients who have abandoned walking; those who have walked possess enhanced transfer, and other, abilities.

We have never regretted performing the appropriate surgery to enable standing; we have, on occasions, regretted that we have not performed such surgery on those thought to be permanently incapable of walking. Later these children have proved to have much more intelligence than was first anticipated; they have commenced walking and we have been faced with rigid deformities that are difficult to correct. The surgery necessary to enable standing is simple surgery – soft tissue releases which can be performed at hip, knees and feet under one anaesthetic.

Even those children who would seem certain to have impaired intelligence should not have their limb disabilities ignored. It might be argued that they are even more in need of motor independence than is a child of normal intelligence. A child with an intelligence quotient below 50 may be capable of walking, feeding themselves and dressing themself.

AT WHAT AGE SHOULD DEFORMITY BE CORRECTED?

The treatment of deformity of spina bifida is largely operative and this surgery is best carried out after the spinal lesion is well healed and when the child is thriving. Then hip deformity may be minimized by posturing the baby, and foot deformity partially or completely corrected by tenotomy of the tendo Achillis and the application of well-padded plasters. Only for equinovarus deformity is operative surgery indicated in the first 6 months of life.

A general plan of the timing of orthopaedic management is set out in *Table 4.1*. This plan dovetails in with other management – closure of the spinal lesion soon after birth, atrioventricular shunt operation in the first few months of life and urinary diversion in the 4th year of life.

SHOULD CONSERVATIVE OR OPERATIVE MEANS BE USED TO CORRECT DEFORMITY?

Operative means are generally most appropriate for the correction of deformity in spina bifida. Conservative correction may, even when used with care, produce sores in anaesthetic areas. After operative division of tight structures the plaster merely holds the part in the correct position without pressure on the skin.

The surgery required may be minor. Tenotomy of the tendo Achillis followed by serial plasters may enable correction of talipes equinovarus. In general, we cannot agree with Gucker (1964) who advocates correction of deformity by a series of plaster casts.

Furthermore, conservative correction will require a longer period of plaster immobilization than operative; this is more likely to lead to aggravated osteopenia and fractures.

Chapter 5

Pressure Sores and Pathological Fractures

John S Barnett and Malcolm B Menelaus

PRESSURE SORES AND CHILBLAINS
Malcolm B Menelaus

Introduction

Pressure sores are a significant problem in the management of these children. They occur in about 40% of patients (*Table 5.1*) and are most frequently situated over the sacrum, over the ischial tuberosities and on the feet. Occasionally, pressure sores are seen on the feet at birth. Hayes and Gross (1963) reported an incidence of 48%. Once pressure sores occur in anaesthetic skin they become indolent and may prevent the child from wearing calipers or boots for quite a long period and may thus considerably interfere with walking.

Hay and Walker (1973) found that the plantar pressures in 78 feet of children with spina bifida were, with few exceptions, higher than those in normal

Table 5.1 The incidence of pressure sores in 168 patients (aged 3 years and over) with myelomeningocele

Level of lesion present	Pressure sores not present	Pressure sores present
Lower thoracic	10	12
Upper lumbar	11	16
Lower lumbar–upper sacral	43	61
Lower sacral	1	14
Total	65 (39%)	103 (61%)

children of the same age. This is probably because the feet are generally smaller in myelomeningocele and increased plantar pressures with anaesthesia leads on to trophic skin ulceration. Chilblains are generally encountered in the winter months and occur most frequently on the hallux and less often on other toes and the heel.

It is of utmost importance to avoid pressure sores due to skin anaesthesia. Plaster of Paris is generally used only to maintain a position which has been achieved by soft tissue operation. In those few instances where serial plasters and wedged plasters are used to correct deformity, then felt pads are placed on pressure points. There will be no pain to warn the surgeon of pressure on the skin or skin breakdown so he or she must be on the lookout for serous ooze into the plaster and for any evidence of blistering or infection under the plaster. Considerable care must be taken in the fitting of orthoses so that there are no sites of undue pressure. Parents must be instructed to inspect the skin daily and to treat any incipient ulcer with respect and to cease putting the child into orthoses and boots until the pressure area has healed or the surgeon has been consulted. Once the patient reaches the age of co-operation, they will be able to do 'push-ups' as they sit at school and take weight from one buttock to the other. Any child who spends prolonged periods sitting is provided with one of the appropriate cushions designed for paraplegic patients.

Chilblains are of less significance as they tend to heal when the cold weather ceases. A course of tolazoline hydrochloride (Priscol) or other vasodilator may be tried but there is considerable doubt as to its effectiveness. Severe burns are seldom encountered but one of

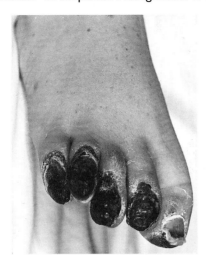

Figure 5.1 Gangrene of the toes presumably due to exposure to cold. The parents were unable to give a satisfactory explanation yet this child had always been well cared for.

our children lost two toes due to burns from some heated cotton wool which had been wrapped about her chilled feet. Sometimes the cause of the gangrene is uncertain (*Figure 5.1*).

A pressure sore may reflect pressure due to deformity that requires correction or to orthoses that require modification. An example of the former is the indolent ulcer which inevitably forms under the base of the fifth metatarsal in a varus foot. This ulcer will not heal until the pressure distribution under the foot has been equalized. This may be achieved by a moulded insole or by surgery to make the foot plantigrade.

If an operation is necessary to make the foot plantigrade then ideally the child should be prevented from taking weight on the affected foot until the ulcer has healed and only then should surgery be performed. Nevertheless, on several occasions the ulcer has failed to heal despite prolonged non-weightbearing, then healed after correction of the deformity by triple arthrodesis.

Flail feet can be associated with areas of increased pressure; such feet commonly have a mobile calcaneovalgus deformity and the greatest part of the child's weight is taken on the heel or merely on the medial portion of the heel producing an ulcer on the instep. Lateral inlay triple arthrodesis spreads the load of weightbearing in these circumstances allowing the ulcer to heal. Some surgeons reject fusion procedures in spina bifida patients because they believe that mobility of the foot is a safeguard against pressure sores. We have not been troubled by pressure effects following triple fusion, indeed triple fusion is one of our most effective weapons used against established sores (Olney and Menelaus, 1988).

THE PATHOLOGY AND MANAGEMENT OF PRESSURE SORES
John S Barnett

Although the child with spina bifida has much in common with the adult paraplegic patient, there are significant differences in the presentation of pressure sores. Whereas most adults with traumatic paraplegia develop a pressure sore at some stage of their life, and frequently within a few months of their injury, it is uncommon for the child with spina bifida to develop pressure sores until he or she reaches school age. The only exception to this rule is ulceration overlying an extensive kyphosis which may occur as early as 2 years of age. Guttman (1955, 1973, 1976) has emphasized the role of pressure in the development of ulceration, and it is understandable that in the early years of life, when nursing care is in the hands of dedicated parents, the position of the child can be changed easily and frequently to avoid localized pressure. In addition, the natural activity of the young child will normally contribute to postural change and the relief of pressure over a particular area.

A study of spina bifida children admitted to the Royal Children's Hospital with the primary diagnosis of pressure sore shows that the majority of the sores are caused by pressure from an external appliance such as a caliper or splint, or follow the application of plaster for a surgical procedure. The remainder occur over any bony prominence from prolonged sitting or lying in one position. The ischial and sacral regions are especially prone to ulceration, but the characteristic trochanteric sores of the adult paraplegic are not common in young children.

As in other congenital lesions where the child rapidly learns to adapt to his or her disability, so in spina bifida there is every opportunity to teach the child the principles of skin care and prevention of ulceration. Most children tolerate long periods of limited activity and can be positioned to allow an incipient trouble spot to be relieved completely from pressure until the danger of ulceration has passed. Unfortunately, the older child may forget these principles in his or her eagerness to participate in normal schooling and sporting activities. Prolonged sitting at school, ill-fitting shoes and failure to check appliances may lead to pressure sores.

Because of the lack of sensation in the lower limbs, the child with spina bifida is prone to home accidents, and particularly to burns from proximity to heating appliances, or from hot liquids. Such apparently simple accidents can readily lead to full thickness skin loss and prolonged morbidity.

Pathology

The pathological changes in the tissues consequent upon local pressure have been well described (Guttman, 1955; Bailey, 1967). The earliest effect is a transient circulatory disturbance, manifested by local erythema and oedema. Such a situation is reversible and is a useful warning sign for the patient or his or her attendants.

If pressure is unrelieved, cutaneous damage extends through the phases of blistering and loss of superficial epithelium, to deep dermal loss and eventually to full thickness skin loss. Tissue damage of this extent is not reversible, but if the loss can be confined to the skin, the formation of granulation tissue can be encouraged and the wound may heal by local epithelial spread from the wound edges, or the denuded surface can be closed by routine skin grafting procedures.

Continued pressure or the intervention of infection rapidly converts the area of skin loss into a deep ulcer, with destruction of the subcutaneous fat and eventual involvement of the underlying bony prominence. In the acute stage, damage to the subcutaneous tissues may be far more extensive than that to the overlying skin, and in the absence of definitive treatment a large undermined ulcer persists (Nola and Vistnes, 1980).

Infection plays a large part in the subsequent progress of the ulcer and culture of the area usually reveals a mixture of organisms, including staphylococci, coliforms, proteus and, occasionally, pseudomonas organisms. Prolonged infection leads to periostitis, heterotopic bone formation in the adjacent soft tissues and, rarely, to the development of osteomyelitis and bone necrosis. The extensive undermining of the skin may develop into sinuses that extend for some distance along tissue planes and emerge in distant areas. Such a situation is not uncommon in the ischial region, with the opening of the sinus in the perineum.

In those areas where a bursa overlies a bony prominence, a bursitis may develop in response to local pressure without skin damage. The fluid in the bursa may at first be sterile, but infection usually supervenes and converts the bursa into a closed abscess, which then discharges through a small sinus in the skin belying the underlying extent of the damage.

Contributing Factors

While it is acknowledged that pressure is the prime factor in the formation of ulcers, other agents contribute to their formation, extension and persistence. Absence of sensation is invariably contributory and lack of mobility in the legs implies that pressure cannot be relieved by normal intermittent changes in sitting posture. Incontinence of urine and faeces may also aggravate the problem. The former can be well controlled by an ileal conduit but faecal soiling is difficult to control, resulting in maceration of tissues and local infection. These local factors are of particular importance in sacral and ischial sores, and become of paramount importance in the surgical closure of such defects.

Of more direct importance are the original scars on the back resulting from the repair of the meningocele. In addition, the bony prominences which result from the kyphotic and scoliotic deformities so common in this condition may be closely related to the meningocele scar, and with the abnormal posture and altered dynamics, these areas are readily subjected to pressure and frequently develop infection. Such areas are also prone to pressure in the postoperative period when patient mobility is limited, and where restraining plaster spicas or jackets have been used. Pressure sores may also develop over the prominence of some form of internal fixation used in the management of spinal deformity.

Prevention

Constant supervision of all pressure areas, especially those relating to plasters, splints and cushions for wheelchairs, should prevent development of pressure sores. The earliest indication of redness is an absolute warning that pressure must be avoided. In the early stages, blistering of the skin and even small areas of full thickness skin loss will heal without surgery if the affected area is completely relieved from pressure. Local dressings appropriate to the stage of ulceration assist in re-epithelialization or healing by wound contracture. Conservative management must of necessity interfere with the daily routine and activities of the child, and if the sore is in the ischial or sacral area he or she should not be allowed to sit and must revert to the prone position on a frame or trolley. In most cases this will mean interruption of schooling, or alternatively, deferment of treatment until the next holiday period. Sound healing cannot be expected in less than 4 weeks, so that even for a superficial ulceration there will be a considerable absence from school. For this reason it is not uncommon to find that treatment is limited to infrequent dressings so that schooling can continue. Such a programme is rarely successful and leads to extension of the ulcer into the deeper tissue. Operative treatment must then be instituted.

Preoperative Investigations

The general condition of the child is assessed, and the haemoglobin concentration estimated. If the ulcers are extensive and heavily infected the serum proteins should also be estimated, although it is unusual in the child to find a significant protein deficiency. However, it is not uncommon to find a degree of anaemia, especially if there has been continuing blood loss during debridement and preparation of the ulcer, and any significant anaemia should be corrected prior to operation.

X-rays are taken to show the underlying bony prominence and to determine the presence of osteomyelitis or heterotopic bone formation in the adjacent soft tissues. Extensive sinus tracts can be outlined by the injection of Lipiodol.

The child is positioned so that pressure over the sore is eliminated, and a programme of turning to avoid prolonged pressure on other areas is worked out and practised prior to operation, to accustom the child to the routine which is necessary after operation.

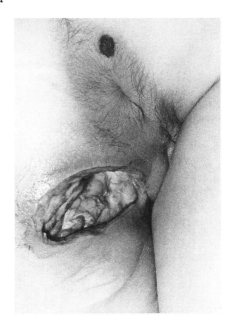

Figure 5.2 An extensive pressure area overlying the left ischial tuberosity with considerable tissue necrosis.

Preparation of the Wound

Before the wound can be closed surgically it must be free from slough and show clean granulation tissues in the walls of the ulcer. Cultures should show minimal bacteriological involvement and preferably be free from certain organisms (especially staphylococci and pseudomonas) before surgery is undertaken.

To convert a sloughing ulcer into a clean wound ready for closure, there is no substitute for careful frequent dressings, packing of the cavity, and debridement with scissors. At the first dressing all necrotic tissue is cut away, and any undermined pockets and sinuses are opened up. The wound is then packed with a single gauze strip soaked in saline or betadine, care being taken to pack firmly into all recesses of the ulcer. This pack is changed 4–6 hourly depending on drainage, and at each dressing any loose slough is debrided with sharp scissors to the point of bleeding.

Removing the slough and establishing drainage improves the wound dramatically. Within a week or 10 days the wound should be free from slough and clean healthy granulation tissue lines the ulcer cavity. Swabs taken at this time should confirm the clinical impression of minimal bacteriological contamination.

Closure of the Pressure Sore

If permanent healing is to be achieved, certain basic principles must be observed. The lining of the ulcer must be completely removed to prevent subsequent seroma formation and the underlying bony prominence should be reduced or eliminated. The wound must be closed in depth to provide a thick layer of soft tissue between the skin and the underlying bone; the skin defect is closed either by direct suture or local flap; and some form of efficient wound drainage must be employed to prevent the accumulation of haematoma or seroma, as such an event can result in complete failure of the operation.

Following careful preparation of the ulcer, complete excision of the lining membrane renders the area surgically clean and there should be no hesitation in proceeding to primary closure (*Figures 5.2–5.4*). In large flat areas and even where bone covered with granulations may be showing in the wound, there may be some advantage in closing the wound by a split skin graft. In areas not normally subject to pressure, this graft may be all that is required, but in most ulcers the graft can be regarded as a temporary measure (*Figures 5.5–5.9*). It will, however, have the advantage of providing a closed wound for the subsequent repair, and contracture of the graft will diminish the size of the defect and make secondary closure considerably easier. Few ulcers require such a two-stage repair, but there are occasions when it may be helpful.

Blood loss may be considerable during the repair of large ulcers because of poor vasomotor control. Blood should be available, and an intravenous infusion should be running throughout the operation. In large ulcers requiring extensive debridement where haemostasis is difficult to obtain, packing the cavity for 24–48

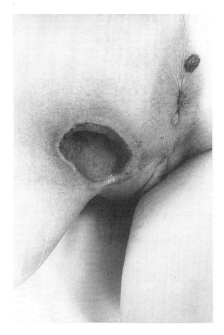

Figure 5.3 Ten days later, the ulcer is clean and ready for direct closure.

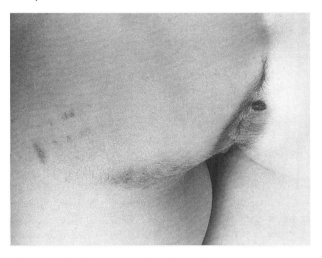

Figure 5.4 Three months after closure.

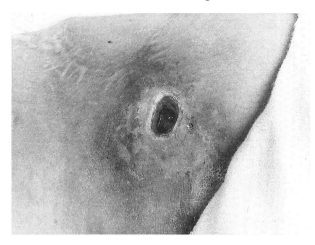

Fig. 5.5 A pressure sore which appeared adjacent to, but not through, a scar lying below and lateral to the left gluteal fold.

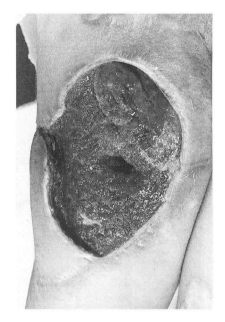

Figure 5.6 A large flat ulcer which resulted from loss of a poorly designed advancement flap.

hours followed by delayed closure may offer the best chance of obtaining primary healing.

Operative Procedure

Excision of the lining membrane is facilitated by the use of the 'pseudotumour' technique described by Guttman (1955, 1973, 1976). The ulcer cavity is packed with a single layer of gauze soaked in Bonney's blue or similar colouring agent, and the mouth of the ulcer closed with a few sutures. The ulcer margin and the wall of granulation tissue can then be excised by sharp dissection around the pack and any break in the lining is immediately noted by exposure of the coloured pack. As the base of the ulcer is approached, that portion adherent to the bone can be removed cleanly, taking only the scar tissue attached to bone, or a small sliver of the bone surface.

It is in the approach to the underlying bone and the method of closing the ultimate defect that differences arise between spina bifida children and the adult paraplegic. In the latter case, removal of bone in some areas may be minimal and will leave a broad flat surface, but areas such as the ischial tuberosity and the greater trochanter may require more radical removal of bone to prevent secondary pressure areas arising.

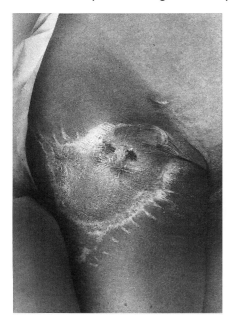

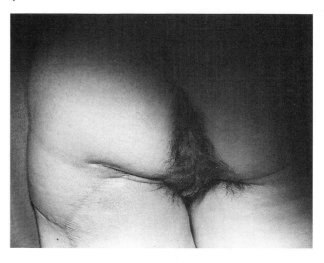

Figure 5.9 The appearance 6 months after operation.

Figure 5.7 The appearance following the covering of the defect with a split skin graft. This procedure was designed as a temporary measure.

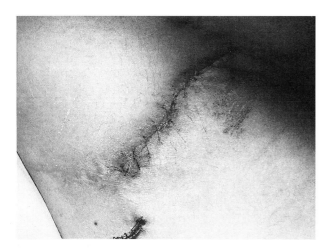

Figure 5.8 The appearance following excision of the graft and direct wound closure.

In the child, a more conservative approach should be employed, and provided there is no bone infection, removal of the adherent ulcer base and judicious rounding of the prominent bone will be sufficient. It seems far too radical a procedure to remove a segment of bone in the young child, and the results of conservative surgery have been justified in the long term.

Most authors advocate formal flap closure of pressure sores in order to provide fresh tissue and avoid a suture line over the bony prominence. However, transposed or rotated flaps also lack sensa-

tion and confer no greater protection than the original tissue. The subcutaneous tissue cannot resist pressure unless it is contained within fibrous pockets, as in the heel pad, but such areas are limited and not available for transfer. In addition, flap closure is complicated and prejudices adjacent areas which may be required in the future. 'It is an illusion to believe that a new surface will prevent the recurrence of a sore' (Bailey, 1967).

Therefore, there is considerable advantage in children in a simple direct technique using local tissue. Bailey (1967) has shown that most ulcers are surrounded by lax tissues which can readily be brought together by direct suture. If a portion of the fibrous capsule of the ulcer is used in the repair, a good depth of tissue can be brought over the bone. There is sufficient evidence of recurrent ulceration occurring through skin adjacent to a scar rather than through the actual scar, and of long-term clinical success of direct repair to justify this method in the child, at least in the first instance. It has the obvious advantage of conserving tissue and creating only a single scar, and thereby avoiding a secondary donor defect. The adjacent tissue remains unscarred and available for future use if necessary.

Direct closure of the ulcer depends on the availability of local tissue, wide undermining to free the layers of scar and muscle which are adherent in the sides and base of the ulcer, and the use of part of the fibrous capsule to provide a strong layer that will hold sutures and support the subcutaneous tissues. The deeper layers of the wound are closed in depth over the bony prominence using 3–0 Dexon or monofilament stainless steel wire, and there should be complete apposition of these layers to prevent the formation of any dead space where a haematoma could collect. The skin is then closed with interrupted nylon sutures, or a continuous wire suture which can be retained for several weeks, and which provides good support for the skin while spreading the tension along the whole suture line.

The most important part of this technique is the use of continuous wound suction, which is maintained until drainage has virtually ceased. It is important that the drain tube has access to all layers of the wound and that it is kept functioning throughout the postoperative period. The tube is brought out obliquely through normal adjacent tissue. The drainage bottle is changed daily at a set time, and the amount of drainage charted. The loss may be heavy for the first few days, but gradually diminishes as it becomes serous. When the drainage has decreased to a few millilitres in 24 hours the tube is removed; this may not be until the 10th or 14th day postoperatively.

In some circumstances, direct closure may be considered unsuitable and use can then be made of a local flap. The rotation flap is preferred, as the donor site can usually be closed directly (*Figures 5.10, 5.11*). The buttock provides a satisfactory and safe flap for most sacral sores, while for the ischial region a flap may be rotated upwards from the posterior thigh (Hurwitz *et al.*, 1981). Trochanteric sores lie in an area which is relatively short of tissue, but a flap from the lateral surface of the thigh can be transposed into the defect, with direct closure of the donor area (Nahai *et al.*, 1978; Hauben *et al.*, 1983).

Pressure sores on the foot or the malleoli can usually be closed by small local transposition flaps with split skin grafts to the donor site.

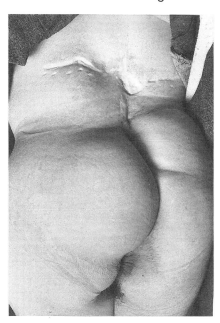

Figure 5.11 The appearance 1 year following closure by rotation flap from the left buttock.

It is essential that the flap be designed with a broad base, that it rotates easily into the defect, that the flap be generous enough to allow it to lie freely in the base of the ulcer and not tent across the wound leaving a dead space, and that the site of the secondary defect be chosen to avoid future problems.

In deep ulcers there may be insufficient local tissue to fill the cavity, and in some areas it may be possible to detach an adjacent muscle from its insertion and turn it into the defect. There are some doubts about the efficacy of this muscle mass in the long term, as a degree of atrophy is certain to occur, and furthermore, muscle in itself offers very little resistance to pressure. It has been established by anatomical dissection that muscle does not occur over bony prominences. It has also been established that muscle transferred in a myocutaneous flap to a weightbearing area will become wasted, giving rise to local depression (Daniel and Faibisoff, 1982). Use of muscle to fill the cavity may therefore be only a convenient manoeuvre at the time of operation, with little permanent cushioning effect.

The popularity of myocutaneous flaps in other areas of plastic surgery has prompted the use of these flaps to cover pressure sores. They can be designed to include a major muscle with its blood supply, with the overlying subcutaneous tissue and skin being supplied by perforating arteries (*Figures 5.12, 5.13*). The most common myocutaneous flaps include the gluteus maximus flap which covers the sacral area (Parry and Mathes, 1982), the extended gluteal thigh flap and the biceps femoris flap for ischial sores, and the tensor

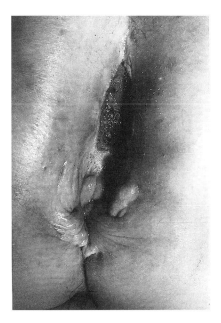

Figure 5.10 An extensive and deep pressure sore with loss of the coccyx.

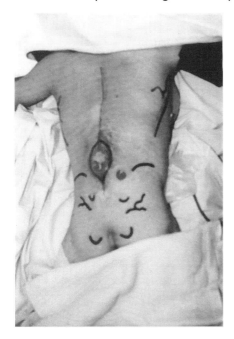

Figure 5.12   Ulcer in the thoraco-lumbar region.

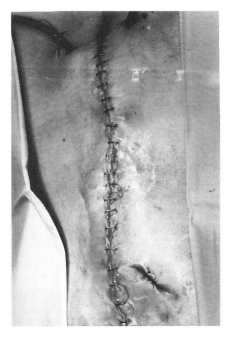

Figure 5.13   Closure of the ulcer using multiple myo-cutaneous advancement flaps.

fascia lata flap to cover trochanteric sores. These axial pattern flaps are safer and more predictable than random pattern flaps, but whether muscle transferred with its blood supply prevents recurrent ulceration remains to be seen.

There is no doubt that the prime cause of pressure sores in spina bifida is the absence of sensation, and much effort has been expended in devising operations to bring sensate flaps into the area. In 1974, Dibell reported the use of a long flap, innervated by the 10th intercostal nerve, to cover a small chronic ulcer of the sacrum in a 2-year-old child. The operation involved four stages, and the ulcer remained healed for at least 2 years. However, such instances where a long sensate flap is available for transfer are not common.

One area where this is sometimes possible is in closure of sacral, ischial and trochanteric ulcers. Myocutaneous flaps incorporating the tensor fascia lata muscle or the gluteus maximus muscle can also contain the lateral femoral cutaneous nerve and the posterior cutaneous nerve of the thigh respectively, with their origin above the level of sensory loss. These flaps easily transfer to the ischial or sacral regions and provide sensation to the reconstructed area (Cochran et al., 1981; Hurwitz et al., 1981; Krupp et al., 1983).

Daniel et al. (1976) have reported the use of island flaps (*Figures 5.14–5.16*), and have also extended the concept with the use of an interposition nerve graft. This may involve the innervation of a myocutaneous flap with a sural nerve graft linked to an intercostal nerve (Shively et al., 1980), or even to the innervation of a free microvascular flap by a nerve graft from the nearest available sensory nerve. The few published reports of these procedures indicate that when the flap does achieve sensation through the nerve graft, the recurrence rate of ulceration is substantially reduced (Dibell et al., 1979; Mackinnon et al., 1985).

However, this procedure is largely limited to pressure sores in the ischial, trochanteric or sacral

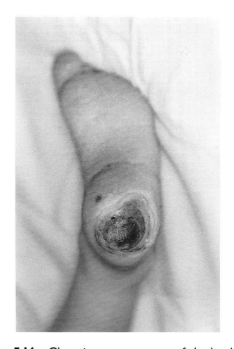

Figure 5.14   Chronic pressure sore of the heel.

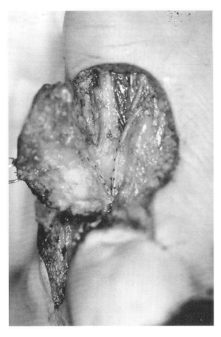

Figure 5.15   Elevation of an island flap from the sole of the foot with its associated neurovascular bundle.

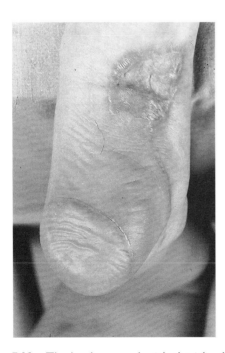

Figure 5.16   The heel covered with the island flap.

without orthoses, and who present late with deep sinuses of the sole of the foot or the plantar aspect of the great toe. Although it is often possible to debride and cover these defects on the foot with local or even distant flaps, they will not have sensation and the necessity to prevent weightbearing during the postoperative period severely restricts activity, which is not well accepted by these children. In addition, some of these patients may have had many orthopaedic procedures in an attempt to improve their ambulation, but in doing so, produce scars which may prejudice the blood supply of useful local flaps and so necessitate the use of free microvascular flaps (*Figures 5.17–5.19*). On the other hand, the ability to move tissue with a nerve supply so far distally is extremely limited and the surgery fraught with complications. It is in this group of patients, therefore, that attention to detail of prevention is so important, with close supervision of footwear and splints.

    If split skin grafts are used either as a definitive

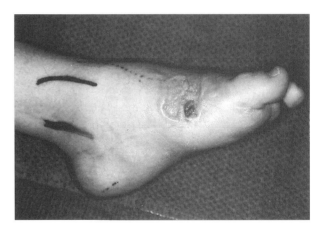

Figure 5.17   Chronic scar and ulcer following multiple operations on the foot.

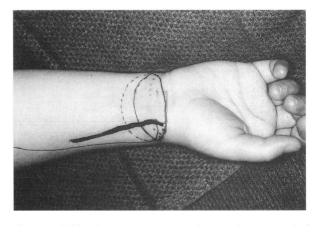

Figure 5.18   Preoperative markings for a radial forearm flap.

area, and is limited by the availability of an intact and functioning nerve of reasonable size, and the length of sural nerve graft which may be required (Coleman and Jurkiewicz, 1984).

    There is an important group of patients with a low spinal lesion and sensory loss on the foot, who have a disproportionate incidence of pressure sores, probably because of their ability to ambulate with or

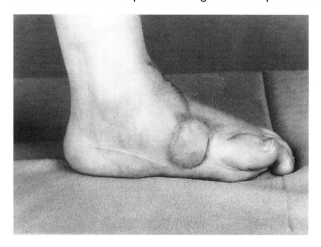

Figure 5.19   The forearm flap transferred to the foot by microvascular techniques.

form of repair or for closing the secondary defect of a transposition flap, the donor area for the graft must be considered very carefully before operation, preferably with the child wearing his or her orthosis. The postoperative position that the child must adopt is also noted, and the area chosen for the graft should not be subject to pressure, and should not be in proximity to any portion of the brace.

It is traditional to apply a firm dressing and this is important in children. Some compression is beneficial in reducing oedema and controlling haemorrhage, but must not be sufficient to produce areas of local pressure. In those wounds closed by direct suture, the dressing can assist in relieving tension on the suture line and limiting unnecessary movement.

The dressing must be carefully applied and attended regularly, so that the elastic compression does not damage the surrounding skin. Some wounds require protection from soiling, especially around the buttock area, and the dressing must be adequate to cover the wound and completely seal it, as an inadequate dressing may be worse than none at all. Preoperative bowel preparation and a low residue diet will help minimize soiling in the postoperative period.

Postoperative Care

No surgery for pressure sores in children succeeds unless the problem of movement is overcome. Older children can be taught to avoid taking pressure on the operative site, and not to make movements that place a shearing strain on the repair. Unfortunately, younger children soon forget their instructions and, unless restrained in some manner, continually move the upper part of their body in their eagerness to see and

take part in everything going on around them in the ward. As their paralysed legs generally remain as positioned, great strain is placed on the suture line and breakdown is inevitable. Restraints must therefore be used, with attention to the prevention of secondary problems. Intelligent positioning of children in the ward so that they do not need to turn around for their entertainment, and suitable occupational therapy, does much to prevent excessive movement.

Pressure on the wound must be avoided, and the routine of turning which was devised and practised before operation is instituted to avoid pressure on other areas.

In the absence of complications, the wound should be healed within 2 weeks, when the sutures can be removed. If continuous wire has been used the suture can be retained for quite long periods to ensure sound healing. Usually about 4 weeks should elapse before allowing normal movement and local pressure. Pressure on the repair, as in sitting, should be gradual, starting with a few minutes at a time and the contact points inspected by the nursing staff for signs of pressure. If no redness occurs, the period of weightbearing can be increased gradually.

Complications

Wound breakdown is almost exclusively related to haematoma formation and excessive movement. Careful haemostasis, meticulous wound closure and prolonged drainage with a catheter which has access to all layers of the wound minimizes the development of haematoma. If this unfortunate complication occurs, the haematoma discharges through the wound and secondary infection follows, with varying degrees of wound breakdown. If the haematoma is confined to the upper layers of a wound repaired by direct closure a shallow breakdown may result and it is possible that this could heal without further operative treatment. More commonly, the breakdown extends into the deeper layers and either a major wound disruption occurs, or a cavity in the depths of the wound drains through a small sinus. A wound breakdown of this extent requires packing and debridement to prepare the wound again for secondary closure. It should be possible to perform direct closure a second time, although on some occasions tension in the area may be too high, and some form of local flap repair has to be considered.

Similarly, if the initial repair has been by a local flap, haematoma is a significant problem, particularly if the flap does not adequately fill the cavity. Poor flap design with embarrassment of the circulation, or suture of the flap under tension, results in more direct wound breakdown. If the initial flap was generous in its proportions, it may be possible to extend the base and further rotate the flap and salvage the situation. However, if the flap was small and badly designed there is usually a complete loss, and tissue from another area has to be found to close the defect secondarily.

Postoperative infection may be a problem, and it is usually secondary to haematoma and wound breakdown. This assumes that the preoperative preparation has been complete, that the wound satisfied the criteria for closure and that all the lining of the ulcer was removed at operation. There is occasionally some cellulitis of the wound edge, but this usually subsides after a few days. Antibiotic cover should be provided according to preoperative cultures and sensitivities.

Rehabilitation after Surgery for Pressure Sores

When the ulcer is healed, patients must be re-educated in the care of their wound to prevent recurrence, and their future programme is carefully considered in all aspects. Each activity and possible source of pressure and trauma is examined. Wheelchairs, splints and braces are inspected to ensure they do not cause pressure. A timetable for sitting in the chair is worked out, and the children or their teachers instructed in the importance of lifting their buttocks off the cushion frequently and inspecting the pressure areas at intervals. Any early signs of pressure must be noted and the source of pressure eliminated. Superficial abrasions must be treated promptly and adequately, with resumption of normal activities on a graduated basis following complete healing of the area.

The key to success in the prevention of pressure sores is early and repeated education and eternal vigilance.

TROPHIC EFFECTS ON BONE AND JOINTS
Malcolm B Menelaus

The leg bones in spina bifida become slender and osteoporotic due to paralysis and disuse (Alliaume, 1950). Pathological fractures occur in about 20% of those with paralysis in the lower limbs (*Table 5.2*). This incidence is slightly lower than that reported by Norton and Foley (1959). Fractures may occur after removal of a plaster hip spica; the upper and lower ends of the femur are most often involved. Because of absent sensation, the fracture commonly presents several days after it has occurred. The uninitiated clinician will

Table 5.2 The incidence of pathological fractures in 168 patients (aged 3 years and over) with myelomeningocele

Level of lesion occurred	Fracture occurred	No fracture
Lower thoracic	9	13
Upper lumbar	8	19
Lower lumbar–upper sacral	14	90
Lower sacral	–	15
Total	31 (18%)	137 (82%)

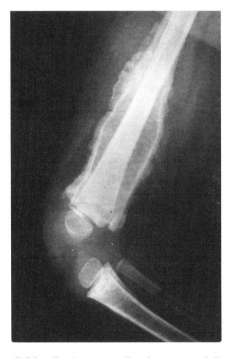

Figure 5.20 Exuberant callus formation following an undisplaced fracture of the lower femur. The presenting features were swelling in the absence of pain, as is commonly the case when there is extensive anaesthesia.

suspect infection as the limb is red, hot and swollen. A typical pathological fracture with hyperplastic callus formation is shown in *Figure 5.20*. Thompson *et al.* (1964) describe similar examples. An unusual condition affecting the os calcis and associated with a fracture of that bone is demonstrated in *Figure 5.21*. Stern *et al.* (1967) describe a case of bilateral tibial and fibular epiphyseal separation in spina bifida. Burney and Hasma (1963) drew attention to the high incidence of epiphyseal separation in spina bifida. Evardsen (1972) has described injuries to the growth plate itself. The lesion is characterized by broadening and loosening of the physis (*Figure 5.22*), possibly due to the repetitive

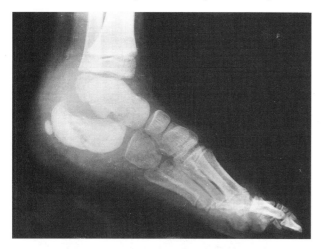

Figure 5.21 Lateral radiographs of the foot of a child with extensive paralysis and anaesthesia and swelling of the heel. X-rays showed a pathological fracture of the calcaneum followed, 1 year later, by avascular necrosis and distortion of the bone.

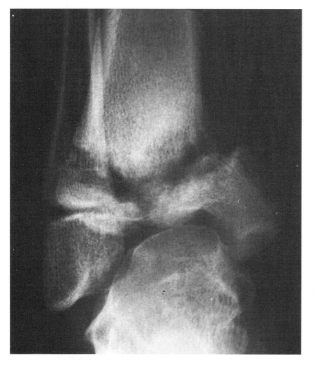

Figure 5.22 Radiograph of a child who presented with a swollen ankle. Note the irregular height and shape of the epiphysis, the broad epiphyseal line and some new bone formation medial to the tibial metaphysis. These changes are due to chronic trauma to the epiphysis. The dome top to the talus was not associated with limited movement of the subtalar joint.

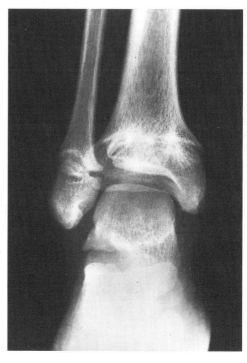

Figure 5.23 Spontaneous fusion of lower tibial physis in a girl aged 11 years (L5 lesion) without a history of trauma.

trauma of daily walking activity and to passive joint movements. Spontaneous growth plate arrest may occur (*Figure 5.23*). These, like the other changes described in this chapter, are presumably due to the absence of protective afferent sensory information.

We have observed several children who have developed chronically swollen knee or ankle joints following injury. There is frequently an effusion in the joint and over growth of the lower femoral or lower tibial epiphyses. Following lower femoral epiphyseal injury with residual valgus deformity, remodelling does not invariably occur in myelomeningocele patients.

Asymptomatic loss of joint space may be seen in patients with myelomeningocele (*Figure 5.24*). Frankly neuropathic joints are also seen (*Figures 5.25–5.27*), which in our experience may be painful.

Osteotomies in spina bifida patients, notably those of the tibia, often exhibit radiological delayed union or non-union. This appearance should be ignored and weightbearing encouraged once the osteotomy is clinically sound. Radiological union may not occur for up to 12 months.

An unusual cause of pathological fracture in spina bifida is renal rickets (*Figure 5.28*), which may occur due to complex biochemical disturbances associated with urinary obstruction and infection. Displaced upper femoral epiphyses may result and there is commonly gross knock-knee deformity in these rickety children. Deficiency of vitamin C has also been implicated as a cause of bone changes in spina bifida in Sheffield (McKibbin *et al.*, 1968). However, radiologi-

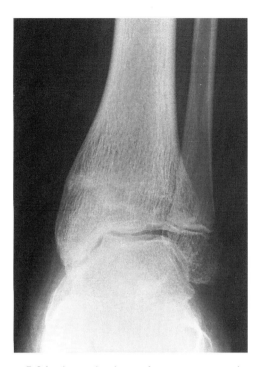

Figure 5.24   Irregular loss of joint space at the ankle in an active girl aged 17 years. There is paralysis below the first sacral level and she has not had foot surgery. There are no symptoms and only slight restriction in the range of ankle movement.

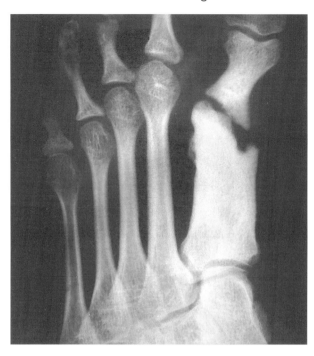

Figure 5.26   Painless hypermobile metatarso-phalangeal joint of hallux in a boy aged 12 years (L5 lesion).

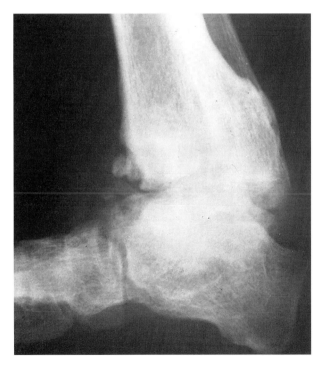

Figures 5.25   Radiograph of the ankle of a 15-year-old girl with paralysis below the fourth lumbar segment. She had undergone triple arthrodesis 3 years previously. The ankle was sufficiently painful to require arthrodesis.

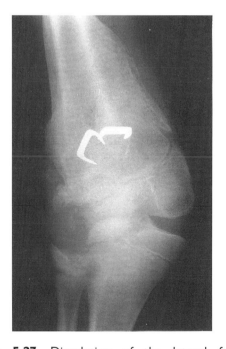

Figure 5.27   Dissolution of the lateral femoral condyle in a boy of 12 years with gross knock knee deformity and an unstable knee. Previous osteotomy has partially corrected the deformity.

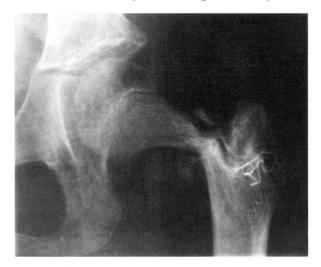

Figure 5.28 Fracture of the attenuated neck of the femur in a child who had undergone posterior iliopsoas transplantation 10 years previously. The fracture is not adjacent to the site of implantation of the tendon (which is in relation to the wire suture). This girl had renal rickets.

cal appearances of infantile scurvy have not been seen in Melbourne. Coxa vara and femoral neck fractures may be encountered (*Figures 5.29, 5.30*). In one of our

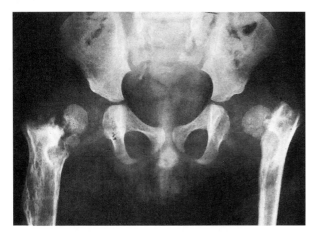

Figure 5.29 Radiograph of the pelvis of a boy presented at the age of 4 years. There is bilateral coxa vara and hip dislocation, an unusual combination. The coxa vara of the right hip resembles the infantile variety. There is evidence of past trauma to the right upper femoral shaft and it is probable that the appearances of the femoral necks is post-traumatic. Cineradiography of the right hip displayed that movement was taking place at the site of the defect in the right femoral neck. (Radiograph provided by Dr Ned Murray Grove of Burlingame, California, to whom acknowledgment is made.)

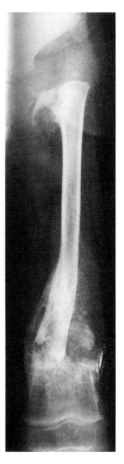

Figure 5.30 A 3-year-old boy with coxa vara, a defect in the inferior portion of the femoral neck and an old fracture of the femoral neck. He has a lesion at the 12th thoracic neurosegmental level and there is a recent fracture of the supracondylar region. Both fractures united satisfactorily.

children a femoral neck fracture resulted in painless non-union.

Efforts should be made to prevent the occurrence of pathological fractures. Multiple operations on the lower limb should be performed at the same time or in quick succession to avoid prolonged immobilization. If it is impracticable to carry out this condensed regime then operations should be staged many months apart so that bones have an opportunity to recalcify. Furthermore, although we may set out to perform several operations in quick succession (1–2 weeks apart), we frequently have to alter our plan because of the necessity for revision of an atrioventricular shunt, intercurrent urinary infection or because of pathological fractures themselves.

The following is an example of condensed management, designed to avoid prolonged immobilization and consequent fractures. Soft tissue release operations are performed on both feet at one sitting, major hip

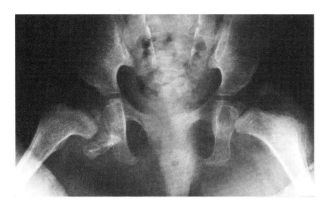

Figure 5.31 Soft tissue calcification about the hips following open reductions combined with anterior release procedures. On the left side subperiosteal bone formation indicates the common complication of pathological fracture, in this case at the trochanteric level.

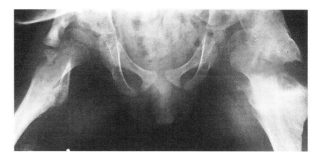

Figure 5.32 Extensive bone formation about the hips of a child who had undergone bilateral anterior release procedures for fixed flexion deformity. There is 60° range of flexion at either hip.

surgery is performed on one hip 2 weeks later followed by similar surgery to the second hip 2 weeks later. A period as short as 10 weeks in a double hip spica is then possible. Soft tissue release operations are commonly performed on both hips, both knees and both feet at the same sitting.

Fractures commonly occur whilst the child is still in hospital following removal of a double hip spica. At this time the nursing staff and physiotherapists must employ great care in handling patients as they are carried to and from the physiotherapy department in the posterior half of the bivalved spica until stiff joints have been mobilized. There is no evidence that activity should be restricted in spina bifida children as a prophylactic measure against pathological fractures; in fact, the best protection against fractures is activity.

The principle of treatment of pathological fractures is that there should be minimum immobilization of the child, compatible with union of the fracture in good position. Usually the fracture is relatively undisplaced and stable so that a short period in traction or continued ambulation in a plaster cylinder will suffice. There is frequently delay in the diagnosis of a fracture and initial X-rays may then show callus formation sufficient to allow activity.

Soft-tissue calcification and ossification may occur in spina bifida as in paraplegia from other causes (*Figures 5.31, 5.32*) and be associated with gross stiffness of the affected joints. This is a valid reason for avoiding surgery on the hips of children with high-level lesions.

Chapter 6

Orthotics

David Phillips

Almost every child with spina bifida is capable of standing and some form of ambulation with the aid of an orthosis. While not all children will walk as their primary mode of mobility, orthotics can provide those using wheelchairs an alternative. The upright posture is encouraged in children with spina bifida, as weight-bearing through the lower limbs retards osteoporosis (Rosenstein *et al.*, 1987) and is thought to help bowel and bladder function, reduce flexion contracture development and improve the self-image of the child. Childhood ambulation, even though temporary, improves adult transfer ability (Mazur *et al.*, 1989). Orthotics are instrumental in achieving this posture and it is their prescription and use that is discussed in this chapter.

THE ROLE OF ORTHOTICS

Orthotics perform several functions for the spina bifida child; a single orthosis may perform one or all the functions listed below, depending on the circumstances. The role of orthotics includes:

* to improve function;
* to aid mobility;
* to improve posture;
* to protect recent surgery or fracture;
* to prevent the development of joint contracture;
* to provide a mobility alternative to a wheelchair.

ACCEPTANCE OF ORTHOSES

Children with myelomeningocele are highly accepting of orthoses during the first 10–14 years of life, enjoying the extra mobility and function that they provide. Once puberty has been reached, some children will elect to use their wheelchairs only and others may change from community ambulators to household or therapeutic ambulators. This is due to a number of factors: (i) body weight increases dramatically at this time, thus lowering the power to weight ratio, making walking more inefficient and difficult (Ryan *et al.*, 1991); (ii) the peer group will influence their decision as the wheelchair is faster; and (iii) their body self-image becomes more acute. This change is also influenced by the neurosegmental lesion level; a child with a lower lumbar or sacral lesion is much more likely to continue walking than one with a thoracic lesion.

Some children will dislike the restriction to movement that extensive bracing demands, and thus will prefer to use lesser bracing even though their gait will be disadvantaged.

As children are introduced to orthoses very early in life for standing and later walking, their acceptance rate is very high, as it is certainly easier for them to explore their environment through the use of supportive devices.

AGE OF BRACING

Orthotic treatment in spina bifida children is commenced early in life: once the infant shows interest in pulling to stand then appropriate orthoses are prescribed. Prior to this event, orthoses are sometimes used for postural reasons: knee and hip contractures frequently increase rapidly at this age and can be kept in extension through the use of stiffened wrap-around splints and prone lying. Tappit-Emas (1994) advocates the use of a total body orthosis incorporating the lower limbs, the infant placed in a position of antideformity during periods of recumbency.

As the child develops and function increases the amount of bracing required is often reduced. A child of 6 years of age may not require as extensive bracing as he or she did when aged 2 years, due to learned postural control, the influence of surgery, greater balance and upper limb strength.

Standing is usually begun at 9–15 months in standing frames, depending on the child. Low-lesion children with hip flexion contractures are stood earlier, before the child is showing an interest in standing, to help stretch the contracture. Orthotics are used at this time to keep the lower limbs in the correct biomechanical alignment. Once the child is ready to start standing independently and then progress to walking, more appropriate orthoses are prescribed to achieve this, with a view to overbracing rather than underbracing, to provide stability and balance. The bracing can be reduced as goals of mobility are achieved, allowing a positive progression of the child's function. Walking may be introduced as early as 15 months, or as late as 4 years, depending on the motivation, physical abilities and intelligence of the child.

BIOMECHANICS OF ORTHOSES

The principles of orthotic application in spina bifida with respect to biomechanical control of the lower limbs and spine does not differ greatly from those of other conditions or orthopaedic problems. To control the motion of body segments, the basic orthotic principles of three- and four-point pressure systems are used. Opposing forces, whether antero-posterior, medio-lateral or oblique, are exerted through the orthosis to hold or guide the segment into its desired position. These forces are applied to the body through the orthosis to skin interface. The child with spina bifida with some degree of anaesthesia requires special consideration in the provision of orthoses. The child may be unaware of undue pressure or friction on the skin and so breakdowns remain an ever-present risk. An exact fit of an orthosis is essential, not only to convey the forces to the appropriate part of the body, but also to avoid excess pressure, especially over bony prominences. Because of anaesthesia, the forces used on body segments may not be as high as those used for sensate skin.

The anatomical axes of joints may sometimes be difficult to determine due to dislocation or deformation. The hip joint axis should be taken at the superior border of the greater trochanter, and it should be noted if the hip subluxes, as it will affect the placement of mechanical joints. On weightbearing, an unstable hip usually subluxes superiorly, causing leg length inequality. In an orthosis such as a reciprocating gait orthosis (RGO), this discrepancy will greatly affect the ability of the child to use the orthosis successfully. Tibial torsion affects the axis of the ankle joint, causing a deviation

from the normal 7° of toe out from the line of progression, and leads to abnormal rollover of the foot. The medial surface of the foot experiences greater loads than the normal and, in addition to weak muscles, this places extra stress on the medial structures of the knee.

When there is fixed deformity, orthoses must be designed to accommodate them. Consideration must then be given to what biomechanical effects this has on the rest of the body. For example, if there is a unilateral equinus deformity, the heel must be built up on that side to keep the hip–knee–ankle line vertical and the contralateral side must also be raised to avoid leg length inequality in the orthosis.

ORTHOTIC MANUFACTURE

The bulk of orthoses for spina bifida are custom made. This is due to the highly individual nature of the problems associated with the condition and the need for exact fit of an orthosis in order to avoid pressure problems. Once an orthosis has been prescribed, measurements of the appropriate body segments are taken by the orthotist in the form of negative plaster casts or careful tracings with measurements noted on special forms. In the case of metal orthoses, casts are not usually taken. For hybrid metal/plastic designs, casts and tracings are necessary. When casting a patient, care must be taken to position the limb or trunk in the desired position of the final orthosis for a correct fit. Minor modifications can be performed on both the negative and positive casts. For less complicated orthoses such as ankle–foot orthoses (AFOs) or foot orthoses, only one fitting is necessary. For more extensive braces, two fittings are needed, one to ensure the fit is correct before finishing the brace for delivery to the patient. As the child grows, the orthosis must be adjusted accordingly; it is therefore fabricated with this in mind. Plastic sections can be widened by spot heating; metal sections can be lengthened through the use of sliding bars, or by moving the metal along the plastic sections. In this way, extensive orthoses can be made to last several years, with regular adjustment. AFOs need replacement on average every 1.5 years (Supan and Hovorka, 1995)

PRESCRIPTION OF ORTHOSES

The orthotist, orthopaedic surgeon and physiotherapist are all involved in prescription of orthoses. Complex cases are best handled with all three present, to avoid confusion and provide the best device for the situation.

The prescription of the appropriate orthosis for the spina bifida patient relies on a combination of many factors, all of which must be taken into consideration to varying degrees. The most important factors determining prescription are:

- the spinal level of the neurological deficit;
- the voluntary muscle power in the lower limbs and trunk;
- the range of motion of joints and orthopaedic deformities;
- the goals of mobilization;
- age.

Other factors include the following:

- motivation
- spinal alignment
- spasticity
- balance
- upper limb function
- skin condition
- sensory deficit.

In general, orthoses are provided to allow activity appropriate to the age of the child: standing at 9–15 months, leading to ambulation if possible after that.

SACRAL LESIONS

Many children with sacral lesions do not require the use of orthoses. Some require minimal bracing to support posture or improve gait. Sacral level children can ambulate without the use of crutches or other gait aids. Gait aids, standing frames and wheeled mobility devices are discussed in Chapter 7.

Foot orthoses, with trimlines distal to the malleoli, are often prescribed for sacral myelomeningocele. Foot deformities requiring treatment in this group include cavo-varus, pes planus, plano-valgus and metatarsus adductus. The transverse arch of the foot is often depressed. Orthoses used to treat minor foot deformities include arch supports, varying from soft to rigid, University of California Biomedics Laboratory (UCBL)-type shoe inserts (*Figure 6.1*) and shoe modifications. Children in this group have reasonably well-balanced musculature around the hips and knees but are lacking in gastro-soleus and foot intrinsics. As a result the biomechanical alignment may be abnormal at the foot, requiring stabilization or correction if possible.

Valgus at the subtalar joint, if correctable, may be treated with the use of moulded medial arch supports or UCBL-type inserts depending on the severity of the valgus. By supporting the medial longitudinal arch, and/or gripping the calcaneus, the tibia is externally rotated, lessening the degree of valgus. Posting and wedging the hindfoot may also be necessary to achieve

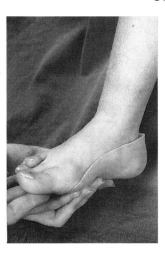

Figure 6.1 The UCBL shoe insert can be used to control mild medio-lateral instabilities of the hind foot.

realignment. A depressed transverse arch may be supported by incorporating a metatarsal dome into the support or insert.

Varus at the subtalar joint is much more difficult to treat than valgus, as there is little area on the foot to direct the appropriate forces. Lateral wedging, whether internal or external to the shoe may help, as may a lateral float on the sole of the shoe. Cavus in the foot cannot be treated satisfactorily with an orthosis. Metatarsus adductus is treated through the use of straight-last shoes, or an extended medial wall on a UCBL.

For those children with weak plantarflexors, an AFO may be indicated to prevent a crouch gait due to excessive dorsiflexion during stance. A solid ankle AFO is used in these cases. For those with weak dorsiflexors, the associated foot drop and high stepping gait can be controlled by using a leaf-spring AFO (Banta *et al.*, 1990). Foot deformities as mentioned before can be controlled by incorporating the appropriate modifications into the AFO as for foot orthoses, but can be better controlled due to the longer lever arms involved.

LOW LUMBAR LESIONS (L4–L5)

Children with low lumbar lesions usually have weak hip extensors and good hip flexors, good quadriceps and some hamstring activity. Hip flexion contracture is common. Internal or external rotation of the lower limb is often present, along with various foot deformities.

Unbraced, a child may be able to maintain an erect posture without crutches or a gait aid but will find ambulation difficult. The standing posture is usually one of dorsiflexed ankles, flexed knees and hips with external rotation or plantarflexed ankles, hyperextended knees, flexed hips and a hyperextended lumbar spine. The lumbar spine extends to compensate for hip flexion contracture to try to keep the centre of gravity between the feet.

Unbraced ambulation is high in energy cost due to loss of several determinants of gait, and the body weight being supported by the upper limbs if using a gait aid. Limited control of foot placement and stability also increases the energy cost. Bracing aims to provide a more stable base of support through controlling the lower limbs and to help control the progression of the limbs in gait. In addition, some orthoses aim to bring the centre of gravity back over the feet.

The young child with a low lumbar lesion will rarely require the extended use of a standing frame when upright posture is commenced. Solid ankle AFOs combined with simple canvas wrap-around splints for knee extension are usually enough to control the lower limbs and provide a stable base. Once ambulation is begun, however, the orthotic support should be reconsidered.

Children with low lumbar lesions with weaker quadriceps, but reasonable hip extensors, will need some form of knee support. Solid ankle AFOs are sometimes sufficient to provide enough support to the knee (*Figure 6.2a,b*). Ground reaction AFOs (GRAFOs) can also be used successfully here. The GRAFO consists of a solid ankle AFO, set in 3–5° of plantarflexion, with an anterior section over the proximal tibia and distal patella. During early- to mid-stance, the GRAFO provides an extension moment to the knee, keeping it stable, while the high trimlines help medio-lateral stability. The GRAFO is particularly suited to L4–L5 walkers whose quadriceps fatigue easily. GRAFOs allow the child to rest against the anterior sections, conserving quadriceps strength. Medial extensions on AFOs, proximal to the condyle, can help prevent a valgus attitude of the knee during gait.

Children with weak or absent hip extensors and hip flexion contractures are often prescribed a reciprocating gait orthosis (RGO) (Yngve *et al.*, 1984) at an age where they are ready to ambulate independently, generally around 2 years old. They will walk well in an RGO due to strong hip flexors driving the extension of the contralateral hip through the reciprocating mechanism.

The RGO provides several benefits at this stage:

- guidance of the lower limbs;
- a stable base of support;
- a four-point pressure system to keep the hips extended;
- training in reciprocal stepping.

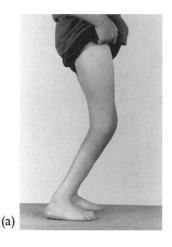

(a)

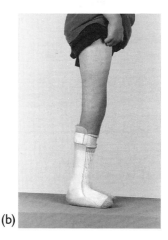

(b)

Figure 6.2(a,b) An AFO has been prescribed to support a crouching stance and gait in this 10-year-old patient with an L5 lesion.

At appropriate points in the child's development he or she can 'graduate' out of the RGO to lesser bracing if possible. This can be a result of strengthening muscles, reduction of contractures and better balance or through surgical procedures, such as muscle and tendon releases and rotational osteotomies of the lower limbs. The use of reciprocating orthoses is discussed later in the chapter.

For those with internal torsion of the lower limbs causing difficulty in placing the foot correctly for weight acceptance in stance, it may be necessary to provide a hip–knee–ankle–foot orthosis (HKAFO). Two types may be used, a dynamic 'twister' design or a static design. Twister orthoses incorporate a flexible cord of polyurethane attached between AFOs and a pelvic band. When the AFOs are donned an internally rotating force is put on the polyurethane, so that when the child stands and walks, the cord will try to return to its original untensioned state and thus externally rotate the lower limbs. Twisters can be 'tuned' to allow the appropriate amount of rotation force, but cannot be

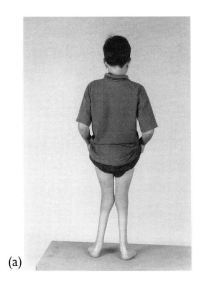

(a)

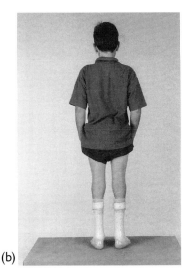

(b)

Figure 6.3(a,b) Severe but correctable valgus at the knees and subtalar joints, corrected by the use of GRAFOs.

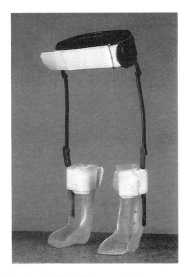

Figure 6.4 An HKAFO used in younger children with low lumbar lesions to help guide the progression of the lower limbs through swing to allow an appropriate position of the foot for acceptance of weight. Internal rotation may be able to be controlled by replacing the metal uprights with tensioned polyurethane cord.

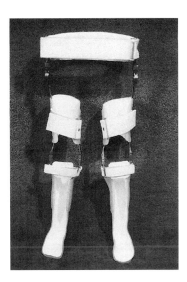

Figure 6.5 An HKAFO with hip and knee locks, used to stabilize the lower limbs for weightbearing.

expected to place the foot in the correct position in every step, due to their flexible nature. Twisters may place undue stress on the knee due to ligamentous laxity that is often present, and their use should be considered with this in mind.

HKAFOs with metal uprights also control the progression of the lower limbs but in a more rigid fashion. AFOs are connected to a pelvic band with light weight lateral uprights (*Figure 6.4*). Hip and knee joints, allow motion. Hip extensor and quadriceps strength and hip flexion contracture determine the need for locks on these joints. The most common setting for L4–L5 patients is for free knees and hips. If the quadriceps are weak but do not warrant a knee lock then posteriorly offset knee joints may be used. These allow a more stable knee joint in extension as the

mechanical knee joint lies behind the anatomical, reducing the need for quadriceps action to keep the knee extended (*Figure 6.5*). The uprights guide the lower limb through swing phase and prevent medial on lateral deviation of the hips, knees and ankles. The Polymedic walkabout unit (*Figure 6.6*) may also be used as a device to help guide the progression of limbs, with added stability around the knees. The lumbo-sacral binder that attaches to the walkabout unit may or may not be used, depending on the trunk control of the child. The

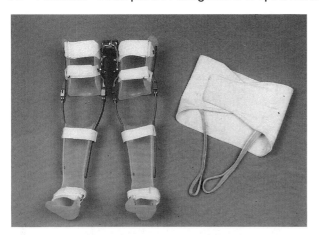

Figure 6.6   The walkabout system: a limited motion joint links a pair of KAFOs, providing much greater stability than an unlinked pair. The lumbosacral binder provides some trunk support.

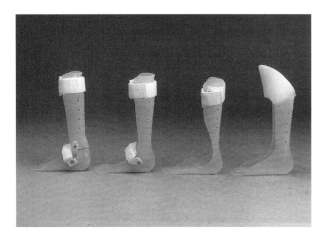

Figure 6.7   Different types of AFOs used in the treatment of spina bifida: Articulated, solid ankle, leaf-spring and ground-reaction (GRAFO).

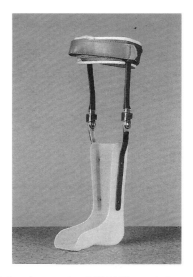

Figure 6.8   A standard KAFO with knee locks and an AFO section. A knee pad (not shown) would provide a posteriorly directed force to prevent knee flexion.

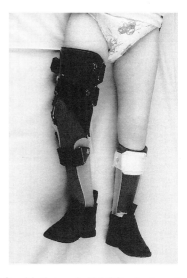

Figure 6.9   Unilateral KAFO designed to prevent gross knee valgus during stance in an asymmetrical low lumbar lesion. The knee joint is free, allowing flexion in swing. There is also a fixed flexion deformity of 15° in the right knee. The AFO is dorsiflexed slightly to compensate for this, keeping the hip–knee–ankle line vertical.

walkabout joint may be easily removed as the child progresses. Various AFOs are shown in Figure 6.7.

For children with weak quadriceps who are unable to keep knees extended in an upright posture, knee–ankle–foot orthoses (KAFOs) may be used (*Figures 6.8, 6.9*). There are a great many variations in design of KAFOs; metal, plastic, carbon or glass fibre, and combinations of these are possible. The KAFO needs to be designed with a consideration of the individual problems of each patient. Designs can include anterior or posterior plastic shells, AFOs, various knee strapping arrangements and different mechanical knee joints.

Children with low lumbar lesions do not necessarily use a gait aid. At a young age a forward rollator or Kaye walker may be used before progressing to

forearm crutches and then possibly to no gait aid. It is most likely that some form of gait aid will be used, however, for a more efficient gait.

HIGH LUMBAR LESIONS LI–L3

Spina bifida children with L1 L3 spinal defects will need to use orthotics if any sort of efficient ambulation is intended. Weakness of the antigravity muscles and associated flexion contractures of the hips and knees prevent the child from standing unbraced without taking the majority of weight through the upper limbs. For energy efficient standing and ambulation, orthoses must at least support the knee, but in most cases the hip and possibly the trunk as well.

The KAFO, in its various designs, is often used on patients with good hip flexor strength and good trunk control. The knees are prevented from collapse during stance by a posteriorly directed force from a knee pad or anterior plastic shell on the KAFO. AFOs are attached to control or accommodate any foot deformity that may be present. In the young child, wrap-around splints or three-point pressure orthoses over and proximal to AFOs are sometimes enough to allow stance. These can be used until the child can independently stand when a more permanent orthosis is prescribed. Standing is initiated a little earlier for these children, to try to reduce the development of hip and knee contractures. HKAFOs can be used for ambulation, but a reciprocating orthosis is used more often, whether it is a RGO, hip guidance orthosis (HGO) or walkabout. These orthoses provide the four-point pressure system necessary for an upright posture but allow reciprocal motion of the lower limbs, for a more efficient gait than a swing-through gait.

The thoracic–hip–knee–ankle–foot orthoses (THKAFOs) are used when the child is unsuitable for reciprocal ambulation but upright posture and mobility is desired. These consist of metal uprights with hip and knee locks attached to AFOs or shoe stirrups. The uprights are connected through metal pelvic and thoracic bands or a thermoplastic spinal section, depending on the support needed (*Figure 6.10*).

THORACIC LESIONS

For children with lesions of T12 and above, there are few options available for standing and walking. Spinal deformity is more prevalent, which can affect balance and complicate orthotic fitting. Many children will be non-ambulators, electing to use a wheelchair only for mobility. Paraplegic children require extensive bracing to maintain the upright posture, and can ambulate using a reciprocal or swing-through gait.

The young paraplegic child can be stood in the same standing devices that include the trunk as mentioned previously, but unlike lower lesioned children, they will not progress to lesser bracing as they develop. A standing frame or parapodium (*Figure 6.11*) will be followed by either THKAFOs, swivel walkers or reciprocal gait orthoses. The current treatment is to proceed from the standing frame straight into an RGO

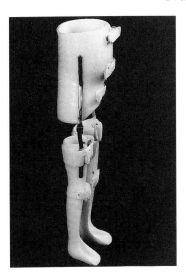

Figure 6.10 A THKAFO with plastic KAFOs and thoracic section, to provide total contact support and thus minimizing the risk of pressure sores.

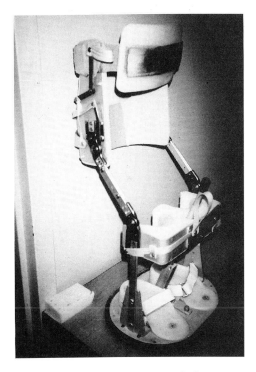

Figure 6.11 A parapodium, used for non-mobile standing, with the advantage of being able to sit without removing the device.

if suitable, or to THKAFOs if a reciprocal gait is not possible. The swivel walker (Rose and Henshaw, 1972) consists of a parapodium-like standing device mounted on a pair of angled swivelling bases (*Figure 6.12*). By shifting body weight from side to side, the bases progress forwards. The swivel walker is used when upper limb function is poor, but mobilization is still

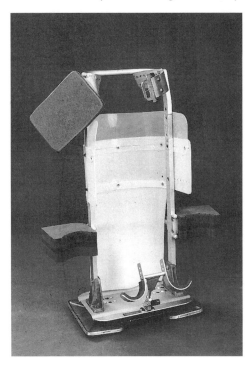

Figure 6.12 A swivel walker, used for hands-free mobility, for those unable to use a gait aid and reciprocal orthosis, or for a transition device from standing to ambulating.

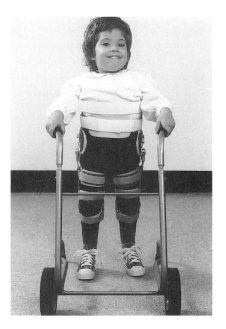

Figure 6.13 A thoracic lesion child standing with the aid of an RGO and forward rollator.

intended or as a transition device from standing to ambulating in a reciprocating orthosis (Banta *et al.*, 1990). Though awkward, the swivel walker provides a means of upright, hands-free ambulation to those unable to handle a gait aid. All orthoses keep the child upright by way of anteriorly directed forces at the heels and buttocks, and posteriorly directed forces at the knees and chest.

RECIPROCATING ORTHOSES

Reciprocating orthoses have been used with spina bifida children for two decades, and have provided a more energy-efficient alternative to a swing-through gait. Hip extension is activated through the use of contralateral hip flexion in children with active hip flexors, or by trunk extension and a diagonal weight-shift for paraplegic children. There are several designs of reciprocating orthoses available for use with the spina bifida patient. They include the RGO (*Figure 6.13*) and its derivatives, the HGO (*Figure 6.14*) and the walkabout. The RGOs work by linking the hip joints in such a manner that flexion of one hip joint causes contralateral extension. The HGO and walkabout allow independent movement of the limbs.

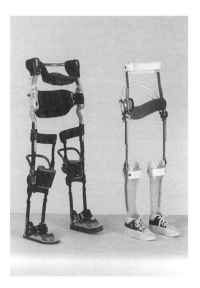

Figure 6.14 HGO and RGO. The HGO, on the left, is much more rigid than the RGO, allowing heavier or obese patients to ambulate with more efficiency.

The RGO has several designs, which are mainly variations on the reciprocating mechanism: the variations are the double-looped cable RGO, the horizontal cable RGO, the advanced RGO (ARGO), the linear bearing RGO and the isocentric or rocker-bar RGO (*Figure 6.15*). There is little difference in prescription criteria for these designs and the choice of mechanism is largely decided by the personal preference of the orthotist. It must be noted, however, that the isocentric

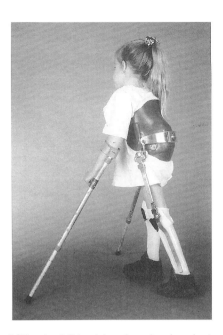

Figure 6.15 A child with a low lumbar lesion ambulating using a rocker-bar RGO design. Note the accommodation of the thoraco-lumbar kyphosis built into the orthosis.

design has been found to be slightly more efficient than the original design when looking at the physiological cost index (Winchester *et al.*, 1993).

RGOs are suitable for children with any neurological lesion, as long as there is good strength in latissimus dorsi and the upper limbs. Hip and knee contractures up to 30° can be tolerated, as can minor spinal and foot deformity. Obese children have difficulty with RGOs as they deform the lateral uprights on stepping and thus require a greater effort to clear the swing leg. The cable-activated RGOs are suitable for young children, and children as young as 18 months have been successfully fitted. The isocentric RGO can be used once the child is large enough for the componentry. RGO componentry is also available with abduction joints, allowing brace-on catheterization, which encourages all-day use of the orthosis.

The HGO, or 'parawalker', is a rigid THKAFO with frictionless hip joints that have selected ranges of motion set into them. It is prescribed for heavier children, and those with significant spinal deformity where there may be difficulties fitting an RGO. The HGO often replaces the RGO as the orthosis of choice between the ages of 7 and 10 years. It is at this age that weight and spinal deformity commonly increase, for which the HGO is better suited (Phillips *et al.*, 1995). It is the most energy efficient of the reciprocal gait devices (Jefferson and Whittle, 1990) due to its rigidity. A disadvantage of the HGO is its bulky appearance. The walkabout system is suitable for children with no hip

flexion deformity, and provides a stable base for the trunk to balance (Kirtly, 1992). Good abdominals, and a flexible lumbar spine are desired for efficient ambulation. The walkabout seems to be most suitable for children with active hip flexors whose lower limbs require a great deal of guidance in swing and stance.

Spasticity of muscles around the hip joint is a contraindication for any reciprocal orthosis.

POSTSURGICAL AND CORRECTIVE ORTHOSES

There are associated problems and deformities in spina bifida that are sometimes treated conservatively, such as foot deformity, fractures and knee flexion deformity.

In the case of fixed deformity, orthotics cannot be expected to reduce the contracture but can be used to prevent further progression of the deformity. Orthoses can also be used to hold and protect surgically corrected deformities and to protect and support fractures.

Equino-varus is a common deformity of the foot and ankle in spina bifida. Orthoses used to maintain position after surgery or prevent progression of deformity include AFOs and a specially designed orthosis which holds the foot in the antideformity position of dorsiflexion, eversion and metatarsal abduction (*Figure 6.16*). An outrigger attached to the footplate is connected to the proximal calf band by a strap to hold the foot in position. A posterior joint lined up with the anatomical subtalar joint allows eversion and dorsiflexion. These orthoses can be custom manufactured or assembled from preformed components. AFOs can be custom moulded in a position of antideformity. Neither can be used for ambulation and are generally only used on young patients after surgery.

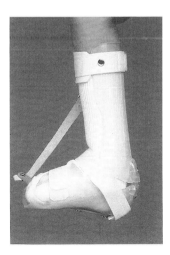

Figure 6.16 Orthosis designed to place a talipes equino-varus foot into a position of antideformity.

For knee flexion control after posterior knee release or to prevent a contracture from developing further, a simple three-point pressure orthosis can be used, fabricated with aluminium uprights, padded polyethylene cuffs and a lambswool four-point knee pad. The brace is easily applied for night use. Three-point orthoses can also be made using fibreglass or spring steel uprights to apply a more dynamic extension force on the knee.

Fracture bracing of the lower limb for spina bifida children usually consists of low temperature thermoplastic shells moulded directly to the patient. High temperature thermoplastic can be used if the fracture is slow to heal or results in non-union or pseudo-arthrosis. Velcro closures hold the shells in place. These can usually be incorporated into the child's normal orthosis with some modification if standing or ambulation is to continue while the bone heals. For stable fractures orthoses have some advantage over plaster in that the insensate skin can be easily checked for pressure problems. Tibial and femoral fractures can be treated with orthoses, but fractures in the upper third of the femur are not suitable for orthotic treatment due to the short lever arms involved and can be managed better in a hip spica or a prone trolley with no external support of the fracture.

Postoperative spinal bracing is often required after spinal fusion. The patient is cast on a casting frame once he or she is stable after surgery but not yet mobilized. A foam-lined polyethylene bivalved jacket is then fabricated to provide the necessary support to the spine. The shells are fastened with velcro closures.

SPINAL ORTHOSES

Orthoses used in the treatment of spinal deformity or instability in myelomeningocele differ from those of other conditions or orthopaedic problems. The role of orthotics here is to support the spine, and not to correct deformity. Bracing the spina bifida spine has no effect on the progression of the deformity, but often improves the function of the child, whether sitting or walking. The main spinal deformities associated with spina bifida are scoliosis, kypho-scoliosis and lumbar lordosis. Asymmetrical curves may cause difficulties with wheelchair use or walking and bracing is indicated when spinal deformity interferes with normal activities. Bracing can be used to help function at any age.

There are several types of orthoses that can be used: the Boston brace; the bivalved jacket; the posterior shell; the soft jacket; and the lumbo-sacral binder.

Spinal deformity usually only affects children with thoracic and high lumbar lesions, and these can be divided into walkers and non-walkers. The walkers use their spinal bracing in conjunction with THKAFOs or reciprocal orthosis, and are of the Boston, bivalve jacket or posterior shell design. The spinal brace may be incorporated or separate to the lower limb bracing depending on whether the child requires support when sitting out of it. For non-walkers, the commonest support prescribed is the soft jacket, made out of plastic reinforced foam of various densities. This provides an adequate support without the rigidity of high-temperature thermoplastics, which can easily cause skin breakdown in this group. Bivalved jackets are also used, but for larger, heavier patients who deform the soft jacket excessively. Skin breakdown is the major concern when using spinal orthoses in spina bifida and care must be taken to avoid this. Pressure on the skin cannot be as high as for normal corrective spinal bracing. The correction given to the braced weight-bearing spine should not exceed its supine shape as casted for brace fabrication. No derotation correction should be built into the brace (Banta et al., 1990)

Lumbo-sacral binders are very occasionally used on patients with weak abdominals and lumbar lordosis, to support posture in wheelchairs.

Chapter 7
Physiotherapy and Occupational Therapy

Catherine A Abery and Jane L Galvin

PHYSIOTHERAPY
Catherine A Abery

Introduction

Movement is an important factor in the development of many other systems in the human body. Through movement a child is able to explore and gain information about his or her environment. It is known that learning is affected when movement and exploration are limited (Tappit-Emas, 1994)

Physiotherapists are expert in the assessment and management of movement disorders. Their training provides them with a sound understanding of normal and abnormal movement, and teaches a variety of assessment and treatment techniques to facilitate the development of gross motor skills. The therapist is in a unique position to advise, educate and monitor the child's progress. This will ultimately assist the child with a movement disorder to gain physical independence.

The physiotherapy programme aims to stimulate the motor development of the infant through handling, positioning and play. The increased sensory input through these activities is believed to facilitate the motor output and thus facilitate development of gross motor skills (Shepherd, 1975). Physiotherapy will enable a child to experience a greater diversity of movement skills than would otherwise be possible. This will enable the child to achieve gross motor milestones that they would have been slow to develop on their own, and will facilitate optimum physical independence.

In addition to a detailed assessment of abilities, the physiotherapy programme also involves teaching the child or family some enjoyable, practical, useful activities, to be performed at home, keeping in mind their lifestyle and other commitments. These activities will be explained, demonstrated and taught in the physiotherapy sessions. Co-operation is therefore essential in order to achieve the aims of the physiotherapy programme (*Figure 7.1*).

The physiotherapist will have an intimate relationship with each child, as an individual and as part of a family unit. This relationship is an integral part of a successful physiotherapy programme. This relationship is established over time and is partly due to the amount of time he or she will spend with the child and family and partly due to the therapist, child and family working towards similar goals. These goals will reflect

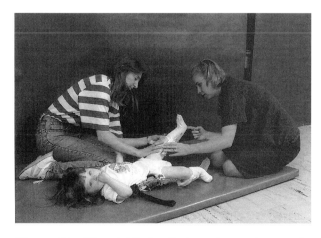

Figure 7.1 The child's family is an integral part of a physiotherapy programme – teaching mother to don the RGO.

those required by a child functioning effectively in their home, school and working environments.

The development of gross motor skills of children with spina bifida is affected by many other factors than lesion level (Hoffer *et al.*, 1973; De Souza and Carroll, 1976; McDonald *et al.*, 1991). However, lesion level appears to be the major determinant of walking ability. It is acknowledged that age, the presence of spasticity, upper limb co-ordination difficulties, intellect, motivation, the presence of scoliosis or contractures, neurological deterioration due to syringomyelia, hydromyelia or tethering, shunt function, skin breakdown, obesity and social circumstances all play a role in the physical abilities of a child with spina bifida (Hoffer *et al.*, 1973; Asher and Olsen, 1983; Stillwell and Menelaus, 1983; Samuelsson and Skoog, 1988; McDonald *et al.*, 1991). The skilled physiotherapist should be able to recognize the factors that could adversely affect the child's gross motor functioning, and in turn, liaise with the appropriate team members about their management.

The physiotherapist must communicate and liaise effectively with the wide variety of professionals who deal with each child with spina bifida. The relationship with these team members – the paediatrician, the orthopaedic surgeon, the neurosurgeon, the orthotist, the occupational therapist, the social worker and the continence specialist – is crucial when striving for a successful-outcome for each child. This team should be able to respond to the individual needs of each child, as the child moves through the different stages of growth and development.

Physiotherapy Assessment

The physiotherapy assessment of a child with spina bifida is very detailed, as many factors need to be assessed. The assessment is fundamentally the same for children with spina bifida of all ages. The factors which need to be assessed are:

- muscle strength of both upper and lower limbs;
- range of movement of all joints of the upper and lower limbs, including contractures and static positioning of joints;
- spinal abnormalities;
- tone;
- sensation;
- upper limb co-ordination;
- gait pattern;
- use of orthoses/gait aides/standing equipment;
- gross motor skills;
- transfer skills/wheelchair skills.

Since 1979, the Royal Children's Hospital has used the International Myelodysplasia Study Group

(IMSG) assessment to assess children with spina bifida, and other neural tube anomalies (Shurtleff, 1986). This is a standardized assessment form which can only be used in accredited centres by trained physiotherapists. This assessment is completed initially in the neonate, at 6-monthly intervals to 2 years, then annually around the child's birthday following this. Assessments are completed at other times if there are concerns regarding deterioration in function.

Muscle strength

The commonly used grading system of a neonate, of absent, weak and full strength muscle contractions is accurate in predicting future muscle strength. Using the Oxford scale, the result is usually within one grade of future strength at maturity (McDonald *et al.*, 1986). Some muscle groups have been shown to be more reliable than others; tibialis anterior, gastronemius and quadriceps are the most reliable, while the toe flexors and extensors, peroneus longus and brevis, iliopsoas, sartorius and quadratus lumborum are the least reliable indicators of future muscle strength (McDonald *et al.*, 1986).

The Oxford scale of grading muscle strength involves five grades of strength:

0 = no power
1 = flicker of contraction felt but minimal or no movement at the joint
2 = across gravity movement
3 = against gravity movement
4 = against gravity movement plus resistance
5 = normal strength.

The IMSG assessment of muscle strength uses the Oxford scale but also includes four other grades:

6 = a transferred muscle
7 = a spastic muscle
8 = an abnormal movement
9 = unknown.

Assessing the muscle strength of a child with spina bifida follows a consistent routine: (i) observation; (ii) positioning; (iii) facilitation; and (iv) applying resistance if necessary. Prior to assessing each individual muscle group, much can be gained from observing the semi-naked child move and play when positioned into either prone, supine, sidelying, or sitting, and when standing, walking, jumping, hopping or performing other functional activities. Evidence of contractures and atrophy of muscle bellies will indicate gross deficiencies in the strength of individual muscle groups.

Facilitation of lower limb movement in a baby can occur through stroking, tickling or touching of the sensate areas. In an infant or young child the facilitation will involve toys and games. Once the child is over the age of 5 years it is possible to assess very accurately the muscle strength of each individual muscle group, as at this time the child will usually follow specific simple instructions (McDonald *et al.*, 1986). It is necessary for comparative purposes to note the perceived accuracy of the muscle chart.

When performing a muscle chart, it is not difficult to assign a value of 0 when a muscle is not functioning or a 3 when the muscle is able to contract against gravity through most of its range. More difficult, however, is distinguishing between grades 1 and 2 or grades 4 and 5. The difference between grades 1 and 2 lies in the amount of movement of the joint the muscle contraction causes. Grades 4 and 5 are assessed with hands on resistance through the joints range and/or observation of the child functioning in a weightbearing position, such as walking or jumping. Grade 5 is assigned to a muscle group if the muscle functions in a normal way, and often the most accurate method of assessing this is to apply a functional test.

The validity or accuracy of a muscle chart is affected by many factors such as the expertise of the examiner, and factors associated with the child. The child's age, their ability to follow simple instructions and to voluntarily contract an individual muscle group and their level of alertness at the time of the assessment will all affect the validity of the muscle chart. Prior to a feed is an ideal time to muscle chart a baby. It is preferable if an experienced therapist is performing the muscle chart and the same therapist performs serial muscle charts over time.

The range of movement of all upper and lower limb joints

Each joint is moved gently through its full range and measured with a goniometer. The axis of motion is standardized according to strict criteria for the IMSG. The static position of each joint may indicate a contracture, and this is recorded. The stability of the knee, the presence of a hip dislocation and any foot deformities are also noted (*Figures 7.2, 7.3*).

Spinal abnormalities

Any spinal abnormality is noted in the assessment including evidence of a scoliosis, kyphosis including a congenital scoliosis or lordosis, and the region of the abnormality. Any child with a new spinal anomaly or a child with a spinal anomaly that has altered rapidly over a short period of time should be reviewed by the orthopaedic surgeon.

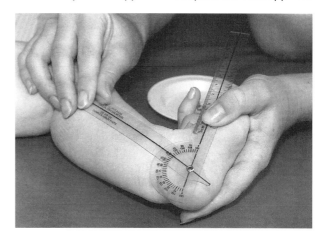

Figure 7.2 A goniometer is used to measure the range of all lower limb joint movements – measuring ankle dorsiflexion.

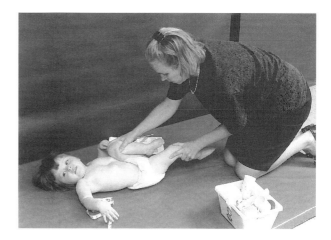

Figure 7.3 Assessing the fixed flexion deformity of the right hip using the Thomas test.

Tone

The presence of spasticity will alter the treatment and prognosis of patients with spina bifida. Children with spasticity tend to be less likely to walk than those with flaccid paralysis, they spend more time in hospital and require more surgical procedures. These children also have more contractures, more difficulties with orthotic fit and impaired personal dressing and hygiene skills (Mazur and Menelaus, 1991). Spasticity is frequently seen in children with spina bifida due to associated central nervous system anomalies, such as tethering and syringohydromyelia.

Involuntary muscle action can be indicated by either muscle action when a child is asleep, continuous muscle action that does not vary according to the child's activity or level of alertness, spasticity that is able to be felt as resistance when the joint is moved through range, an apparent contracture, or increased reflexes. During a muscle chart each muscle group is tested for spasticity.

Sensation

Though it is difficult and time consuming to assess accurately the sensation in a neonate or young child, a general picture can be obtained by applying a sharp instrument or touching or tickling the limb and watching for an immediate response. The reliability of such a test improves as the child matures and can accurately communicate a verbal response. This way a picture can be illustrated of the sensate and insensate areas, which can be used as a guide for the parents and other professionals treating the child.

Upper limb co-ordination

A detailed assessment is performed by the occupational therapist. The physiotherapist can perform tests of muscle tone, diadokinesthesia, proprioception, kinaesthesia, muscle and grip strength using a dynometer, to establish a baseline of upper limb function.

Gait pattern

The gait pattern of the child is recorded according to the following criteria: two-, three- or four-point gait, the presence of gluteal lurch, or walking on heels with poor balance. The posture of the lower limbs in gait should also be recorded: windswept to the right or left, or feet in or feet out, toes in or toes out. Any general comments on the child's gait are recorded in the physiotherapy assessment, and this provides a baseline with which to measure change over time. A more detailed assessment of the gait pattern is performed in the gait laboratory.

Hoffer's classification system of walking ability is used to distinguish between those children who are community, household, non-functional/exercise walkers and those who are non-ambulant (Hoffer *et al.*, 1973). The household or community walkers are distinguished from the other groups due to their ability to transfer independently. Nine years appears to be the critical age before which functional ambulation is usually attained (Hoffer *et al.*, 1973). With younger children it is necessary to clarify whether the child is walking inside or outside, at the home or school. This is in order to modify the environment as necessary. Any gait aides currently in use are also recorded.

Orthoses

Any orthoses the child is using should be noted and these orthoses should be checked for fit, as frequent adjustments are necessary for growth. Similarly, any gait aids and standing devices are noted and checked for height, wear and tear. The ability of the child to don and doff the orthoses is also assessed.

Gross motor skills

There is no standardized, objective developmental test to examine the gross motor skills of children with spina bifida. As previously stated, children with even low lesions may have delays in their gross motor abilities. Children with different level lesions will progress along an individual gross motor path.

The assessment entails placing the child in different positions, such as supine, prone, sidelying, kneel standing, standing and walking, and watching the child function in these positions. Features such as balance, equilibrium reactions and protective extension, head control and the ability to maintain a posture or transfer between two positions are examined. The posture of the limbs is also examined in each of these positions. Frequently, it is necessary to facilitate the child to perform a movement by providing the motivation to do so through the use of toys and games.

Careful observation by the physiotherapist enables an evaluation of the strengths and weakness of the child's gross motor development. The skills the child is able to perform and the skills the child is not able to perform are noted. The physiotherapist will analyse these results and from this, they will be able to formulate accurate short-term goals for the child. The physiotherapist will be able to advise the parents on ways to facilitate the skills which a child is having difficulty achieving. The correct timing to introduce orthoses, and the choice of orthoses, will also become evident.

Wheelchair skills

The correct age to introduce the use of a wheelchair and type of wheelchair to be introduced will be determined by many factors, and will differ markedly according to the level of lesion. This decision is usually a joint one between the child, family and physiotherapist. There are many different types of wheelchairs available for children with spina bifida, so a detailed examination of the child's size, sitting balance, transfer skills and home and school environments needs to be undertaken before a decision is finalized. The wheelchair will need to be assessed and reassessed regularly for size and wear as well as suitability for the environment in which it is used. The use of a reciprocal gait orthoses or parawalker will need to be taken into account when ordering a wheelchair for a child with spina bifida, and an allowance must be made in width and depth when measurements are taken.

The child's ability to transfer to and from the wheelchair, from the floor and the bed, toilet, floor and from a standing posture will need to be assessed if appropriate to the child.

Assessment Findings Requiring Referral

Regular physiotherapy contact over time places the physiotherapist in a unique position to identify difficulties that may require specialist referral.

Spinal cord tethering

The experienced physiotherapist who is consistently performing these detailed assessments is likely to pick up the early signs of spinal cord tethering. These signs may be an increase in spasticity, a rapid change in a contracture or a scoliosis, an increase in the number of falls a child may experience, or increased balance difficulties, a deterioration of the gait pattern, back or leg pain, changes in sensation or muscle strength, or changes in the bowel or bladder pattern. The neurosurgeon treating the child should be informed of the changes, particularly if they are felt not to be a consequence of natural progression or change over time.

Syringomyelia/hydromyelia

The assessment performed by the physiotherapist may also be likely to pinpoint changes characteristic of syringomyelia or hydromyelia. These changes may be a rapid decrease in grip strength or strength in lower limbs, a change in sensation or gait pattern, or a rapid increase in scoliosis. If these changes are found on assessment, the neurosurgeon should be informed.

Shunt malfunction

The signs of shunt malfunction are varied. When a child with a shunt is being treated regularly by a physiotherapist, the therapist may be able to note some of the likely signs of a shunt malfunction, and refer the child to the neurosurgeon for assessment.

Pressure areas

Most children with spina bifida will suffer from a pressure area at some stage during their lifetime. The pressure area may have been caused by crawling on rough surfaces, touching hot surfaces, or pressure from ill-fitting orthoses. It is imperative these areas are treated early, and signs of onset require urgent action.

Fractures

Pathological fractures are a frequent occurrence in patients with spina bifida (Menelaus, 1980). There is commonly heat and swelling without pain or a history of injury, so that infection is at first suspected (Menelaus, 1980). Confirmation of a suspected fracture may be made by the treating orthopaedic specialist.

Hip dislocation

Some of the signs and symptoms of hip dislocations include asymmetry of posture, decreased range of hip abduction, hip, thigh or groin pain, leg length inequality and a positive Barlow's test. If a hip dislocation has not been previously diagnosed, the child should be referred to the orthopaedic surgeon. Not all hip dislocations require treatment in the child with spina bifida. The management of a dislocation varies according to the child's level of mobility and degree of paralysis.

Scoliosis

Evidence of a scoliosis or the rapid deterioration of a scoliosis should by documented and the child reviewed by the orthopaedic surgeon and possibly the neurosurgeon. Scoliosis is known to be associated with spinal cord tethering or syringohydromyelia.

Physiotherapy Management

The motor development of children with spina bifida, with even low lesions of paralysis, is frequently delayed (Wolf and McLaughlin, 1992). This delay, which increases with age, is due to many factors: upper limb co-ordination and strength deficiencies, hypotonia or hypertonia in the trunk, upper limbs and the lower limbs, inefficiencies in balance and automatic reactions, the delayed development of fine motor and manipulative skills as well as the biomechanical and cognitive impact of hydrocephalus.

Hydrocephalus and the associated increase in head size and weight is likely to delay the development of head control. Adequate head control is one of the prerequisites for the development of visual control. Adequate head control and trunk control are necessary for the development of rolling, sitting, kneeling, standing, walking and other gross motor activities.

Balance reactions, including equilibrium reactions and the protective extension response necessary to prevent or break a fall, are often delayed in children with spina bifida. It is unknown whether the cause of these delays is central in origin, or is the result of a number of peripheral factors. The effects of both hydrocephalus on the developing brain, and the presence of the Chiari malformation in the majority of children may well be a central cause of balance difficulties. Paralysis in the trunk and lower limbs, as well as the lack of proprioception and sensation in the lower limbs, will adversely affect equilibrium reactions and therefore balance reactions. For example, the child with L3/4 myelomeningeocele without hip extensor control will have difficulty learning to sit. Delays in balance will adversely affect the development of fine motor control and manipulation because of the child's need to use their arms for balance for a much longer period, thus compromising the child's ability to explore and play using their hands.

Early management

The physiotherapist is initially involved with the child with spina bifida in the neonatal unit, either before or after the lesion is closed. If the child is referred before the back is closed, a baseline of motor functioning is established, which may be more accurate than an immediate postoperative assessment. A postoperative assessment may be adversely affected by the lethargy of the baby postanaesthesia, and swelling around the closure site.

The aims of physiotherapy for the neonate with spina bifida include:

- Gain the confidence and trust of the family. Establish a rapport with the parents so they feel comfortable to ask questions with regard to the likely motor progress and ability of their child.
- Perform an initial assessment.
- Discuss the aims and benefits of a physiotherapy programme on the child's motor functioning and discuss a plan for physiotherapy intervention.
- Formulate a treatment plan of positioning and or range of movement exercises, if appropriate, to be performed by parents at home.

In this initial period the physiotherapist will explain the effects of motor and sensory function and hydrocephalus on the child's motor functioning. The therapist should be able to give the parents an idea of the likely sequence of gross motor skills that their child will acquire. They will then begin to grasp the differences in gross motor development from other children.

The most important feature of the early communication between the physiotherapist and the parents is to be realistic with motor expectations and to focus on the positive aspects of what the child will be able to do,

not what the child will not be able to do. Most parents wish to learn how they can encourage the child's motor development and are very willing to participate in a very simple programme of positioning and/or range of movement exercises, as this often gives them a sense of being able to do something positive for their child.

A neonate with spina bifida should experience a variety of postures, for example prone, supine, sidelying, propped over a shoulder, propped in a supportive chair, and not be positioned and coddled in just one position. It is the variety of positions that will stimulate the development of head and trunk control which is often slow to develop in a child with hydrocephalus.

If there is a specific contracture that is felt to be greater than the normal flexion contractures of a neonate, then gentle range of movement exercises for that joint and/or positioning may assist in decreasing the contracture. All neonates have a limitation of hip extension, knee extension and ankle plantarflexion, as well as elbow extension and shoulder abduction. These limitations are believed to be due to the position of the foetus *in utero* in the third trimester.

A general description of the sensate and insensate areas in the child's lower limbs needs to be discussed in order to give the parents an understanding of the practical implications of anaesthetic skin. Issues such as protection from heat and cold and the inability of the child to feel pain in the affected areas will usually result in discussions relating to appropriate clothing to protect the limbs, appropriate footwear, moderate temperature in the bath or shower and the importance of regular skin inspection. The family can assist the child to develop a body image inclusive of their anaesthetic areas by touching, stroking, massaging, tickling and placing the denervated areas in the child's sight.

Parents will often ask what they can do to strengthen the weak muscles. Using play to touch, tickle and stroke the sensate areas, the neonate will be stimulated to move. Tactile, visual and auditory stimulation are the 'strengthening exercises' for a neonate. Placing the baby in a variety of positions will give the innervated muscle groups an opportunity to move against gravity, across gravity and with the assistance of gravity. The child needs time spent without being tightly wrapped with multilayers of clothing. They need to be able to move freely, in a warm and stimulating environment. The parents should be encouraged to decrease the assistance given when handling the child in order to stimulate the child to control their own head and trunk. The child should be challenged rather than coddled, during play, handling and other activities of daily living, as this attitude assists in achieving the eventual goal of physical independence.

The physiotherapy programme will include activities which are part of a child's normal daily routine such as feeding, carrying, playing, positioning and bathing. When a child is having a bottle, the child will usually fix on their mother's eyes. If the mother slowly moves her head then the child will be encouraged to follow with her eyes. Similarly, if a child has a limitation of hip abduction, then carrying the child over one hip will assist the flexibility of this hip joint. Many of the games parents play with their children can be used as part of the child's programme, for example swaying when singing to improve trunk control, flying like an aeroplane to stimulate head and trunk extension.

The development of floor skills

This period of development is characterized by increasing head and trunk control, rapid changes in hand function and the initiation of independent mobility. The aims of physiotherapy in this period include:

- prevent contracture and deformity;
- facilitate head and trunk control and balance reactions in a variety of positions;
- facilitate independent mobility by providing the appropriate motivation, equipment and environment;
- advise on the appropriate aids to encourage use of the upper limbs.

Preventing contracture and deformity
Any joint whose range of movement is less than the normal range of movement for a child of comparative age should be managed with either a simple range of movement exercises performed by both the parents and therapist, by orthotics, including the use of plaster of Paris or by positioning. Rarely in these early years is surgery required to control contractures. Most of the early contractures are due to the position of the baby *in utero* and naturally tend to decrease with time.

Positioning can be used to enhance range of movement. Positioning in prone is preferable for those children with hip flexion contracture, and a tendency to kyphosis. Within the first year standing in a standing frame may be used to stretch the hip flexors. Many children with thoracic lesions will develop a hip flexion and external rotation contracture of their hips. In the early months, a tubigrip sleeve fitted around both legs and as high as the waist may be used at sleep periods to restore range of movement.

Range of movement exercises need to be performed regularly during the day if they are to be effective. A routine of range of movement exercises, focusing only on those joints that have a contracture, with nappy changes appears to be manageable for many families. It is not practicable or necessary for each joint to be taken through its full range passively, as most joints are moved many times a day through most of their range during normal activities such as carrying, bathing, dressing, nappy changing, and alternating the child's posture on the floor.

For knee flexion deformities, if simple stretches are not sufficient to restore the range of movement, then either a canvas wrap-around splint, or a three-point splint is used during sleep periods in the day and overnight. Occasionally, serial plastering may be required if the range of movement is not restored using either range of movement exercises or splinting. These plasters must be well padded, and changed weekly for the period of plastering, which is usually a month. Knee extension contractures as seen in many children with L3 and L4 lesions do not seem to be an ongoing problem, as the contracture usually tends to decrease with time. Therefore, intensive management does not seem justified.

The calcaneus deformity seen in the child with a L5/S1 lesion, can be managed with range of movement exercises, orthoses or serial plastering. If the joint is easily correctable into a neutral position, then the deformity is postural in nature and is likely to correct with time. If, however, the joint cannot be easily corrected into a neutral position or requires force to maintain a corrected position, then serial plastering or orthoses will usually be indicated to control the deformity. Equinus deformities are usually only seen in those children with spasticity in the gastrocnemius muscle, or those children with a degree of talipes equino-varus deformity. The early management of these deformities follows the above criteria.

The facilitation of gross motor skills
Placing the child in a variety of positions such as sidelying, prone, supine, propped sitting and sitting will give the child the opportunity to improve their head and trunk control. These positions may need to be modified and some ideas are listed below:

- *Prone:* a pillow, rolled towel or foam wedge may assist a child with hydrocephalus to negate some of the effects of gravity. A weight or hand on the buttocks may help stabilize the pelvis of a child with unopposed hip flexor activity. There are also many other fun ways a child can experience prone, without being directly positioned on the floor, such as lying across the parent's lap, or lying on the parent's stomach (*Figure 7.4a,b*).
- *Supine:* a pillow and towels can again be used to position a young child into supine. Other ideas include resting the child supine on the parents lap or in a bouncinette or fraser chair in a reclined position.
- *Sitting:* a child will develop interest in their surround-

(a)

(a)

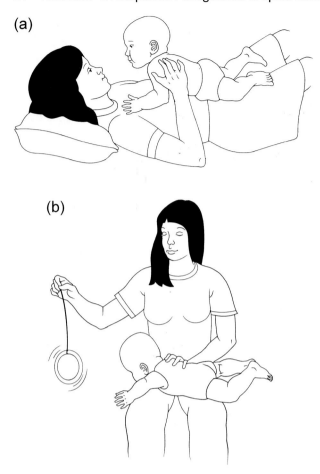

(b)

Figure 7.4(a,b) Ideas for encouraging the prone position to improve head control in a child with hydrocephalus.

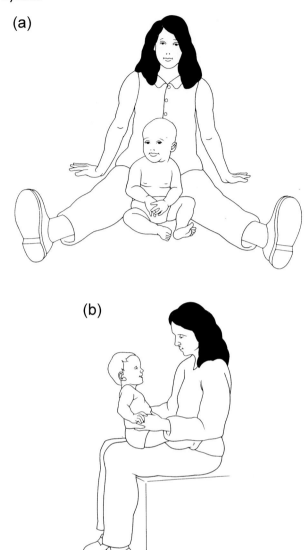

(b)

Figure 7.5(a,b) Ideas for supported sitting to improve trunk extension and balance which is commonly delayed in children with spina bifida.

ings if they are upright, initially propped with assistance and later sitting independently. Cushions can be used to support a child initially, as can the corner of a couch or the corner of a cardboard box. Sitting the child in the crook of the therapist or parent's knee or between their legs when in a long sitting position can also be another alternative. For those children with significant delays in head and trunk control and balance, a corner chair can be used. Once the child has achieved static sitting balance, the use of a roller with the child sitting astride, swings, rocking horses and games played in sitting can be used to develop the child's dynamic sitting balance. The therapist will use toys to encourage reaching and propping both forwards, sideways, and backwards (*Figures 7.5a,b, 7.6*).

- *Rolling:* rolling is usually initiated by the head, arms, trunk and then the legs. If the lower limbs are paralysed, or the child has poor head control, then the child will have difficulty learning to roll. A

significant portion of children with spina bifida will also be apprehensive when rolling because of the loss of control as they move from one position to another. Thus, in the physiotherapy sessions and at home, rolling can be encouraged with toys and gentle assistance.

- *Transfer from lying to sitting:* when learning this skill, children usually pull up on a cot or furniture to sit up from a supine or prone position. The physiotherapist may opt to break this skill down into its component parts and practice these individually: reaching out of the base of support, sitting balance and rolling, as well as weightbearing through the upper limbs.

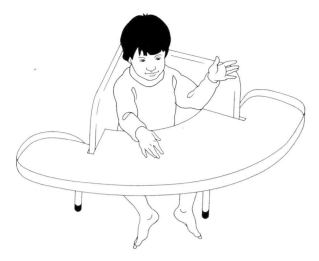

Figure 7.6 A corner chair can be used for safe supported sitting – so the child can practise bilateral hand function.

It is the motivation to achieve a skill or perform a task, and stimulation from the environment that will give the child the practice controlling his or her head and trunk against gravity. Through this interaction the child will practice repeatedly the head and trunk control necessary to interact with the stimulus. The positive outcome of the interaction will provide the child with the positive reinforcement to try the task again. The child should ideally be in an awake and happy state. Noises, voices, faces, touching different textures and surfaces in a variety of positions, cuddling and massaging all provide important early sensory input. This sensory input will stimulate appropriate motor output and will encourage the child to use the innervated muscles. The child will progress from interacting with their eyes, to interacting with their hands. Thus the motor control progresses in a cephalo-caudal direction.

In this early period a playgroup setting is an ideal environment to provide this sensory input. The child will watch and learn from other children. The playgroup setting also provides an environment where the parents can view other children with spina bifida at various stages of development. The playgroup also provides an informal setting for the parents to discuss the more practical issues affecting their child.

Hydrocephalus will affect the ability of the child to learn, practise and repeat a gross motor skill. The experienced therapist must be aware that hydrocephalus does affect the short-term memory, motivation, initiation, sequencing, upper limb co-ordination, concentration, perception, fine manipulative control, spacial orientation and figure ground discrimination. The physiotherapist may need to provide an enormous amount of motivation to encourage a child to perform

and practice a task. The task may have to be repeated over and over again before it is memorized, or the task may need to be broken down into simple portions. For example, learning to sit from a supine position may need to be taught in steps such as: (i) supine to sidelying, which is a component of rolling involving cervical flexion and rotation followed by trunk rotation; and (ii) rising from sidelying using hip flexion, trunk flexion and weight bearing through arms to a sitting position which involves sitting balanced outside a base of support.

The facilitation of independent mobility

Before achieving independent mobility, the child must have the necessary head and trunk control, be able to support weight and shift weight from side to side with their upper limbs and/or their lower limbs and must have the will or motivation to move towards a stimulus. It is the stimulus which provides the encouragement to move, not the actual movement itself. If a child is consistently handed every toy they show an interest in, then there is very little motivation for the child to move. The child requires a stimulus to move and often some assistance to commence independent mobility. Some ideas for assisting mobility are the use of a towel under the stomach to assist weight shift forward, or the use of a scooter board or prone trolley. Later, for children with higher lesions, a chariot may be used (*Figure 7.7*).

Children with spina bifida will move in a number of different ways; some will roll, some will commando crawl, some will crawl in a reciprocal fashion, while others will bottom shuffle. The child will move in the easiest way, depending on their degree of paralysis and amount of contracture or deformity. The age at which the child will begin to move will vary from child to child.

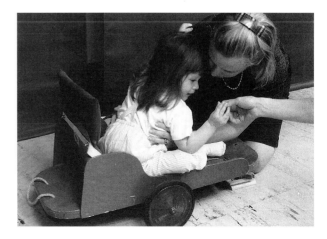

Figure 7.7 Introducing a chariot to assist mobility for a child with thoracic myelomeningocele.

A home environment which provides the appropriate stimulus to encourage the child to move will assist in achieving independent mobility. Spending time playing with the child on the floor, providing the child with toys appropriate to their level of development and providing the child with achievable goals are some of the factors which will assist, as will an environment which gives the child a sense of achievement through positive reinforcement. The positive reinforcement may be verbal encouragement, a hug, or it may be the use of an appropriate toy.

Independent mobility enables a child to learn about their environment. As the child learns to move away from and back to their known environment, the child will develop a sense of security. It also allows a child to develop an awareness of space and a sense of their body and how their body relates to their environment.

The development of upper limb skills

For many babies with spina bifida, the development of upper limb skills is inhibited by the lack of head and trunk control and later sitting balance. The arms are needed for support in the sitting position, and can therefore not be involved in the development of fine motor skills. For these children, often the emergence of hand dominance is delayed. Therefore for many children, especially those with thoracic and high lumbar lesions, it is necessary to provide a stable trunk from which the arms can reach and grasp. Some simple ideas can assist, such as placing rolled towels under the shoulders of a neonate to protract the shoulders, positioning the child with a flexed cervical spine using a pillow or towels so the child can view the object, propping the child in a stable seat or bouncinette, or sitting in a fully supported chair such as a corner chair.

The physiotherapy programme will focus on the weightbearing ability of the upper limbs, and their strength and endurance. The involvement in sports such as wheelchair track and field, swimming, and ball sports is encouraged, as these sports will improve the strength of the upper limbs. This strength will assist with transfer skills and wheelchair skills, as well as the use of a gait aide.

Progress to standing and walking

Physiotherapy to encourage standing

All children with spina bifida are given the opportunity to stand. Though the benefits of standing are only beginning to be scientifically investigated, it is believed that standing will slow down contracture and deformity development, and will slow down the development of osteoporosis by providing weightbearing forces, especially in children who will not progress to walking

(Anschuetz *et al.*, 1984; Rosenstein *et al.*, 1987). Standing is also believed to assist bowel and bladder function through the effects of gravity, and standing will also stimulate head and trunk control. Standing will also improve the self-esteem of the child.

There is no literature to assist the decision as to how much standing is necessary to achieve some of its benefits. We incorporate daily standing into the child's routine at home. Standing is commenced in the first year, when the child has shown some floor mobility skills, and is beginning to show interest in pulling to stand. Thus the child has demonstrated the appropriate trunk and head control and balance reactions in a sitting position. Children with significant hip flexion contractures will commence standing earlier than this in order to stretch their hip flexors.

There are many different ways a child with spina bifida will achieve standing. Children with lower lesions will pull to stand on their own. Children with mid-lumbar or low lumbar lesions may require the assistance of orthoses such as wrap-around splints or ankle foot orthoses, while children with high lumbar or thoracic lesions will require the assistance of a standing frame (*Figure 7.8*). The physiotherapist will guide the child and family through this period, providing the appropriate equipment to commence safe standing, authorizing the appropriate orthoses to enable the child to stand, and providing the opportunity in the physiotherapy sessions to practice standing. Skills such

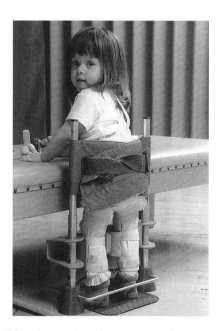

Figure 7.8 A standing frame is used to allow standing in a child with a thoracic myelomeningocele within their first year.

as kneel standing against a piece of furniture, or the ability to perform a sit-to-stand transfer, may need to be practised prior to the commencement of standing. These skills encourage equilibrium reactions and trunk control and the child can experience weightbearing through the upper and lower limbs. Once static standing has been mastered, the child will learn to weight shift to the side, then in a diagonal direction before walking is achieved. This is usually practised through play. The child will build up their endurance in standing and improve their balance in this position in readiness for walking.

Physiotherapy to encourage ambulation
The progress of children with spina bifida from standing to ambulation will vary according to the degree of paralysis. Many factors affect a child's ability to ambulate: age, height, the presence of hydrocephalus, the presence of spasticity, musculoskeletal-deformities such as scoliosis or contractures, obesity, motivation and social circumstances (Hoffer *et al.*, 1973; Stillwell and Menelaus, 1983; Knutson and Clark, 1991). Generally the prognosis for walking is directly related to the level of lesion (Knutson and Clark, 1991). There is a small population of children who will not walk at all – those with severe hydrocephalus, spasticity or gross contractures. It has been shown that walking, even if later abandoned, encourages independence especially in transfer skills (Mazur *et al.*, 1989). Despite the high cost in terms of time for the therapist, family and child and the financial cost for the orthoses, most children are given the opportunity to walk.

The physiotherapist has a guiding role to ensure that all the factors that may adversely affect the child's physical mobility, including walking, are minimized. The physiotherapist will assess each child and with the child, family and other team members discuss realistic goals for mobility and ambulation. Effective communication through this period with the team members involved with each child including the orthopaedic surgeon, the neurosurgeon and the orthotist, is often crucial to the child's ability to attain the goal of independent mobility. The physiotherapy sessions will be directed towards preventing contracture and deformity, selecting the appropriate orthotics and equipment to achieve the goals and problem solving. The sessions will provide practice for the child's gross motor skills with the necessary assistance provided initially by the therapist and subsequently taught to the parents. The sessions are enjoyable for both the child and family, as all the activities involve toys and games.

Ambulation of children with thoracic and high lumbar myelomeningiocele. The developmental sequence of this group of children is predictable. All will be significantly delayed in the acquisition of basic gross motor abilities such as rolling or sitting. All will require splinting up to the chest level for efficient ambulation, and all will require a chariot and subsequently a wheelchair for long-distance mobility. The development of ambulation orthoses, such as the parawalker, the dual cable reciprocal gait orthoses (RGOs), the isocentric orthoses and the advanced reciprocal gait orthoses (ARGOs) has enabled a much higher proportion of children with this level of paralysis to achieve community ambulation (Yngve, 1984; Winchester *et al.*, 1993; Davidson, 1994). In some centres the rate of community ambulation has been as high as 52% (Charney *et al.*, 1991). A reciprocating gait orthoses is more energy efficient, and the child can walk more quickly than using bilateral knee–ankle–foot orthoses (KAFOs) or hip–knee–ankle–foot orthoses (HKAFOs) (Flandry *et al.*, 1986; McCall and Schmidt, 1986).

A multidisciplinary clinic involving the orthopaedic surgeon, the orthotist, the child's local physiotherapist and the specialist physiotherapist will recommend the use of one of the types of reciprocating gait orthoses. At this stage some of the children may require surgery, such as hip flexor lengthening procedures, knee flexor lengthening procedures, or one of the many procedures to the foot to produce a plantigrade foot position (McCall *et al.*, 1983).

The criteria for selection for each of the reciprocating devices includes the assessment of contractures and deformities, intelligence and motivation, support from the family, local physiotherapy services, the coordination and strength of the upper limbs, spasticity, scoliosis and age.

The full programme of gait training for the (RGO) dual cable system is outlined in the application manual by Fillauer and for the parawalker, once a centre has been licensed by attending a training course organized by an accredited parawalker training centre, a manual outlining the specific gait training principles for the parawalker is provided.

Training will begin prior to the manufacture of the orthoses. Pretraining will include stretching and range of movement exercises, upper limb strengthening, and dynamic standing balance practice to improve equilibrium reactions and build up confidence. The features of a reciprocal gait that require reinforcement are weight shift, bottom tuck or hip extension and the reciprocal use of the hands and feet in a four-point system. Even a child under 2 years can usually learn these tasks (*Figures 7.9, 7.10*).

During the manufacture of the orthoses and at its completion, the physiotherapist will check the alignment of the joints and check the fit of the orthoses with the orthotist. The child and family will spend many sessions in the physiotherapy department, learning to

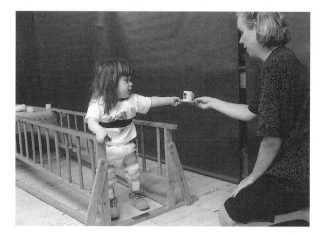

Figure 7.9 Encouraging weight shift, early in the RGO gait training programme.

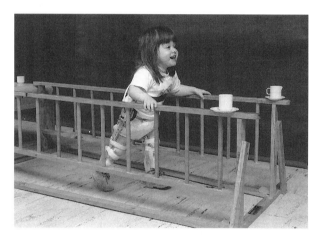

Figure 7.10 Practising independent walking using a RGO in the parallel bars – a 20-month-old girl with a thoracic myelomeningocele.

Later training includes walking on slopes and uneven ground, climbing kerbs and steps and learning to transfer in the orthoses from the ground to standing and vice versa, and from a sitting position to a standing position and vice versa. Transfers require a level of fine motor control and a sequence of movement that is usually not learnt until the age of 4 or 5 years. In our experience the majority of children will never become independent in all aspects of use of RGOs (*Figures 7.11–7.14*).

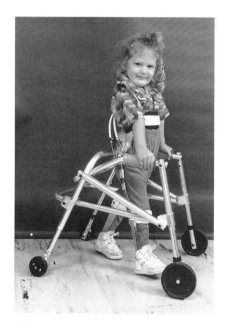

Figure 7.11 Independent walking with a RGO and a Kaye walker – the stance leg hip joint must be fully extended for an efficient gait pattern.

don and doff the orthoses, and learning the features of a reciprocal gait. Ambulation will occur initially in the parallel bars, then the child will progress on to a Kaye posture walker, forward rollator or elbow crutches depending on the orthoses.

Some children require little or no training to ambulate independently, while others may require many months to learn to walk. If the child has strong hip flexor power with little or no hip flexion contracture and has only mild hydrocephalus, then the training time required can be extremely short. The child will progress to a Kaye posterior walker then on to crutches. The main factors affecting the eventual outcome appear to be the presence or absence of a shunt, the presence of a scoliosis, hip flexion contractures and the child's social circumstances (Phillips *et al.*, 1995).

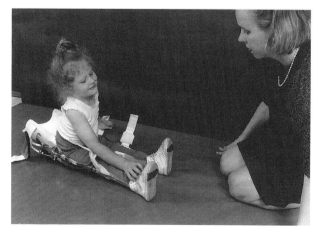

Figure 7.12 The physiotherapist teaching independent doffing of the RGO in a 5 year old with a thoracic myelomeningocele.

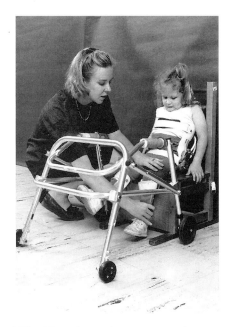

Figure 7.13 The physiotherapist teaching stand to sit transfers in the RGO.

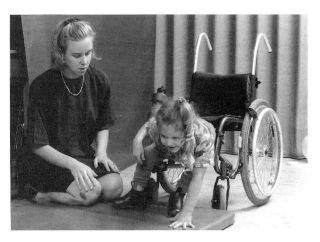

Figure 7.14 The physiotherapist supervising practice of wheelchair to floor transfers in a 5 year old with a thoracic myelomeningocele.

Ambulation of children with mid-lumbar myelomeningeocele. The gross motor abilities of children with mid-lumbar myelomeningocele are variable. Some of the children will use a RGO, some will use a KAFO, some will initially use wrap-around splints and an ankle–foot orthosis (AFO) and some will only use an AFO. A small group of children will improve their level of ambulation while decreasing their orthotic requirements in the early years; however the vast majority will require more orthotic support as they age (Dudgeon *et al.*, 1991). Some children will be long-term community walkers, while others will be household ambulators only. Many factors affect the child's ability to ambu-

late. The level of paralysis appears to be the major determinant (McDonald *et al.*, 1991). The strength of specific muscle groups has been shown to be an accurate predictor of ambulation ability: quadriceps (Schopler and Menelaus, 1987; Dudgeon *et al.*, 1991; McDonald *et al.*, 1991), iliopsoas (McDonald *et al.*, 1991), followed by tibialis anterior, gluteus maximus and gluteus medius strength. The walking ability of children with L3/4 lesions is also affected by contractures and deformities, especially deformities around the hip, such as subluxation or dislocation (Asher and Olsen, 1983). All will benefit from the use of a gait aid initially, though some will dispense with this later. Most children will require a wheelchair for long-distance mobility and a significant proportion will prefer this to ambulation when they reach adolescence.

The physiotherapy management of this group is often one of problem solving for the individual. So many factors will affect the gait of a child and all these factors need to be taken into account when assisting the child to mobilize and subsequently ambulate. Particular muscle groups may require stretching, so positioning, range of movement exercises or orthoses may be ordered to achieve this aim. The upper limbs may need strengthening, so the use of a chariot or prone trolley may be discussed for home. Particular muscle groups may require strengthening, so ideas for strengthening including hydrotherapy, the use of a bicycle and other games may be introduced into the treatment sessions. The child may require parallel bars, a Kaye walker or forward rollator for home use. The child will need to practise standing and walking at home as well as in the physiotherapy sessions, so the parents are shown how best to assist the child to perform these activities. A supportive and motivating environment using toys and games will help to stimulate the child to step and walk.

Ambulation of children with low lumbar and sacral myelomeningocele. Children with low lumbar or sacral lesions are much more predictable with regard to their walking abilities. All will learn to roll, crawl reciprocally, pull to stand, stand without the use of a standing frame, cruise around furniture and finally walk independently. Many will require AFOs and a gait aid to assist walking initially; however, many will progress to independent mobility without the use of a gait aid. Many are long-distance walkers who do not require a wheelchair.

The physiotherapy management of this group involves standing balance work, encouragement to side step and weight shift and thus cruise around furniture and, finally, assistance with stepping in the parallel bars. Most will progress on to a gait aid relatively quickly and will ambulate independently prior to school age.

Later management

Physiotherapy management of school-age children is dependent on need. Some of the aims of a physiotherapy programme for a school age child are detailed below.

Continue regular and thorough assessments

These assessment include all of the factors mentioned above in the assessment section. The gait of a child with spina bifida may change during the school years, and the reasons for the change must be closely assessed. Some of the changes may be due to changes in height, weight and energy expenditure as the child grows, some may be due to the development of a contracture or scoliosis, some may be due to spinal cord tethering or the presence of syringomyelia, and some may be due to a hip dislocation or ill-fitting orthoses. The physiotherapist once again must assess closely, try to determine the cause of the changes or refer to the appropriate personnel. Thus, the role is one of problem solving or trouble shooting. Orthotic requirements, gait aids and wheelchair needs may change with age, so these factors need to be regularly assessed.

The development of an appropriate treatment programme

This programme will reflect the goals established by the child, family and school and may include working on specific independence skills such as transfer skills, or a gross motor programme encouraging general fitness, balance and co-ordination. Specific muscle groups may be targeted for stretching or strengthening, and orthoses may be ordered to assist with the stretching process.

Assessment of the home and school environments

A physiotherapist will provide a thorough assessment and may suggest modifications to encourage independent physical mobility, for example non-slip floor surfaces and appropriate access to both the indoor and outdoor areas for a child using a gait aide or wheelchair, including the classroom, the toileting areas, the library and any other classrooms the child will be attending. The feasibility of wheelchair use versus independent ambulation will need to be discussed and consensus reached by the family, the school and the child. Special equipment in the classroom, such as a modified table, chair or lifting equipment, may need to be purchased. Extra space may be required in the classroom to accommodate gait aides or wheelchairs.

Provide training and resources to staff at the school

Most children with spina bifida attend mainstream schools with the assistance of an attendant in the classroom. This person can assist in achieving the goal of independent mobility by allowing the child to ambulate and transfer independently in the classroom, while being available for assistance if the child is experiencing difficulty. This attendant and others involved in lifting the child will need to be taught the principles of safe lifting.

The physiotherapist can provide valuable support to the school staff, by providing support letters for integration funding. Therapists can also advise on the purchase of appropriate aides and equipment to be used in the school environment.

Encourage participation in physical education and sporting activities

Involvement of children with spina bifida in physical education at school is to be encouraged and the physiotherapist may be able to assist the school in devising ways to involve the child. Sporting activities will improve self-esteem, help to prevent obesity and may improve upper or lower limb and trunk strength. The secondary gains will be in the child's level of independent mobility.

OCCUPATIONAL THERAPY
Jane L Galvin

Occupational therapists work as part of a multidisciplinary team to assist children with spina bifida to develop and maintain their maximum level of independence in all tasks of daily living. Occupational therapy involvement can be broadly summarized as relating to fine motor development and upper limb function, seating and pressure care, and activities of daily living (ADL) including cognitive and perceptual development. Children with spina bifida are typically not referred to occupational therapy until approximately 6 months of age as it is felt that medical issues and the adaptation of the family to a new child take precedence during this time. Earlier referral during the first 6 months of life may be appropriate if the child has been hospitalized for an extended period of time, or if they are showing a delay in development. The level of occupational therapy involvement varies according to the needs of each child but is generally related to the level of the lesion and the presence of hydrocephalus, with or without a shunt. Children with higher-level lesions and hydrocephalus tend to show greater delays in fine motor, cognitive perceptual and self-care development and as a result will tend to require greater input from occupational therapy services.

Fine Motor Development

Children with spina bifida frequently show functional delays in upper limb development in comparison with their peers. These delays have been shown to be directly related to hydrocephalus, the results of which are frequently seen as ataxia, motor planning difficulties and delayed neurological maturation (Turner, 1986). These delays are further compounded by decreased experiences of movement, related to reduced lower limb function and delayed development of balance reactions and independent mobility.

Henderson and Pehoski (1995) identify the importance of early movement experiences and exploratory play in developing fine motor skills.

The need to use one or both hands to maintain sitting balance reduces the potential for bilateral play at mid-line and for exploration in children with spina bifida, and thus limits their opportunity to gain these early experiences of play and manipulation of toys. This can also be a contributing factor to delays in visual perceptual development, as spatial concepts are often ill defined and the child's perception of the world is limited by difficulty moving within and between positions (Holgate, 1990).

Playgroups are an important part of occupational therapy intervention in the pre-kindergarten years and focus on development of fine motor skills and visual perceptual skills. Children should be encouraged to play in a variety of different positions to provide differing perspectives of the world and to challenge the perceptual system. Positions such as lying prone over a bolster, supine on a wedge, sitting in a corner chair or tumbleform, or standing supported in an RGO provide an opportunity to improve perceptual skills through viewing the world from different angles. Supported positions such as these also encourage development of fine motor skills by freeing up the hands from their support role to allow play at mid-line and further exploration or manipulation of toys. Parents and therapy staff can co-actively guide the child's hands so that a task is completed successfully and an end result achieved. Activities such as posting blocks in containers, finger feeding and banging toys encourage development of fine manipulative skills. Resistive activities that encourage development of upper body strength should also be encouraged from an early age as children will frequently be relying on their upper bodies to assist with mobility in propelling wheelchairs, using walking frames and transferring to and from different surfaces. It is important to provide exposure to a variety of tactile sensations to provide new sensory experiences and to reduce the impact of tactile defensiveness that is frequently related to hydrocephalus. Playing outside provides an opportunity to explore the different textures of grass, dirt, sand and water which helps to increase the child's awareness of the sensory world. Playgroups also frequently include activities such as finger painting, water play and other messy games to provide tactile experiences of differing textures and temperatures.

As children enter school age, handwriting often presents a problem due to a combination of fine motor and visual motor problems (Ziviani, 1987). The use of thicker pens or textas or an adapted pen grip can sometimes improve the ease with which a pen is grasped and the quality of the script; however, handwriting is frequently slow and laborious and children often struggle to keep up with the amount of writing required, particularly as they progress into and through high school. Contributing to difficulties with handwriting are visual memory and visual motor difficulties, which often make copying written work from the blackboard difficult as children have difficulty recalling the shape and pattern of the information written on the blackboard. Visual perceptual difficulties also create difficulties in transferring images from the blackboard into a written form in workbooks. The use of a sloping work surface reduces the need to change visual focus from vertical to horizontal and can provide an easier and more supportive position for handwriting. The use of computers is also an excellent compensatory tool which addresses the need for immediate visual feedback. The occupational therapist can provide assessments of the child's physical and cognitive functioning and make recommendations regarding the most effective type of computer, and specific programs or adaptations to benefit the child. The use of computers can also compensate for decreased speed and quality of handwriting by allowing the production of a neat and legible finished product.

Seating and Pressure Care

Children who use a wheelchair as their primary means of mobility are at increased risk of developing pressure areas and skin breakdown. The main reasons for these are spending long periods of time in a wheelchair or other stationary sitting position, and reduced sensation in the lower half of the body. Other contributing factors include bowel and bladder accidents, reduced circulation to the skin, and poor posture due to scoliosis. Children with lesions above L3 will spend the majority of their waking hours in a sitting position, due to the limited function in their lower limbs, and are especially at risk of developing skin breakdown. It is essential that all children are seated in a comfortable and supportive chair which allows them stability to use their hands and arms for other play or work activities. Seating systems for the wheelchair, bath, school and car need to be assessed to ensure that they are providing appropriate support and that they are not contributing to potential pressure areas. The role of occupational therapy includes assessing the child's sitting posture and daily routine to identify aspects that might contribute to skin breakdown. All children should be pressure tested over their bony prominences while sitting in their wheelchairs and using a variety of cushions to determine which provides the most appropriate form of pressure relief. Parents and children should also be provided with written information, following a teaching session, on skin care and pressure relief. Following a research project at the Royal Children's Hospital this system was introduced and appears to have been successful in reducing the number of inpatient hospital days caused by skin breakdown (Johnson, 1995). It is also recommended that the occupational therapist be present at the wheelchair clinic where a child's initial wheelchair is prescribed. This helps to ensure that the wheelchair and cushion form a complete package to fit the child and prevents the need to make multiple adjustments later.

Pressure mattresses, ranging from high density foam to dynamic air flow systems are prescribed to prevent skin breakdown in children with high-level lesions who also have anaesthetic skin and reduced ability to roll from side to side while sleeping.

Occupational therapists are also involved in selecting and modifying car seats to allow safe transport in the car. National and State safety regulations should always be consulted prior to making any changes to a car seat; however, the addition of high density foam padding to accommodate a scoliosis, reduce pressure over a lesion site or to provide greater trunk and head support is generally acceptable as it does not alter the inherent structure of the car seat.

For kindergarten or school-aged children, it is important that they have a supportive chair and a table that is at an appropriate height to allow them to complete table-top tasks. Reaching up high or bending low compromises both their fine motor and visual perceptual skills and should be avoided by the provision of suitable equipment that is fitted to the child's needs.

Activities of Daily Living

Children should be encouraged to assist with self-care tasks and to become independent as they become more physically able. Depending on the level of the lesion, balance in sitting is often a limiting factor in initiating and achieving independence with dressing tasks. Practising while lying in bed, seated in a chair, or leaning against a firm surface often provides a feeling of security to allow the child to explore with their hands and to begin to assist with dressing. Children will generally learn to undress before they learn to dress and should be encouraged to assist where possible, for example pulling off socks or helping to pull their arms out of sleeves.

Children with hydrocephalus frequently have difficulty explaining the relationship between shapes and objects and with spatial perceptions such as near and far. Difficulty with concepts such as these often makes it difficult to grasp the spatial concepts involved in dressing as in advice to put your feet 'through' the holes, pull the jumper 'over' your head. Children with spina bifida generally perform better on verbally orientated tasks and because of this it is often helpful to emphasize the verbal components of the task by having the child talked through the action ('I put my leg into the hole'), thus making the task controlled by the verbal left side of the brain rather than the more visual right side (Sobkowiak, 1990).

As mentioned above, children with spina bifida generally develop the ability to sit unsupported later than their peers. In the bath, with the added buoyancy of water, children will require additional support to maintain an upright position. Commercially available bath seats provide an opportunity for the child to sit safely in the bath, while allowing their hands to be free to play with the water and toys. The use of bath seats also reduces the potential for parents to sustain back injuries while transferring their child into the bath, or when assisting with bathing. Seats with safety belts and non-slip surfaces are recommended to prevent children slipping forward out of their chairs and to provide added support for trunk stability.

As the child becomes older and more independent with self-care and mobility, modifications may need to be made to the home to allow the child to access all areas without assistance from parents. The major area of difficulty is generally in the bathroom and often major renovations are required to allow independent access. If a wheelchair is able to be placed alongside the bath, a bath or bath chair can be used, with a sideways transfer being used to transfer from the wheelchair to the bath board. If the bathroom is inaccessible to a wheelchair, the entire bathroom may need to be redesigned to accommodate a wheelchair or other adaptive equipment. The renovations most frequently made are to replace a walk-in shower stall with a non-slip stepless shower base that is then fitted with a shower seat and a hand-held shower spray. This type of shower base is useful for two reasons: if the child is ambulant but unsteady, the removal of the step can increase safety getting in and out of the shower and the provision of a seat allows the child to rest, or sit to wash the lower half of the body if becoming fatigued or feeling unsteady on their feet. For children in wheelchairs, the stepless shower base also provides increased access to the shower as door entrances are generally wider than standard showers. With the seat in a folded down position, children can transfer independently on to the seat and use the shower spray to assist with washing.

It has often been helpful to modify the arrangement of kitchen cupboards so that items used most frequently are placed at or below bench height to allow the child easy access to all areas. For the family or adolescent considering moving to a new or different home, it is important to consider the height of benches and other work surfaces to ensure that all surfaces and cupboards can be accessed from a wheelchair, if necessary, or when standing.

As children become adolescents and young adults, the occupational therapist becomes involved in preparing them to live independently of their parents, whether that be in supported or independent accommodation. Hydrocephalus and the presence of a shunt often leads to difficulty with high-level cognitive skills such as planning, problem solving, initiation and sequencing, which can have a negative impact on the adolescent's ability to complete grocery shopping, home management and other community living tasks that are skills necessary for independent living. Activ-

ities such as menu planning, budgeting, banking and home management are all skills that may need to be developed to allow the adolescent to live independently. The occupational therapist can be involved in helping the adolescent develop these skills and in structuring their day to ensure that all tasks are completed. As in childhood, an occupational therapist can assist in modifying the home environment to ensure access, but is also frequently involved in conducting work site visits to modify work stations and job demands to increase the potential for independence in the workplace.

Occupational therapists are also involved in completing driving assessments, to determine whether a person has appropriate motor, visual perceptual and cognitive skills to drive a car, and to make modifications to the car if necessary to compensate for decreased lower limb function.

As part of the allied health team, occupational therapists work to ensure that each individual with spina bifida is able to achieve the highest level of independence possible. As outlined above, for the person with spina bifida this encompasses regular assessment of fine motor and visual perceptual skills to monitor their development and provision of aids or equipment to maintain physical safety and independence.

Chapter 8

Gait

Catherine M Duffy, Shane A Barwood and H Kerr Graham

INTRODUCTION

The study of normal gait has developed rapidly during this century since the advent of moving pictures and instrumented gait analysis (Sutherland, 1988; Perry, 1992). The study of pathological gait is also advancing rapidly, especially in cerebral palsy and more recently, in spina bifida (Gage, 1991; Vankoski *et al.*, 1995). An excellent introduction has been published by Gage in 1991 and the reader is referred to this work for clarification of terminology and more detail on areas which can only be mentioned briefly here.

GAIT ANALYSIS

Gait analysis is the study of how body segments move in relation to each other during walking and may be divided into several important components.

Temporospatial Parameters

Temporospatial parameters are velocity, step length, stride length and cadence. These measures can be obtained by simple means and do not require a gait analysis laboratory.

Kinematics

Kinematics is the study of motion in terms of displacement, angles and velocities, without regard to the forces behind the events. When normal motion is plotted as angular displacement against time, characteristic plots are generated at each joint level and in each plane. Kinematic data can be measured in various ways but the most practical is by a photographic system that tracks markers directly attached to the walking child.

Kinetics

Kinetics deals with ground reaction force (GRF) measurements by force plates from which can be calculated joint moments and powers. External moments are produced by the GRF and internal moments by muscle action.

Electromyography

Electromyography (EMG) measures the timing and intensity of electrical activity within muscle. Recordings can be made from the surface of muscles by recording the signal from a large area through the skin or using fine wire electrodes inserted directly into the muscle. The utility of surface EMG is limited by interference or 'cross talk' from signals detected from adjacent large muscle groups and fine wire EMG by its invasiveness. In upper motor neurone lesions such as cerebral palsy, disorders of timing are common and EMG an important component of clinical gait analysis. In the (mostly) lower motor neurone disorder of spina bifida, disorders of muscle timing are usually secondary compensations and not part of the primary pathology, for example prolonged firing of the quadriceps during stance in children with 'crouch' gait. This information is readily available from a study of kinematics and kinetics and the role of electromyography is limited.

Energy Expenditure

Energy expenditure is the energy cost of walking which may be measured indirectly by measuring oxygen consumption and carbon dioxide production during walking. Normal walking conserves energy by a constant interplay between storing potential energy as the centre of mass is elevated with each step, followed by conversion to kinetic energy as the centre of mass undergoes a controlled fall. The vertical and horizontal displacements of the centre of mass of the body follow a sinusoidal curve and are equal and opposite. If we walked with stiff limbs our centre of mass would have to rise and fall 9.5cm with each step. By using co-ordinated pelvic, knee and ankle motions this is reduced to 4.4cm and is important in conserving energy.

Abnormal gait is frequently characterized by a relative failure of these mechanisms and is energy expensive. The stiff knee gait in cerebral palsy and the Trendelenburg gait in lumbar level myelomeningocele are characterized by large centre of mass oscillations which greatly increase energy consumption. Many teenagers are unable to sustain these increased demands without becoming excessively tired. Despite successful walking as younger children, some will increasingly need to use a wheelchair in high school.

Measurement of the energy cost of walking may therefore be the single most important parameter in assessing the efficiency of pathological gait. Various direct and indirect methods are used. The simplest is to measure the heart rate and velocity of walking and to derive the PCI or 'physiological cost index'. This calculation has been used as heart rate and oxygen uptake may be linearly related, but there are many limitations to this simplistic approach which have been discussed elsewhere (Corry *et al.*, 1996). The oxygen used during walking can be measured directly by various means. Until recently the equipment was cumbersome and better suited to normal subjects in controlled laboratory conditions. Portable, light weight telemetric systems are now available which are capable of giving reproducible results in children with motor disorders, using their normal aids and orthoses.

By measuring oxygen uptake during walking, we can derive two key values to describe the efficiency of gait. These are *oxygen rate* (millilitres of oxygen, per kilogram, per minute) and *oxygen cost* (millilitres of oxygen, per kilogram, per metre). Many motor disordered children with an inefficient gait simply slow down to keep their oxygen rate within normal limits but their oxygen cost remains grossly elevated compared to normals (Corry *et al.*, 1996; Duffy *et al.* 1996a).

There are three planes in which motion can be defined and studied: sagittal, coronal and transverse. Much can be gained from careful observation of the walking child. However, even the most experienced eye cannot detect the nuances of disordered gait at the three levels of hip, knee and ankle in both lower limbs and in all three planes. Watching patients walk in real time or recording it on video will give some information about kinematics of the subject's gait, but tells us nothing about kinetics.

GAIT ANALYSIS LABORATORIES

Although simple temporospatial gait data may be collected in an informal setting, instrumented gait analysis requires a dedicated laboratory and sophisticated equipment. The three-dimensional kinematic and kinetic data in this chapter were collected using the Vicon gait analysis system in which light reflective markers are placed on fixed anatomical points and are traced by multiple cameras. The cameras collect 50 frames of data per second which are integrated through a software package to yield information regarding the angles through which the joints of the lower limb move in a single gait cycle. Two force plates situated in the centre of the 'walkway' in the laboratory measure pressure exerted through the planted foot, from which is derived information regarding the joint moments and powers. A walking track within the laboratory provides a controlled environment in which to conduct energy studies. The equipment used in our energy studies was the Cosmed K2 and K4.

NORMAL GAIT

The gait cycle is the interval occurring between a foot first making contact with the ground (initial contact) and the next time it contacts the ground. For 60% of this interval the foot is in touch with the ground (stance phase) and for 40% it is off the ground (swing phase).

Stance phase itself may be divided into five parts:

- IC = initial contact: foot strikes ground;
- LR = loading response: period of deceleration when shock of impact is absorbed;
- MS = mid-stance: body's centre of mass passes over base of support;
- TS = terminal stance: centre of mass has passed over centre of support and is accelerating as it falls forward to unsupported side;
- PS = preswing.

Swing phase may be divided into three parts:

- IS = initial swing;
- MS = mid-swing;
- TS = terminal swing.

A limitation of gait analysis is that it assumes all gait cycles to be identical for a given individual, which is not strictly the case.

GAIT ANALYSIS IN SPINA BIFIDA (Duffy et al., 1996b)

During normal walking there are 104 muscles controlling 22 joints in the lower limbs. The power for walking is supplied by:

- plantar flexors of the ankle (36%);
- hip extensors (32%);
- hip flexors (22%);
- quadriceps (10%).

In children with spina bifida these muscles have a variable degree of paralysis depending on the level of lesion.

Most children with thoracic and high lumbar levels require high-level bracing to walk, precluding useful gait analysis. However, all children, are capable of having their temporospatial parameters and energy consumption studied.

Children with lesions of level L3 and below are capable of gait analysis but fixed deformities make the examination difficult. Study of foot and ankle motion is limited by ankle–foot orthosis (AFO) dependence and marker placement is difficult in deformed feet. Strict adherence to a marker placement protocol is required if reliable and reproducible results are to be obtained.

Many children with spina bifida are dependent on the use of crutches or other walking aids for walking (Lourenco et al., 1992). The use of such aids makes it difficult to assess kinetic activity as at least part of their body weight is transmitted through the walking aid, thus impairing ability to measure the ground reaction force.

SAGITTAL PLANE KINEMATICS AND KINETICS

Our kinematic and kinetic studies of children with spina bifida have shown that the higher the neurological level the greater the deviations from normal and the wider the range of abnormality found. Consistent patterns were noted, which become more exaggerated as the neurological level ascends. This is best illustrated by the kinematic changes of 'crouch gait' (*Figure 8.1a,b*). In children with sacral level lesions a slight increase in dorsiflexion at the ankle was a consistent finding with a reduction in power generation by the gastrosoleus complex in late stance. There was also a slight increase in knee flexion and hip flexion over normal. As the neurological level ascends, the crouch gait pattern becomes much more severe (Duffy et al., 1996c).

Pelvic Tilt

In normal gait the pelvis is tilted forward (anterior tilt) by about 10° throughout the gait cycle, controlled by gravity, inertia and the hip flexor and extensor muscles. With the higher levels of spina bifida lesion, the anterior tilt increases. Children with a low lumbar level spina bifida lesion have weak hip extensors strongly outweighed by their hip flexors, often resulting in fixed flexion contracture. The excessive degree of hip flexion found in these children is accompanied by increased anterior pelvic tilt. The presence of weak hip extensors in their own right reduces the ability to restrain forward motion of the pelvis, even in the absence of fixed flexion contracture.

Hip Flexion and Extension

The main muscles controlling the hip are the extensors and abductors in stance and the flexors in swing. The former, supplied mostly at S1, are weak or paralysed in spina bifida but the latter, supplied at L1,2 are likely to be strong. Maximal input from the hip extensors occurs from late swing through to loading response. Flexor muscle activity begins in terminal stance and continues into initial swing. In children with spina bifida, however, where the usual motor for walking (the ankle plantarflexors) is likely to be deficient, the hip flexors must provide much of the power for walking and are found to be much more active.

Maximum hip flexion normally occurs at terminal swing then, after initial contact, it is decreased by the extensors. Maximum hip extension occurs at terminal stance, which is initial contact for the opposite limb. There is increased hip flexion in all children with spina bifida at initial contact and terminal swing. There is also decreased hip extension at terminal stance. Normal hip extension reaches 2.5°, while for the spina bifida children it barely reaches 0°. The overall amplitude of motion (approximately 40°) of hip flexion and extension remain the same for children with spina bifida and normal children.

Knee Flexion and Extension

The knee kinematic consists of two flexion waves, the first occurring at loading response as the stance limb accepts body weight, controlled by eccentric

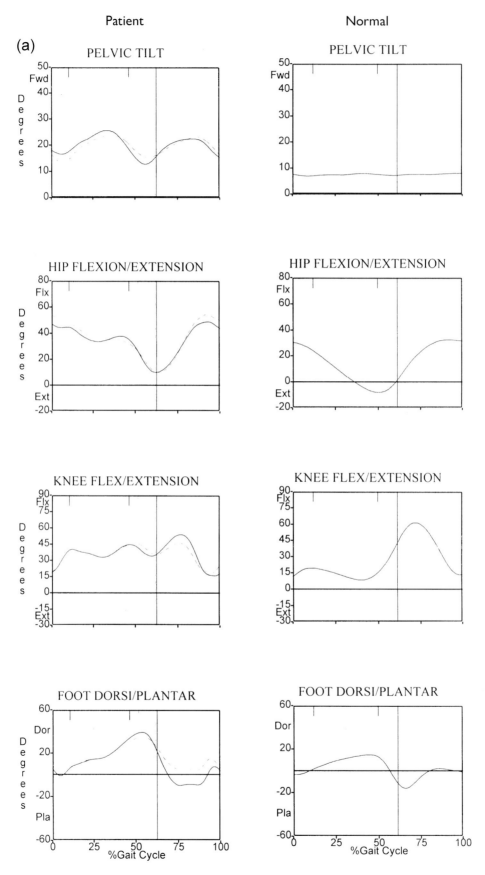

Figure 8.1   (continued opposite)

(b)

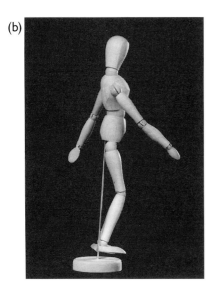

Figure 8.1 (a,b) Crouch gait in spina bifida. Sagittal plane kinematics in a 12-year-old boy with L5 level spina bifida. The left column are the patient's traces with the right limb shown as a solid line and the left limb as a dotted line. The right column are the traces from a normal child of the same age and sex. The vertical line separates stance (0–60% of the gait cycle), from swing (60–100% of the gait cycle). The pelvic trace shows a 'double bump' pattern with marked anterior pelvic tilt. At the hip level, extension is incomplete and the pattern is abnormal. The knee shows excessive flexion throughout stance and swing. At the ankle level the pattern is exaggerated and in the calcaneous range. Conclusion: these are the typical sagittal plane kinematics of 'crouch gait'. The model in (b) illustrates this pattern.

contraction of quadriceps and gluteus maximus. Maximum flexion in loading response is of the order of 15°. The second flexion wave commences as the knee is pushed forward, by gastrocnemius, at terminal stance in preparation for swing. During swing, knee flexion is maintained by the short head of biceps (initial and early swing), popliteus (mid to late swing) and the hamstrings (late to terminal swing). Maximum knee flexion in swing is of the order of 70°. All of the muscles involved in initiating knee flexion are supplied distally and are likely to function poorly in children with spina bifida. Early knee extension is normally a passive phenomenon in which no active muscular activity is required. In the latter part of swing knee extension is brought about by the action of the quadriceps and gluteus maximus. Despite having normally functioning quadriceps, children with spina bifida do not extend fully in terminal swing and have a more flexed knee at initial contact than normal children.

There is much greater knee flexion during stance in all children with spina bifida than in normal individuals, despite the fact that for most of the children studied, the quadriceps are working normally. Although some children have a knee flexion contracture the major reason for inadequate extension in midstance is likely to be weakness of paralysis of the gastrosoleus (see below).

Ankle Motion

Normally, the initial contact is made with the heel leading and the ankle in a neutral position. The ankle then plantarflexes until the foot is flat and dorsiflexes as the body passes over the foot. At terminal stance the heel begins to rise under the influence of the soleus and gastrocnemius and this is followed by a period of rapid plantarflexion which occurs largely passively, the ankle being held by strong plantarflexors in a position of plantarflexion, as the foot and tibia roll forward over the forefoot. Children with spina bifida have strongly functioning dorsiflexors but weak or paralysed plantarflexors and so may often have the ankle in an excessively dorsiflexed position at the time of initial contact. This represents a position of instability. This dorsiflexed position is maintained as the centre of gravity continues forward under the influence of the swing limb and the plantarflexors are unable to restrain the forward motion of the tibia. At terminal stance the heel rise is also less than usual.

Swing phase ankle kinematics in children with spina bifida are relatively normal, reflecting the normally functioning tibialis anterior.

Sagittal Plane Kinetics

The typical sagittal plane kinematics described above are of the child with spina bifida walking in a 'crouch' gait pattern (*Figure 8.2*). During normal walking extension of the lower limb is maintained in mid-stance by the plantar flexion/knee extension couple (PF/KE couple). This mechanism acts after loading response (LR). During LR, the GRF passes behind the knee as body weight is accepted, the knee flexes and is controlled by the quadriceps. Normally, the quadriceps are switched off after LR as the GRF moves in front of the knee and exerts an external extensor moment. Thereafter, a slow twitch activity in soleus is all that is required to keep the tibia from sagging forward and bringing the knee with it into flexion. In children with spina bifida, soleus is either paralysed or weak and so the PF/KE couple does not work effectively and this results in a sustained internal extensor moment being required at the hip and knee and an internal planta flexion moment being required at the

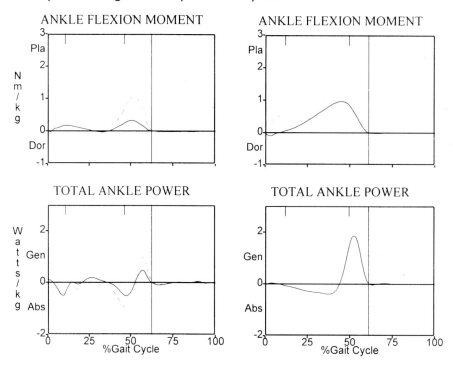

Figure 8.2   Ankle kinetics in spina bifida. Note the patient's flat ankle moment traces and the greatly reduced power generation in terminal stance compared with the normal traces. In these children the 'plantar-flexion, knee-extension' couple is deficient and is part of the reason for the crouch gait. In sacral-level children there is usually a reduction in the ankle plantarflexion moment and power generation even when the calf power tests as MRC grade 5 on manual testing. Posterior transfer of tibialis anterior to the calf may help but a GRAFO may be better.

ankle. Therefore, the quadriceps must remain 'switched on' throughout the stance phase of the gait cycle. In the latter part of mid-stance, the GRF would normally move posterior to the hip joint, exerting an external extensor moment on it and rendering it stable against the iliofemoral ligament of Bigelow. This cannot occur in children with spina bifida whose hips and knees remain flexed throughout stance. The delayed 'cross-over' and shallow nature of the internal hip flexor moment is evidence of this.

Children with L4 and sacral level lesions still exhibit a strong internal plantarflexion moment throughout stance, although it is of lesser magnitude than in normal children. However, even when the plantarflexors in children with sacral level spina bifida test clinically as being MRC grade 5, they often do not function as such and the measured power generation at terminal stance and preswing is very much less than normal. Thus the plantarflexors cannot function as the power house for walking that they are in normal gait. There is also a close relationship between the strength of the ankle plantarflexors and the hip extensors because they share a common level of innervation (McDonald *et al.*, 1991) The combination of weak plantarflexors and hip extensors explains the major

sagittal plane abnormalities in children with lumbo-sacral myelomeningocele (Vankoski *et al.*, 1995).

CLINICAL SIGNIFICANCE OF SAGITTAL PLANE KINEMATIC AND KINETIC STUDIES IN SPINA BIFIDA

In spina bifida 'crouch gait' is ubiquitous, progressive with age and ascending neurological lesion and energy expensive. The maintenance of a balanced extension posture is paramount. The calf muscle, even at the sacral level, generates insufficient power to maintain the PF/KE couple and this may require surgical and orthotic correction. For many children a better balance at the ankle is achieved by a posterior transfer of tibialis anterior to the heel because a deforming force is transferred to become a correcting force. A successful transfer will correct static calcaneus deformity, when combined with an anterolateral release and appropriate postoperative bracing but the transfer cannot correct dynamic calcaneus, in other words 'A boy cannot do a man's job'.

In many children the use of a ground reaction AFO (GRAFO) will be needed to augment the strength of the transfer but this can only work if there is good quadriceps strength and a knee that extends fully. Nothing will discredit the GRAFO more rapidly than trying to use it in the presence of fixed flexion deformity of the knee. The foot must also be braceable or made so by corrective surgery. Lateral tibial torsion and abducto valgus in the foot further weakens the PF/KE couple by dissipating the weak calf power through an unstable foot. Supramalleolar osteotomy for lateral tibial torsion and a variety of hindfoot osteotomies and arthrodeses can be used to correct this form of 'lever arm' disease. Given that there is no muscle transfer which can substitute for a paralysed calf, tenodesis of the tendo achilles to the fibula is another option. In our experience the results are variable. Serial gait laboratory studies are required in order to properly evaluate these procedures.

CORONAL PLANE KINEMATICS AND KINETICS

Children with spina bifida tend to walk not only in crouch but depending on the level of the lesion, with a gross Trendelenburg gait. The latter is the result of the effect of paralysed or weak hip abductors, present in children with L4 and L5 level lesions (*Figure 8.3a,b,c*). The hip abductors (gluteus medius and maximus) normally contract in mid-stance to hold the unsupported (swing) side of the pelvis level. In children with low lumbar spina bifida this mechanism is not possible and the centre of gravity must be moved over the hip of the stance phase lower limb (to negate the external adductor moment and prevent collapse) and the unsupported side of the pelvis 'hiked' up using strong trunk musculature (to effect clearance of the swing phase limb)

Pelvic Obliquity

At initial contact the pelvis is normally in neutral and elevates slightly during loading response and mid-stance as the abductors pay out a little to allow the opposite (swing) side of the pelvis to drop a little. This is an energy-conserving exercise. The stance side of the pelvis then elevates again through mid-stance as the abductors contract to support the swing side of the pelvis. In children with low lumbar spina bifida this control of the pelvis is not possible. In order to support the swing side of the pelvis trunk musculature must be used to bring the whole trunk towards the stance side of the pelvis and maintain the centre of gravity over the stance phase hip. This causes depression of the stance side of the pelvis relative to the swing side throughout stance phase. The amplitude of movement of the pelvis in the coronal plane in children with low lumbar spina bifida is much greater than in normal children. The low lumbar spina bifida children also have their maximum pelvic obliquity at the time of initial contact, rather than at loading response as normal children do.

Hip Abduction

The hip is normally slightly abducted at initial contact but adducts through loading response and terminal stance as the ipsilateral abductors pay out slightly to allow the contralateral side of the pelvis to drop a little. The hip abducts towards the end of stance phase as the opposite side of the pelvis is elevated again. Children with low lumbar spina bifida are unable to so control their hip kinematic and show gross abduction throughout the stance phase. This is a consequence of having the limb 'hiked' laterally during swing which results in an excessively abducted position at initial contact.

It is normal for the ground reaction force to pass medial to the hip and knee, imposing an external adductor moment on the hip and varus moment on the knee, reflected by the internal abductor moment at the hip and valgus moment at the knee. This pattern of activity is seen in normal children and children with sacral level lesions. For children with low lumbar level lesions, the GRF passes lateral to the hip and knee, imposing an external abduction moment at the hip and valgus moment at the knee. Coronal plane kinetics are therefore useful to determine which children are at risk of imposing undue strain on their medial collateral ligaments and developing medial instability and degenerative arthritis.

CLINICAL SIGNIFICANCE OF CORONAL PLANE KINEMATIC AND KINETIC STUDIES IN SPINA BIFIDA

The Trendelenburg gait seen in lumbar level spina bifida cannot be corrected completely surgically or orthotically without unacceptably high bracing. The iliopsoas transfer was introduced to stabilize the hip and improve gait in this group of children but the reported effects on hip stability are variable and most reports are pessimistic about the effects on gait. This is not surprising, given that the iliopsoas has very different length to cross-sectional area characteristics

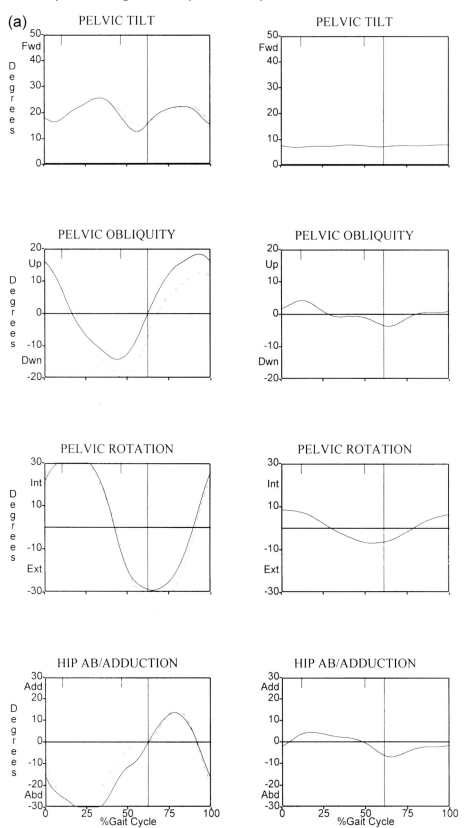

Figure 8.3   (continued opposite)

(b)

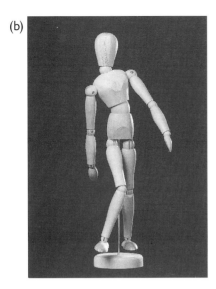

(c)

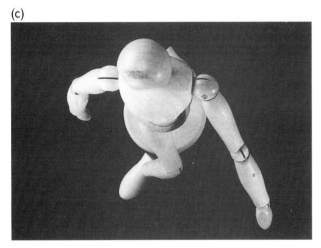

Figure 8.3(a,b,c) Pelvic instability in spina bifida. These are the four 'key kinematics' from sagittal, coronal and transverse planes which illustrate the pelvic instability in spina bifida. From sagittal plane, note the pelvic tilt. From coronal plane, note the massive increase in pelvic obliquity and hip abduction/adduction. These kinematics are also out of phase with the normal pattern. From the transverse plane note the massive 'S' shaped pelvic rotation curves. These are most closely correlated with increased energy expenditure. The model illustrates this pelvic instability from both the coronal (b) and transverse planes (c).

compared to gluteus medius and minimus. Furthermore, the available evidence suggests that the transfer continues to fire in swing, not stance, making the key kinematic deviations of hip abduction, pelvic obliquity and pelvic rotation worse, thereby increasing energy expenditure. The alternative transfers (external oblique to the great trochanter, posterior transfer of the adductors to the ischium) have not been adequately evaluated

by objective means but may prove again to be a 'boy sent to do a man's job'.

The wide range of hip, pelvic and spinal motion required for lumbar-level children to walk in low bracing has important surgical implications. Hip stiffness cannot be accommodated and a mobile dislocated hip is more functional than an enlocated stiff hip. Similarly, arthrodesis of the lumbar spine may be effective in correcting deformity but abolishes the very movement essential for walking. There may therefore be significant conflicts in clinical management priorities for some children; for example continued walking versus scoliosis correction.

At the knee level, the basis for the clinical syndrome of anteromedial instability and degenerative arthritis has now been clearly demonstrated, using coronal plane kinetics (*Figure 8.4*). In the study by Williams and Menelaus 20% of their study population were affected. These patients can be identified during childhood as being 'at risk' and advice given regarding prevention. Some improvement in the knee varus moment can be achieved by correction of torsional problems (medial femoral torsion and lateral tibial torsion) as well as correction of fixed flexion at the knee. However, a radical rethinking of mobility goals for these children may be required. Having gone through an extensive surgical, orthotic and physiotherapy programme to gain independent walking with below-knee bracing, few teenagers will relish once more taking up crutches or reverting to higher bracing. However, the use of crutches may well be the best solution. It would be better to identify these children at an earlier stage and advise them to continue with assistive devices throughout childhood.

TRANSVERSE PLANE KINEMATICS AND CLINICAL SIGNIFICANCE

Pelvic rotation is usually under the control of the adductors and is involved in determining stride length. Maximal internal rotation normally occurs at initial contact and rotation is always in the same direction as overall movement of the limb. Pelvic rotation is neutral at two points in the gait cycle: mid-stance and mid-swing, both periods of double support (*Figure 8.3a,b,c*).

The need to use trunk musculature to lift the unsupported side of the pelvis and swing limb results in an abnormal momentum being applied to the swing limb which results in an excessive degree of internal rotation. There are no strong hip extensors present in children with low lumbar spina bifida to arrest the forward movement of the limb and internal rotation

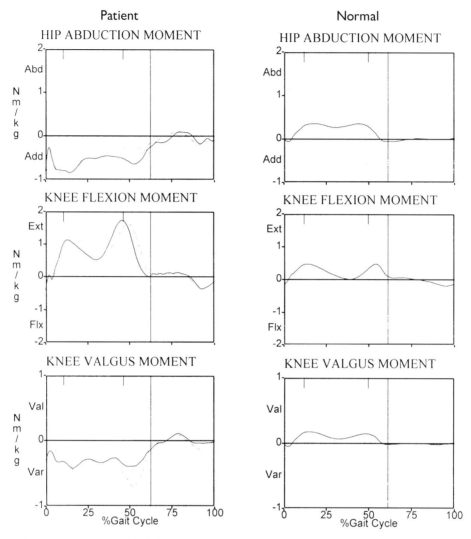

Figure 8.4   Joint kinetics in spina bifida. The patient exhibits an adductor moment at the hip, a greatly increased extensor moment at the knee and a varus knee moment. For comparison, note the normal child's abductor hip moment, normal knee extensor moment and valgus knee moment. The abnormal hip and knee moments are the result of the Trendelenburg gait and may result in knee instability and degenerative changes.

persists until body weight is accepted on to a collapsing knee at loading response. Maximum internal rotation usually occurs at initial contact but in children with low lumbar-level spina bifida it occurs at loading response. The enormous 'S' shaped pelvic rotation curves are characteristic of lumbar level spina bifida because of the need for an additional motor (the trunk musculature) and as a result of having no 'brakes' (hip extensors).

Correction of. transverse plane abnormalities is possible at the knee and foot level by femoral derotation, tibial derotation and foot stabilization. The correction of the bony levers to align the hip, knee and ankle joints with the line of progression, similar to that described by Gage in cerebral palsy, may allow deficient motors to work in a more efficient manner. A reduction in abnormal moments around the knee may be a further benefit.

ENERGY EXPENDITURE

Energy expenditure may be estimated by measuring heart rate and time/distance parameters or by direct measurement of oxygen consumed and carbon dioxide produced during walking (*Figure 8.5*). The use of heart rate as a means of assessing energy expenditure is based on the understanding that there is a linear relationship between heart rate and oxygen consumption. In our gait laboratory we have not used heart rate as a means of assessing energy expenditure because of the limitations of this method. Instead we have used the Cosmed

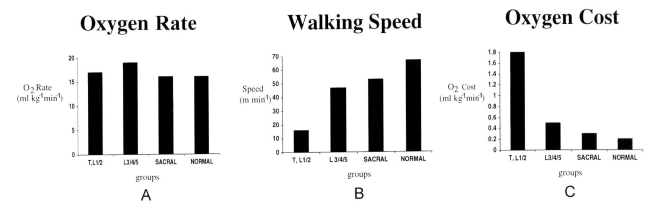

Figure 8.5 Energy studies in spina bifida. Note that the oxygen rate (A) is similar in all groups and not significantly greater than normal. However this normal rate is achieved by a reduced speed (B). The most important parameter is oxygen cost (C). This falls progressively as the neurosegmental level descends but is still raised above normal in sacral level children.

K2 and K4 systems, which are lightweight, portable telemetric systems capable of measuring ventilation per minute and respiratory rate, heart rate, oxygen consumption and carbon dioxide production. We found the system produced repeatable results and was well tolerated by disabled and able-bodied children as young as 4 years old (Corry *et al.*, 1996a).

Oxygen consumption may be measured in terms of oxygen consumed per unit time, *oxygen rate*, which is measured in millilitres of oxygen consumed, per kilogram body weight, per minute ($ml\ kg^{-1}\ min^{-1}$). Oxygen consumption may also be measured in terms of oxygen consumed per unit distance travelled, *oxygen cost*, which is measured in millilitres of oxygen consumed, per kilogram body weight, per metre walked ($ml\ kg^{-1}\ m^{-1}$). Oxygen cost is derived by dividing oxygen rate by walking speed:

$$Oxygen\ cost\ (ml\ kg^{-1}\ m^{-1})$$
$$= \frac{Oxygen\ rate\ (ml\ kg^{-1}\ min^{-1})}{Speed\ (m\ min^{-1})}.$$

We have found that children with spina bifida walk at a rate of oxygen consumption that does not differ appreciably to that of normal children, regardless of the level of lesion. However, they do have a very much greater oxygen cost of walking. We have postulated that children with spina bifida walk at a speed which keeps their rate of oxygen consumption comfortable but in doing so incur a higher oxygen cost. This is in contrast to children with diplegic cerebral palsy who appear to be unable to so reduce their walking speed and walk with a higher oxygen rate than normal (Corry *et al.*, 1996; Duffy *et al.*, 1996a).

Oxygen Cost and Kinematics

Normal walking mechanisms are designed to reduce the excursion of the centre of mass in all three anatomic planes and so to reduce energy expenditure. Children with low lumbar level spina bifida walk with a gross lateral sway, with flexed hips and knees and with marked pelvic rotation. This is energy expensive. We have shown that it is the lateral trunk movement, mandated by the presence of weak hip abductors that has the most influence on the raised oxygen cost found in children with lower lumbar level spina bifida (Duffy *et al.*, 1997) There is a positive correlation between increasing pelvic obliquity, pelvic rotation and hip ab/adduction and oxygen cost.

It could be theorized that stabilizing the pelvis to correct the abnormal kinematic patterns about the hip and pelvis might decrease oxygen cost. However, there is no procedure that has currently been proven to produce this desirable goal. The postero-lateral psoas transfer described by Sharrard (1964b) may result in measurable gains in the strength of hip abduction and extension according to static manual testing but this is not found in dynamic studies. In our study, we found it had no effect on pelvic obliquity and appeared to make pelvic rotation and hip abduction worse (Duffy *et al.*, 1996c). Presumably, this is because psoas, as a swing phase muscle, cannot become a stance phase abductor of the hip. By continuing to function in swing, increased momentum is added to the swing limb, increasing pelvic rotation. On both theoretical and practical grounds, posterolateral psoas transfer cannot reduce the oxygen cost of walking.

Use of Energy Expenditure Measurement

Energy expenditure may be used as an outcome measure for an individual, or a group of individuals, to assess the outcome of therapeutic intervention whether surgery, orthotics or physiotherapy.

For a given individual, expenditure measurements may also be used to help assess whether long-term walking is likely to be a viable proposition. The single greatest predictive factor of long-term ambulation is neurological level of lesion. Children with high lesions will go off their feet, it is usually just a matter of when. Children with sacral level lesions will continue to walk. However, there is a large group of children in the middle with a mid-low lumbar lesions for whom long-term ambulation is possible but not certain.

It is the practice of many centres to encourage all children with spina bifida, regardless of their level of lesion, to walk. This is because of the perceived physical and psychological benefits of the upright posture. Among the physical benefits are included greater independence in transfers and in wheelchair use, fewer fractures and pressure sores, greater development of upper body musculature, and of the central nervous system (CNS) and fewer flexion contractures. A decision may well eventually have to be made, however, regarding when a child with a high lesion should cease the effort of walking or whether a child with a low lesion should be subjected to a programme of intensive surgery, bracing and physiotherapy to remain ambulatory or if wheelchair mobility would be preferable. The cessation of functional walking for children with high- and lower-level lesions often occurs by crisis, at a time when increased functional demands are placed on the child, for example when they switch from primary to secondary schooling. The crisis appears to be the result of a number of obvious factors including increasing age, height and weight, accompanied by an increase in fixed deformities and brace intolerance. After a period of using a wheelchair and without functional walking, the adolescent may be presented to the orthopaedic surgeon as a candidate for further corrective surgery, bracing and rehabilitation in an effort to regain lost walking ability. The less obvious factor, a high energy expenditure, may be the most important factor in determining whether this strategy is appropriate and as a predictor of success. Appropriate monitoring of the child's walking ability and planning for the future from an early age might help to avert the crisis.

It has been shown that energy consumption is a key factor in determining whether a child will continue to walk or use a wheelchair. We propose that serial measurement of oxygen cost in children with spina bifida may allow difficulties with walking to be anticipated early and appropriate plans to be made.

For all younger children with spina bifida, oxygen cost is higher than normal and for children with high level lesions this remains so. For many children with low lumbar and sacral level lesions, however, oxygen cost approaches normal values around the early teenage years. We suspect that it is the children whose oxygen cost does not fall to sustainable levels who will stop walking. For children in the higher level lesions groups a plateauing of the oxygen cost values is likely to herald unsustainable difficulties in walking. We propose that it is not an increase in the oxygen cost of walking as the children become older that puts them off their feet, but a failure for it to fall towards normal, sustainable values.

CONCLUSION

Walking may not be the most efficient or sustainable method of mobility in the community for many children with spina bifida, especially those with higher lesions. It is necessary to set realistic goals in planning for mobility rather than life-long walking for some children. Instrumented gait analysis may help us understand the complexities of pathological gait in spina bifida, how it can vary with neurosegmental level and with time. It may also give valuable insight to the benefits and limitations of our surgical and orthotic interventions.

ACKNOWLEDGEMENTS

Ian Corry MD, FRCS who set up the Mitre Gait Analysis Laboratory and pioneered the use of the Cosmed K2 in children with disabilities.

The Staff of the Hugh Williamson Gait Analysis Laboratory: Bio-Engineers, Elise Cullis and Roland Starr; Physiotherapists, Jill Rodda and Roslyn Boyd.

Chapter 9

The Leg and Foot

Malcolm B Menelaus with Shane A Barwood and H Kerr Graham

Almost every foot deformity that can occur does occur in myelomeningocele, either as a result of the condition itself or of surgical management.

Incidence and Causation of Foot Deformity

The incidence of various foot deformities, at the Royal Children's Hospital, Melbourne, is indicated in *Table 9.1. Table 9.1* also relates this incidence to the neurosegmental level of the lesions present. Previous reports of the incidence of deformity in this condition are by Hayes *et al.* (1964), Sharrard and Grosfield (1968), Lindseth (1976) and Schafer and Dias (1983).

Causation of foot deformity

Sharrard and Grosfield (1968) implied that muscle imbalance was the cause of the deformity and reported that faradic stimulation of the motors of the foot was a good predictor of deformity. We have not been able to reproduce their findings. Furthermore, when assessing muscle power clinically, we were not able to correlate muscle power and paralysis with deformity present. This is indicated in *Table 9.1*. The material in *Table 9.1* is based on work carried out at the Royal Children's Hospital, Melbourne (Broughton *et al.*, 1994) and on studies yet to be published (Frawley *et al.*, 1998). In these studies we indicate that 89% of the feet were deformed in patients with high-level spina bifida in

Table 9.1 Types and incidence of foot deformity in the 596 feet of a consecutive series of 298 children (percentages shown in parenthesis) (Broughton *et al.*, 1994; Frawley *et al.*, 1998)

	Thoracic–L3	L4	L5	Sacral
Equinus	70	20	7	11
Equino-varus	47 } (51)	30 } (31)	5 } (22)	10 } (17)
Equino-valgus	9	3	0	0
Calcaneus	18	48	17	18
Calcaneo-varus	6 } (28)	0 } (38)	0 } (37)	0 } (19)
Calcaneo-valgus	46	17	3	5
Valgus	16	22	8	11
Varus	3 } (10)	5 } (19)	5 } (28)	10 } (17)
Convex Pes Valgus	5	6	2	0
Total with deformity	220 (89)	151 (88)	47 (87)	65 (53)
No deformity	28 (11)	20 (12)	7 (13)	58 (47)
Total	248	171	54	123

which there was no voluntary activity in the motors of the feet. The range of deformities present was in high-level lesions, similar at all neurosegmental levels and the deformity was of a degree that required surgical correction in 78 percent of the deformed feet. Spasticity of the muscles affecting foot posture was present in 59 of the feet with deformity and in none of those with no deformity.

In a consecutive series of 174 children with low-level spina bifida, deformity was present in 76% of the feet. There was a similar incidence of foot deformities in high-level lesions and in L4 and L5 spina bifida patients, regardless of the presence of muscle imbalance. In calcaneus deformity there is a higher incidence of activity in the tibialis anterior together with weakness of the calf but it should be noted from *Table 9.1* that calcaneus deformity occurs in a significant number of patients who do not have this muscle imbalance. In sacral lesions the incidence of foot deformity is much lower. A striking dissimilarity between high-level and low-level patients is that 24% of the former and only 12% of the latter have spasticity present in the lower limbs. Equinus deformity is common in patients with high-level lesions and in patients with L4 lesions. These findings are supported by Dias (1983). It is no longer tenable to attribute foot deformity entirely to muscle imbalance. In view of the number of asymmetrical deformities, many of which could not be explained by spasticity, it seems unlikely that habitually assumed posture is a main reason for the development of foot deformity. Intrauterine posture may be the cause of some deformities and some children have feet resembling those seen in arthrogryposis. Most of the equino-varus feet that are deformed at birth are rigid and difficult to treat (*Figure 9.1a*), whereas calcaneus presenting at birth is pliant.

Management of Foot Deformity

Fixed varus deformity invariably requires complete correction by operation, as complications from bearing weight on a small area of the sole are otherwise inevitable. Partial correction must never be accepted for the ambulatory patient (occasionally foot surgery is to enable shoe fitting in the non-ambulatory).

Flail feet and feet with a mobile deformity frequently merely require appropriate footwear and an orthosis to control the position of the foot and ankle until adolescence. Mobile valgus deformity of the sub-talar joint is commonly complicated by torsional and valgus deformity of the ankle mortice; the deformity is difficult to control by bracing and surgery is necessary to correct the complex of deformities.

Calcaneus deformity tends to be progressive and should be treated surgically. Whenever possible, foot and leg surgery should be performed under the same anaesthetic as other limb surgery, urology or neuro-surgery.

Repeated operations are frequently necessary in the correction of a foot deformity because of inadequate correction, unrecognized muscle imbalance or because of unrecognized spasticity. Sharrard and Grosfield (1968) report that surgery had to be repeated in 14% of the children with foot deformity and that 19% of patients had persistent deformity despite multiple procedures. The author's experience is very similar to this. Sharrard urges the use of faradic stimulation in the assessment of muscle power and performs tendon transfers based on the results of faradic stimulation. Experience in our department leads us to achieve muscle balance by removing motors, even if weakly acting, which produce the deformity. Seldom do we perform tendon transfers as often these fail to function or produce a secondary deformity.

Whilst mobile feet are preferable to stiff feet, the surgeon has no need to fear arthrodesis of the sub-talar and mid-tarsal joints in spina bifida patients (Olney and Menelaus, 1988); indeed triple arthrodesis for children with pressure sores due to varus deformity has for many represented the light at the end of a long dark tunnel. Following a properly performed triple arthrodesis, the pressure sores have invariably healed and if non-union has occurred, it has not been symptomatic. If there is persistent prominence of one metatarsal head (commonly the first metatarsal head) this can be corrected by osteotomy of the base of that metatarsal. The combination of triple arthrodesis and ankle arthrodesis has not been successful in our hands; one or other has failed to fuse or has fused and then the fusion subsequently broken down. Nor need the risk of infection deter the surgeon from performing bony surgery: the author has only observed minor and infrequent soft tissue infection; there have been no cases of postoperative osteomyelitis. Amputation has been necessary twice on teenage patients with a combination of non-union and infection following tibial osteotomy; delayed and non-union are more common than in the patients with normal sensation. The need for amputation is mentioned by Hayes *et al.* (1964).

The risk of ulceration is high in the postoperative period; casts must only be employed to maintain correction achieved by surgery, felt pads must be employed over the patella and tendo achilles and the leg must be frequently inspected postoperatively.

Deep venous thrombosis has been reported as a rare complication following surgery in children with myelomeningocele (Bernstein *et al.*, 1989).

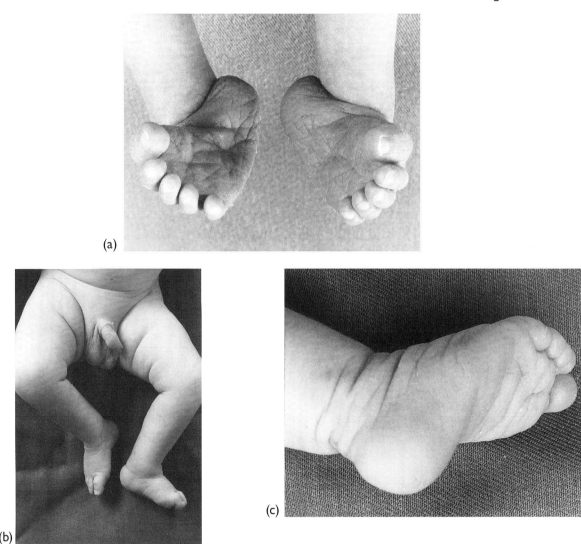

Figure 9.1 (a,b,c)   Equino-varus foot deformity at the age of 5 days (a) and at the age of 8 weeks (b,c). Tenotomy of each tendo Achillis had been performed at 5 days and was followed by serial casts. Note the well-formed and neutral right heel (c).

Equinus and Equino-varus Deformities

The complex of deformities found in talipes equino-varus are commonly seen at birth in spina bifida. It is difficult to determine clinically whether there are active motors present, but long-term follow-up of such children indicates that any muscle power that might be present will not be useful and may be a cause of recurrent deformity; the surgeon may feel free to divide or excise tendons. If the varus is corrected an equinus deformity is generally unmasked. The rigidity of the deformity varies from that seen in the usual form of talipes equino-varus to the extreme rigidity as is seen in arthrogryposis multiplex congenita.

Equino-varus deformity is also seen at a later age, in feet that have been normal or appear normal at birth. In these, muscle imbalance has been a factor in the production of the deformity. A less radical approach to treatment is appropriate in this group, otherwise over-correction of deformity will occur.

Equino-varus deformity tends to recur despite adequate initial correction. Resistance to treatment and recurrence is most common in the arthrogrypotic type deformity. Equino-varus deformity should be treated from birth unless it is improbable that the child will survive. Early management need not disturb the child, the parents or those responsible for closure of the spinal defect. The feet are placed in well-padded plaster casts, which are changed frequently whilst the baby is still in hospital and then at intervals. Conservative methods of management in the neonatal period are of considerable value in minimizing equino-varus deformity, as indicated by Walker (1971). The tendo achilles is divided by closed tenotomy as soon as the varus and adductus have been corrected (*Figures 9.1a–c*). This procedure never produces evident pain as presumably there is anaesthesia of an S1 distribution in these children. Seldom does this casting, plus tenotomy of the tendo achilles, fully correct the deformity and even in those in which full correction is achieved relapse generally occurs so that a soft tissue release becomes necessary. This is usually performed between the ages of 4 months and 1 year, dependent on the general condition of the child and the need for surgery at other sites.

In general, a full postero-medial release is performed. If there is no gross residual equinus, following the previous conservative management, then a Cincinatti approach is employed. If there is considerable residual equinus we prefer a medial incision for the medial and plantar release and a longitudinal posterolateral incision for the posterior release. The surgery performed corresponds to that performed in idiopathic talipes equino-varus except that it is wise to excise a portion of the tendo achilles and tibialis posterior and to aim at a very radical release if arthrogrypotic features are present; seldom does one see over-correction of an arthrogrypotic foot in spina bifida whereas 50% or more of such feet relapse to an extent that further surgery is necessary.

Tendon transfers are not recommended in the management of equino-varus feet in myelomeningocele. The long-term follow-up of such transfers has been disappointing. Tibialis anterior transfer to the mid-dorsum of the foot led to calcaneo cavus deformity in four feet and to cavus deformity in two feet of the nine procedures performed. Five feet which had been subjected to tibialis posterior transfer to the dorsum of the foot were reviewed 9–15 years postoperatively (Williams, 1976); the transferred tendon was found to be weak or non-functioning in all feet. Levitt *et al.* (1974) found that only four tendon transfers were functioning satisfactorily in 20 patients on whom tendon transfers had been performed and attributed the satisfactory results in most of the other children to a tenodesis effect.

If equino-varus deformity cannot be corrected by radical posteromedial release, then lateral column shortening is performed (Evans, 1961) (*Figures 9.2, 9.3*). The shortening may take place in the calcaneum, calcaneocuboid joint, cuboid or cuboid plus base of fifth metatarsal, depending on the apex of the convexity of the deformity.

Recurrent and late-presenting deformity
Recurrent equinus deformity may be a problem and has been treated by hemi-transplantation of the tendo calcaneus (Ogilvie and Sharrard, 1986). We have not found a place for this transfer in spina bifida cystica but have used it in other circumstances.

If deformity recurs, despite radical posteromedial release, then repeat postero-medial release, commonly combined with lateral column shortening, is performed. The procedure is followed by 10–12 weeks in a cast. Since we have been performing more radical postero-medial release procedures, the need for these secondary procedures is lessening. Although we

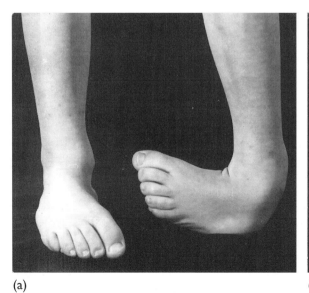

(a)

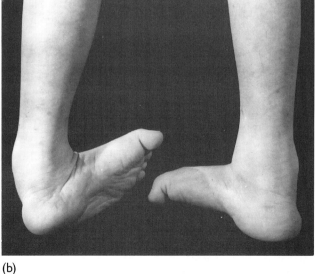

(b)

Figure 9.2(a,b)   The feet of a child who presented for treatment at the age of 5 years. The left foot was in gross varus which masked some equinus deformity and there was a large fat pad where weight was borne on the lateral aspect of the foot.

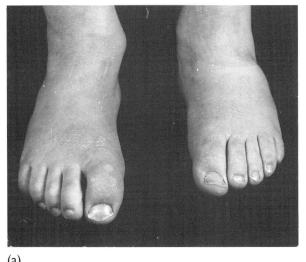 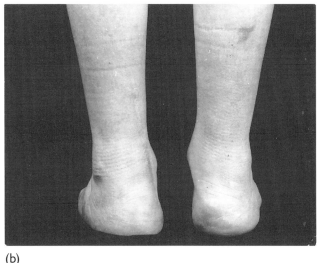

(a)   (b)

Figure 9.3(a,b) The same feet following medial and posterior release of the left foot plus excision of a wedge of bone from the calcaneocuboid joint and subsequent tendon transfer of tibialis anterior laterally. The right foot had tibialis anterior transferred laterally as the only procedure necessary.

have written about the benefits of talectomy in the past we now prefer repeat postero-medial release plus lateral column shortening to talectomy. Whilst talectomy is capable of giving a satisfactory foot, those feet which relapse after talectomy are extremely difficult to manage, whereas postero-medial release may be performed on several occasions and generally gives a better foot in the long term than talectomy.

If a child presents late with severe equino-varus deformity or severe varus deformity then the surgeon's attitude to the problem is tempered by the demands made on these feet and those likely to be made on them in the future. Those children who walk but little may be maintained by conservative measures until the age when triple arthrodesis can be performed. Those who are showing signs of undue pressure on the lateral border of the foot demand surgical management. This management may involve postero-medial release, lateral column shortening or the Verebelyi–Ogston procedure (see below).

Triple arthrodesis is best performed on varus feet at as old an age as possible; namely close to skeletal maturity. If the surgery is performed too early, then the foot is likely to be unacceptably small and one suspects that the high incidence of failure of triple arthrodesis in spina bifida (Hayes *et al.*, 1964) may be avoided by performing surgery at a late age.

Specific procedures in the management of equinus, varus and equino-varus deformity

Posterior release operation

This operation is indicated when there is equinus

deformity too gross for correction by tenotomy alone or for deformity that has recurred following tendo achilles tenotomy. We now prefer a postero-lateral incision lying mid-way between the lateral border of the tendo achilles and the posterior border of the lateral malleolus. Through a vertical incision the sural nerve is exposed and reflected. The tendo achilles is exposed and approximately 1 cm of this tendon is excised. The deep fascia, the posterior capsule of the ankle and subtalar joints, the posterior inferior tibiofibular ligament, the posterior talofibular ligament, the tendon sheath of the peroneal tendons, the medial, interosseus and lateral ligament of the subtalar joint, the flexor hallucis longus, the posterior fibres of the deltoid ligament and the posterior calcaneofibular ligament are divided. The blunt end of the Howarth elevator is passed forward into the ankle joint to raise any adhesions of the anterior ankle capsule from the neck of the talus. The operation as described above represents the most radical procedure; the surgeon will use his or her discretion as to the extent of the procedure to be performed when less of the deformity is present. Post-operatively the foot is immobilized in neutral position for at least 6 weeks.

This operation may be combined with medial soft tissue release (see below).

Medial release operation

This operation is indicated where there is adductus and varus, commonly combined with some cavus and equinus. It is generally performed between the ages of 4 months and 6 years and may be combined with posterior release and lateral column shortening.

The incisions employed have already been

discussed; in general the Cincinatti approach is employed but should there be significant equinus (and in particular in those children over the age of 4 years) then the posterior release is performed through the incision already described, and a medial release is performed through a dorso-medial curved incision from the base of the first metatarsal to the medial border of the insertion of the tendo achilles. All tight structures on the medial aspect of the foot and ankle are divided once the neurovascular bundle has been identified and retracted. The divided structures include the origin of the abductor hallucis, plantar fascia and the origin of the muscles from the tuberosity of the os calcis, the ligaments of the cuneiform–first metatarsal, naviculocuneiform, the talonavicular and the subtalar joints together with a portion of the deltoid ligament, the tendon sheaths and generally the tendons of tibialis posterior, flexor hallucis longus and flexor digitorum longus. It is commonly necessary to combine this procedure with a posterior release operation (as outlined above). Division of the insertion of tibialis anterior may be necessary in addition. We agree with Neto *et al.* (1996) that the use of a K-wire to derotate the talus is important.

When these structures have been severed and the division of ligaments has been extended laterally on to the dorsal and plantar aspects of the foot, it is possible to place the foot in a position of calcaneo-valgus. As the foot is placed in this over-corrected position, the joints of the medial side of the foot may open out (as a suitcase will open when the latch has been unfastened) rather than one bone slide on the other, as occurs in normal joint movement. If this is the case, then lateral column shortening is performed by excision of bone at the apex of the deformity, which may represent excision of calcaneum, calcaneocuboid joint, cuboid or cuboid and fifth metatarsal base. Postoperatively, the foot is immobilized for a period depending on the severity of the deformity, but never for less than 3 months. It is seldom appropriate to perform lateral column shortening under the age of 4 years for fear of over-correction.

To avoid undue tension on the skin it may be necessary to immobilize the foot in an under-corrected position until the wound has healed. At 2 weeks, the plaster is changed and the foot placed in a new padded plaster with the deformity corrected. Generally, this single change of plaster is adequate but if the foot cannot be placed in some over-correction at this time then a further plaster change is performed several days later, and for the grossly deformed foot a series of changes of plaster may be necessary. Using this technique, wound breakdown and other significant complications are rare. In a consecutive series of 100 feet, only two feet of one child were the site of wound breakdown.

This was attributed to too early and too radical post-operative manipulation. It has not been found necessary to perform the V–Y plastic procedures as described by Sharrard (1967a). Nor has the extensive rotation flap described by Walker (1971) been employed. Eight feet had recurrence of deformity of sufficient degree to require talectomy. We have not performed talectomy for recurrent deformity in the past 20 years, but have used repeat postero-medial release procedures.

The difficulty in treatment of equino-varus deformity in spina bifida is stressed by Sharrard and Grosfield (1968). They comment that 22% of equino-varus feet required secondary surgery for this deformity and despite this secondary surgery, 22% of equino-varus feet had persistent deformity at the time of review and were likely to require a further operation.

Talectomy (Menelaus, 1971; Sherk and Ames, 1975; Segal et al., 1989)

This procedure was formerly performed for severe and rigid equino-varus feet. In the past 20 years we have not seen the need to perform talectomy; radical soft tissue release, commonly combined with lateral column shortening, has generally prevented the needs for the procedure. We would prefer to perform repeated postero-medial releases, or the Verebelyi–Ogsten procedure in preference to talectomy because of the difficulty in performing any further procedure should talectomy fail.

Talectomy is carried out through a curved antero-lateral incision and is best performed with a pair of eye scissors which will find the plane of the joints and enable division of ligaments without damage to articular cartilage. The ankle, subtalar and mid-tarsal joints are each opened at an early stage of the operation and all the ligaments of these joints divided as the foot is placed into increasing equinus and varus. The talus can thus be excised without damage to other structures. After the bone has been removed, a portion of the tendo Achillis is excised to prevent recurrent equinus deformity. It may be necessary to shorten the lateral malleolus or to divide the anterior–inferior tibiofibula ligament to enable the calcaneum to lie in the ankle mortice in a position of slight valgus. After the operation, the foot is immobilized in plaster for 6 weeks.

Carroll, in a personal communication, advocates a radical soft tissue release and excision of the cuboid combined with talectomy.

Verebelyi–Ogston procedure (as described by Freeman, 1974)

Freeman suggests that the patient should be under the age of 2 years, however, we have performed the procedure up to the age of 10 years. An incision is made over the neck of the talus and a curette inserted into the

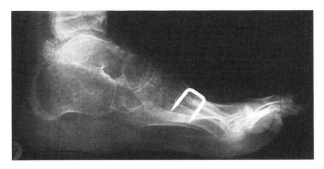

Figure 9.4 The right foot of a 15-year-old boy who has undergone excision triple arthrodesis to correct varus deformity. Postoperatively there was prominence of the first metatarsal head and a small trophic ulcer developed over it; this rapidly healed after dorsal wedge osteotomy of the base of the first metatarsal. The position was maintained with a staple.

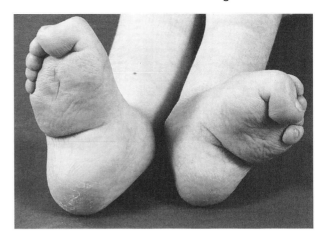

Figure 9.5 Bilateral calcaneo cavovalgus deformity in a boy aged 5 years.

bone. As much as possible of the cancellous bone is curetted to leave a hollow shell and the cartilaginous lateral wall of the bone is incised longitudinally to facilitate its collapse. An incision is then made over the cuboid, which is similarly curetted. The foot is then manipulated into calcaneus and valgus, which leads to crushing of the talus and cuboid. Finally, the heel cord is lengthened by open or closed means.

The procedure is less ablative than talectomy and Freeman reports satisfactory short-term results.

Triple arthrodesis for varus and cavovarus deformities
Unhealed trophic ulceration of the foot is not a contra-indication to this surgery. Postoperatively the position is held by K-wire fixation. The wires are removed and a cast applied at 2 weeks. Satisfactory results, in spina bifida patients, are recorded by Olney and Menelaus (1988) (*Figure 9.4*).

Cavus Deformity

The management of cavus deformity depends on the degree and rigidity of the deformity and the age of the child. Minor deformity in the young child may be corrected by open division of tight plantar structures; a medial release procedure may be combined with this operation. Shanahan *et al.* (1985) describe the long-term results of soft tissue release combined with tendon transfer in the management of cavus deformity.

If there is heel varus and the child is over the age of 4 years, yet too young for triple arthrodesis, then osteotomy of the os calcis (Dwyer, 1959) is appropriate. If the deformity recurs despite radical plantar release and the child is too young for triple arthrodesis, then it may be necessary to osteotomize all the metatarsals at

their bases. Over the age of 10 years, wedge tarsectomy may be performed if there is no heel varus. Triple arthrodesis is carried out if there is a combination of cavus and varus in a patient close to skeletal maturity.

For calcaneocavus deformity (*Figure 9.5*), the os calcis may be osteotomized in such a way as to reduce the vertical alignment of its tuberosity. A wedge of bone is excised from the tuberosity, the base of the wedge lying on the dorsum of the tuberosity and its apex being on the plantar aspect of the tuberosity. When the wedge has been excised, the tuberosity is less vertical. Older children have successfully been subjected to the Elmslie procedure (Cholmeley, 1953).

Specific procedures for cavus deformity

Metatarsal osteotomy
This is appropriate for children with a cavus deformity in which a plantaris deformity of the forefoot is responsible for much of the undue height of the arch. The operation may be combined with other soft tissue or bony procedures for cavus deformity. It is appropriate between the ages of 5 and 10 years. Wedges of bone are excised from the bases of all the metatarsals with the bases of the wedges situated dorsally. There is frequently a pronation deformity of the forefoot in association with plantaris deformity and this pronation deformity can be corrected by this technique.

Dwyer osteotomy of the os calcis for cavovarus
This operation is best performed between the ages of 4 and 8 years. It is indicated for cavovarus deformity in the mobile and growing foot and up to the age of 10 years. It is performed when the degree of deformity is not gross. A wedge of bone, based on the lateral surface of the os calcis, is excised following the technique described by Dwyer (1959) for cavus feet. Excision of

this wedge corrects the varus heel associated with the cavus foot and further correction occurs with growth as, once the heel is in valgus, the arch tends to become flatter with weightbearing. The results of this procedure have been most satisfactory. The operation is not used to correct varus in association with equino-varus deformity as the heel in that condition is generally small and should not be made smaller by excision osteotomy.

Calcaneus Deformity (With or Without Varus or Valgus)

The incidence of this deformity is indicated in *Table 9.1*.

Calcaneus deformity is generally associated with activity of the tibialis anterior muscle in the absence of significant calf function, though this is not invariably the case. In some children the activity of the tibialis anterior is involuntary and in these there is commonly involuntary activity also in the peroneus tertius, causing a valgus drift to the foot (*Figures 9.6, 9.7*). Calcaneus deformity demands treatment as it is invariably progressive. The heel becomes bulky (*Figure 9.8*) and prone to ulceration and there is difficulty in accommodating the foot into normal footwear.

Calcaneus deformity is difficult to control by bracing; the wearing of boots with a solid tongue is as affective as any measure.

There is room for a variety of treatment. Fixed calcaneus deformity requires an anterior ankle release. This procedure, in our hands, is performed through a lazy S-incision commencing proximally and medially and then obliquely crossing the anterior aspect of the ankle to pass distally and laterally. The neurovascular

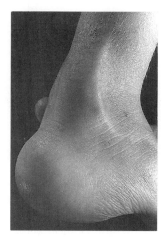

Figure 9.7   The peroneal tendons lying permanently in front of the lateral malleolus and acting as ankle extensors and evertors.

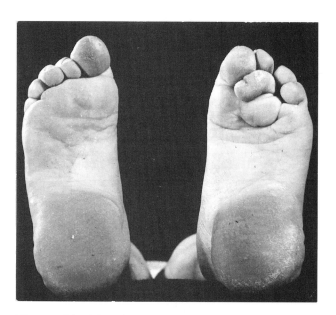

Figure 9.8   The feet of a child who presented at the age of 9 years with untreated calcaneus deformity. The forefoot takes no part in weightbearing and is an embarrassment in shoe fittings.

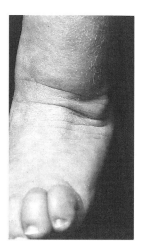

Figure 9.6   Peroneus tertius acting alone as an ankle extensor and forefoot pronator. This is commonly due to an upper motor neurone lesion.

bundle is exposed and then all other structures are divided, from the medial malleolus to the lateral malleolus; if the tibialis anterior is to be transferred as part of the same procedure then it is divided at its insertion and passed up into the wound as a preliminary to a routine tibialis anterior transfer to the heel. It is seldom that this transfer is worthwhile if there is gross fixed calcaneus deformity present; in these circumstances we prefer either to perform peroneal tenodesis or to make the foot flail and rely for stability on the subsequent use of an ankle–foot orthosis (AFO).

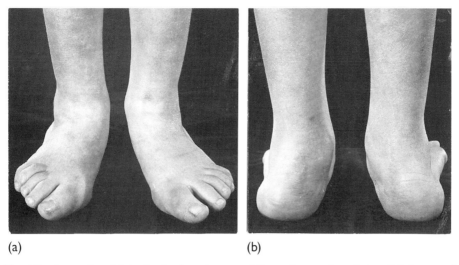

(a)   (b)

Figure 9.9(a,b)   The feet of a child who had undergone bilateral transfer of the tibialis anterior to the heel for calcaneus deformity. There is pronation of the forefoot and valgus of the heel.

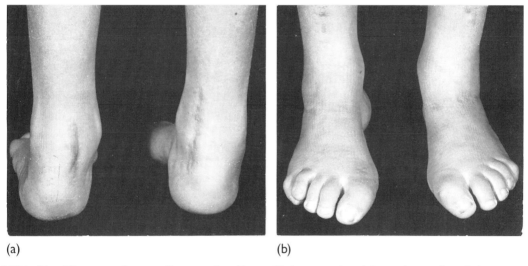

(a)   (b)

Figure 9.10(a,b)   The same feet as illustrated in *Figure 9.9* 4 years after bilateral transfer of the remaining ankle extensors to the heels and subtalar arthrodesis.

If there is spasticity of the tibialis anterior (and other dorsal muscles) then a portion of these tendons should be excised, either as part of an anterior release procedure or as a definitive procedure using a few short incisions overlying the tendons. Spasticity of these muscles can be recognized by continuous activity of the muscles or by reflex activity of the muscle when the child is stimulated in any way. If there is doubt as to whether the activity present is voluntary then it is wise to defer surgery if possible. If the tibialis anterior is of full strength, then we prefer to transfer the tendon to the heel. Our experience has been recorded (Bliss and Menelaus, 1986). Patients who had been operated on over the age of 5 years generally benefited from the operation in that additional surgical procedures were not necessary. It is unusual for the transfer to remain functioning until maturity, but the justification for the procedure is that most who have undergone it do not require an orthosis in the short or in the long term. Complications include the need to lengthen the transfer because of progressive equinus deformity, the development of valgus deformity (*Figures 9.9, 9.10*) and the development of a depressed first metatarsal head which probably represents unopposed activity of an active peroncus longus; this complication may necessitate basal osteotomy of the first metatarsal. Despite these complications we continue to perform the procedure because it invariably prevents progressive calcaneus deformity. Some patients who have undergone the procedure have a degree of calcaneus deformity at maturity that is mild and not troublesome. Banta *et al.* (1981) advocate combination of this procedure with tendo Achillis tenodesis and suggest that the combined procedure restores a more optimal

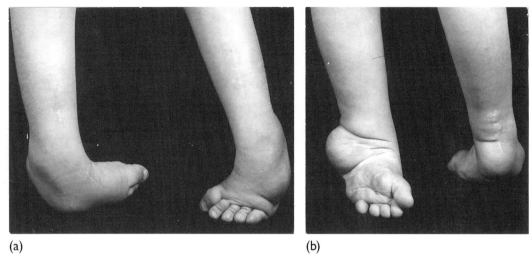

(a)   (b)

Figure 9.11 (a,b)   An illustration of the importance of proper preoperative assessment, and in particular, the appreciation of an upper motor neurone lesion in myelomeningocele. The feet of a child aged 3 years and 6 months who had undergone bilateral transfer of tibialis anterior, extensor digitorum communis and peroneus tertius of the heel, at the age of 1 year and 9 months, for calcaneus deformity. There was some spasm of the tendo Achillis, not recognized before operation, but becoming more marked on weightbearing so that this equinus deformity resulted.

balance to the foot and ankle, basing their comments on gait analysis.

Good results of tibialis anterior tendon transfer have been reported by Georgiadis and Aronson (1990) and by Fraser and Hoffman (1991). However, Janda *et al.* (1984) found the dynamic EMG studies indicated that the transferred muscle usually did not develop the desired phasic contraction during the stance phase of walking and that bracing requirements were unaffected by the procedure and concluded that it is undesirable.

If the anterior muscles are spastic or weakly acting they are divided and the tendo achillis is tenodesed to the fibula, close to the fibular growth plate. Westin and DiFiore (1974) observed that there was stimulation of growth at the lower fibula to a degree which was capable of correcting valgus deformity at the ankle mortice, as a result of this procedure. We would stress that tendon transfer for calcaneus should be deferred to an age when proper assessment can be performed (*Figure 9.11*).

For late-developing calcaneus deformity with a 'pistol-grip' heel, in addition to restoring muscle balance, osteotomy of the os calcis should be performed so that the tuberosity lies less vertically. A wedge of bone is removed from the junction of the tuberosity with the body of the os calcis; the base of the wedge lies on the dorsum of the tuberosity and the apex on the plantar aspect of the bone. When the wedge has been excised the tuberosity can be displaced into a more horizontal position. Over the age of 10 years the Elmslie procedure (Cholmeley, 1953) may be appropriate if there is calcaneo cavus deformity.

Valgus Deformity

Valgus deformity may occur in isolation, in association with plano abductus, in a foot that has formerly had a calcaneus deformity and commonly in association with external tibial torsion; if external tibial torsion is present the forces of weightbearing will lead to or perpetuate valgus of the foot and both conditions require treatment if the deformities are producing a significant problem. Clearly, the deformity should not be corrected if there is doubt as to whether the patient is going to remain weightbearing for a sufficient portion of the time and for a sufficient portion of their lives to produce a problem. If in doubt delay surgical management and control the deformity with an orthosis.

Valgus deformity may occur:

- at the ankle mortice
- at the subtalar joint
- at both the above sites.

Which of these three situations is present may be difficult to distinguish clinically, although if there is valgus at the ankle mortice one commonly notes that the tip of the fibula lies more proximal, in relationship to the tip of the medial malleolus, than normal. Radiographs and weightbearing radiographs of the foot and ankle are necessary. Hollingsworth found that the ankle mortice was the site of the valgus deformity in 22 of 39 feet. Valgus of the ankle mortice is not present under the age of 5 years then increases in incidence. This condition is not seen in unparalysed children with valgus feet and heels. Hollingsworth (1975) indicates that the deformity may increase after the Grice procedure if the graft is taken from the tibia on the affected side. He recommends the fibula as the donor site.

When there is valgus of the ankle mortice, the lower tibial epiphysis becomes triangular in shape with the apex of the triangle situated laterally. There is invariably proximal shift of the lower fibular growth plate. The causation of valgus deformity at the ankle joint has been studied by Dias (1985). He deduced that soleus strength and anatomical continuity of the fibula are important factors in normal growth at the ankle. Any factor that interferes with the balance of forces at the distal fibula physis can cause abnormal shortening of the fibula and lead to valgus deformity at the ankle.

Normally, the fibula growth plate is proximal to the level of the dome of the talus until age 4 years, at that level from 4 to 8 years and distal to it over the age of 8 years. In those with valgus at the ankle mortice the growth place is proximal to the normal for that age.

Westin and DiFiore (1974) note that the stimulation of growth following tenodesis of the tendo achillis to the fibular metaphysis is capable of correcting valgus deformity. Stevens and Toomey (1988) report a stimulating influence in 81% of patients subjected to the procedure.

Ankle valgus can be corrected either by growth plate arrest of the medial portion of the lower tibial plate or by osteotomy. Growth plate arrest of the medial portion of the distal tibial epiphysis, in the correction of valgus deformity, was first described by Burkus *et al.* (1983). They stapled the medial portion of the distal tibial physis and followed 12 of 13 patients subjected to this procedure to maturity. The average correction was 16°. In our institution, we initially used staples but found that they sometimes worked loose and hence prefer a buried screw. Growth plate arrest of the medial portion of the growth plate is a small procedure which can be readily combined with other surgery. The procedure should be performed at about the age of 7 years in girls and 9 years in boys. We produced overcorrection in one boy performed at the age of 9 years and then had to arrest the whole of the tibial growth plate. Close monitoring of growth postoperatively is therefore desirable. The medial growth plate is most conveniently arrested by inserting an AO cancellous screw proximally from the tip of the medial malleolus under image intensifier control.

Should the deformity be too gross or the child too old for medial growth arrest (or should the degree of associated external tibial torsion demand treatment) then supramalleolar osteotomy of the tibia and fibula is performed. Details of this procedure are discussed below. If inlay fusion of the subtalar or subtalar and mid-tarsal joints is to be performed because of the associated subtalar valgus then this may be combined

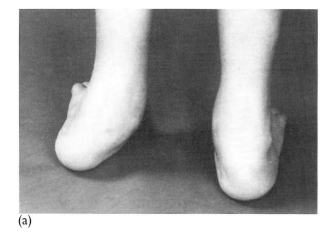

(a)

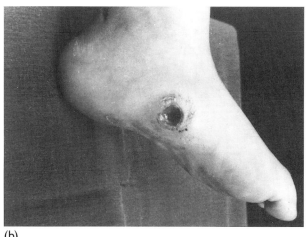

(b)

Figure 9.12(a,b)   Gross valgus deformity of the left foot of a 13-year-old girl with an L5 lesion. Note the pressure sore on the medial aspect of the foot.

with supramalleolar osteotomy (Nicol and Menelaus, 1983) (*Figures 9.12, 9.13*). Malhotra *et al.* (1984) described the techniques and results of supramalleolar osteotomy.

Subtalar valgus deformity, which cannot be controlled by an orthosis or which is associated with a pressure sore on the medial aspect of the heel, in children under the age of 10 years may be treated by osteotomy of the tuberosity of the os calcis followed by a medial shift and medial angulation of the tuberosity into slight varus. We hold the position with a Steinmann pin for a period of 3 weeks and then allow weightbearing in a cast for a further 3 weeks. This represents an alternative to correction and subtalar arthrodesis and we have come to prefer this procedure to subtalar arthrodesis, unless the deformity is gross in which case subtalar extra-articular arthrodesis (Grice, 1952, 1955) may be performed over the age of 3 years and on to maturity. Parsch (1973) has extended the indications for this procedure. The technique described by Brown (1965) has been discontinued because of its

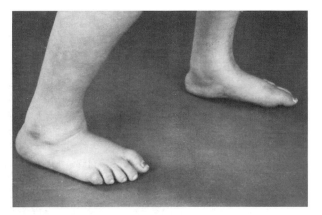

Figure 9.13 The postoperative appearance of the feet of the child illustrated in *Figures 9.2* and *9.3* following lateral inlay triple arthrodesis of the left foot plus supra malleolar osteotomy of the lower tibia to correct external tibial torsion plus ankle valgus.

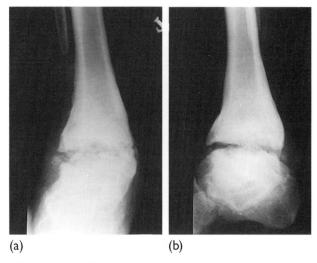

(a)   (b)

Figure 9.14(a,b) Failed ankle arthrodesis with sound fusion of a previous triple arthrodesis. Ankle arthrodesis had been attempted by complete excision of the articular cartilage through lateral and medial approaches combined with a fibula graft. Ten years following the failed fusion this boy continues to be a community walker and has no pain in this ankle.

low fusion rate in our hands. The results of this and similar procedures, in patients with spina bifida, are described by Aronson and Middleton (1991) and by Gallien *et al.* (1989). Over the age of 12 years we prefer to perform an inlay fusion of both the subtalar and mid-tarsal joints by a lateral inlay triple arthrodesis (Williams and Menelaus, 1977). These heavy children if subjected to subtalar fusion alone, tend to develop a plano-abductus deformity of the forefoot.

Ankle arthrodesis plays no part in the management of deformity, valgus or otherwise, in the myelomeningocele patient as the failure rate is unacceptably high. The results of ankle arthrodesis by Chuinard and Peterson (1963) suggest that their method of arthrodesis is likely to be the most suitable if one were forced to perform this procedure. Personal communication with Chuinard indicates that his later results in patients with spina bifida were not as successful as in the earlier published series. When ankle arthrodesis does fail (*Figure 9.14*) there is considerable persistent swelling of the ankle but little pain or instability. Levitt *et al.* (1974) record the same observation; three of the five ankle fusions in their series had failed to achieve bony arthrodesis but were asymptomatic. Hayes *et al.* (1964) report failure in five out of six ankle fusions and in four out of five pantalar fusions in spina bifida. Sharrard and Grosfield (1968) mention the high incidence of failure of ankle arthrodesis and the development of Charcot joints at the site of attempted fusion. Ziller (1974) also reports neuropathic osteolysis following arthrodesis of the ankle joint in myelodysplasia.

Specific procedure for valgus deformity

Supramalleolar osteotomy of the tibia and fibula
We prefer to perform this procedure through two incisions: one vertical incision lying just lateral to the crest of the tibia and a second incision overlying the lower fibula. A transverse osteotomy is performed through the lower tibia at approximately 1–2 cm above the growth plate (depending on the size of the child). A second osteotomy is performed parallel to the valgus ankle mortice and meeting the transverse osteotomy at the lateral border of the tibia. The closer this osteotomy is to the growth plate (without of course disturbing it) the better. A wedge of bone is removed. Through the fibula incision, the fibula is osteotomized obliquely and if necessary a portion of the fibula is excised. The deformity is then corrected. Abraham *et al.* (1996) describe the results of 55 procedures and state that their best results were obtained with over-correction to 5° of varus. Should there be associated external tibial torsion then this is corrected by rotating the foot internally before performing the second lower tibial osteotomy. We now prefer to maintain the position of the osteotomies by crossed K-wires, one entering through the medial malleolus and one through the lateral malleolus. The wires are not buried and are removed at 3 weeks. Plaster immobilization is maintained not less than 8 weeks and until there is sound radiological union which may be as long as 12–14 weeks.

There is an incidence of delayed union and non-union following this procedure. We have treated four patients with delayed union (out of a total of over 100 supramalleolar osteotomies) by the application of an external fixator. Union has eventually occurred in all cases. Lindseth (personal communication) has found a non-invasive electrical stimulator to be of value in these circumstances. Because we believe that supramalleolar osteotomy should be performed as low as possible in the tibial metaphysis (to avoid delayed union and non-union) we have not been attracted to the use of plating following this osteotomy nor have we been attracted to more complex osteotomies as described by Wiltse (1972).

A further complication that may occur following this procedure is wound breakdown with or without necrosis of an area of skin; two of our patients have required a split skin graft. Our impression is that the complication is more likely to occur if the incision, instead of being purely vertical, drifts laterally as it passes distally (to compensate for internal rotation occurring at the osteotomy site in the correction of external tibial torsion). We now resist the tendency to make an oblique incision. Careful retraction of the skin is essential. Parents must be warned of the possibility of these complications.

Triple arthrodesis for valgus deformity

The operation consists of the removal of a precisely measured rectangle of bone from the junction of the talus, navicula, cuboid and calcaneal bones with the foot held in the neutral position. A similar rectangle of cortical bone from the upper end of the tibia is then countersunk into the trough that has been prepared for it. In addition, the subtalar joint is denuded with a

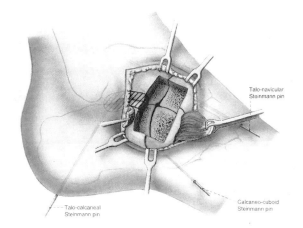

Figure 9.15 The foot is held in the final desired position of plantigrade, slight heel valgus and normal longitudinal arch by an assistant. Stability is obtained by placing two large (4.5 mm) longitudinal Steinmann pins across the talonavicular and calcaneocuboid joints and one pin across the subtalar joint. Each pin is left protruding through the skin to facilitate removal. An oblong, or coffin shaped trough is cut across the midfoot centered at the junction of the talus, calcaneus, navicula and cuboid bones.

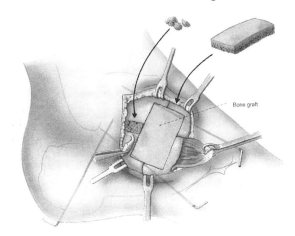

Figure 9.16 A rectangular shaped, corticocancellous graft approximately 2 mm larger in each dimension than the trough is taken from the upper third of the ipsilateral tibia and hammered into the trough in the tarsus to give a tight fit.

narrow osteotome and some medullary bone from the upper tibia punched into this joint (*Figures 9.15, 9.16*).

This method of triple arthrodesis does not shorten the foot. Although the early radiographs may suggest that fusion has not occurred, there has been only two failures in over 100 myelomeningocele patients subjected to this procedure (*Figures 9.17, 9.18*).

The success of this procedure depends on the fact that valgus deformity, unlike fixed varus deformity which requires excision of bone wedges for its correction, can be corrected without bony excision (Williams and Menelaus, 1977; Romness and Menelaus, 1995). Since bone is not excised, the foot retains its length and is more stable after operation than it is following triple fusion for varus deformity. This stability of the foot and the accurate fitting of the rectangular bone graft, which is in compression when the foot is held in the plantigrade position, would seem to be major factors in the high fusion rate.

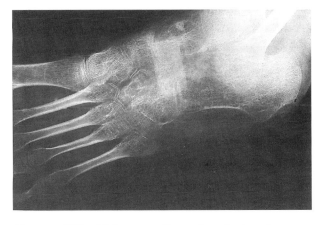

Figure 9.17 Oblique radiograph of the foot on removal of cast at 3 months postoperatively.

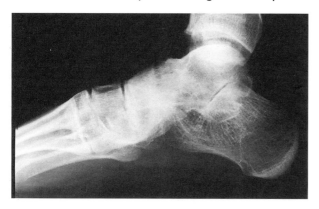

Figure 9.18 Lateral radiograph of the foot 10 years postoperatively.

The operation is indicated for those children, over the age of 10 years and preferably approximately 14 years old, who have valgus deformity of sufficient degree to necessitate braces which might otherwise be discarded or who have valgus deformity that cannot be controlled by braces or polypropylene inserts.

Nicol and Menelaus (1983) describe how this procedure may be combined with supramalleolar osteotomy.

Paralytic convex pes valgus (vertical talus)

The rigid complex of deformities known as convex pes valgus or vertical talus as is seen at birth in non-paralytic states also occurs at birth in children suffering from spina bifida, diastematomyelia and lipoma of the cauda equina. In addition to this rigid congenital deformity there is a less rigid form which develops slowly in the first few years of life. Duckworth and Smith (1974) report several patients who had feet which were normal or near normal in shape at birth and slowly developed deformity – one not until the age of 10 years. We have recorded a very low incidence of this condition; the florid and rigid deformity was present at birth in only four of 359 deformed feet analysed in 1969 and published in the first edition of this book. This is much lower than the 10% incidence reported by Sharrard and Grosfield (1968). Our incidence remains low as we have seen only seven additional feet with this deformity in the 700 children managed since the 1971 report. It may be that we have been alone in not categorizing some feet as having the true deformity, in particular those feet which slowly develop a less rigid deformity and those that have a corrigible subluxation rather than a true dislocation of the talonavicular joint. Those feet that have not been categorized as having true vertical talus deformity have had gross plano-

abductovalgus deformity with a lump on the medial aspect of the sole but have generally not exhibited fixed equinus deformity.

There is another reason why there may have been a low incidence of a deformity in our patients. Early lengthening of any tight extensor digitorum communis, peroneus tertius and tibialis anterior, as routinely performed in our department for fixed calcaneus deformity, may have prevented the late occurring form of the deformity.

Paralytic convex pes valgus is invariably associated with weakness or paralysis of the intrinsic muscles of the foot and may or may not be associated with activity in the dorsiflexors (innervated by the fourth and fifth lumbar segments) and calf (innervated by the first and second sacral segments). There is generally paralysis of the tibialis posterior or that muscle is placed at such a disadvantage by displacement of the navicular that it will not function and its activity is difficult to assess because of the rigidity of the foot. Two instances of the deformity have occurred in legs that have been completely flail and presumably deformity is then due to a residue of intrauterine muscle imbalance. Ralis and Duckworth (1973) described dissections of the feet in young children with this deformity in whom all the leg muscles were paralysed; the most severely atrophied and contracted muscles were on the lateral or tight side of the deformity rather than on the elongated side. It would thus seem that this deformity is not purely due to Stark's type I paralysis (see Chapter 2).

The pathological anatomy of a deformity in two children with myelomeningocele has been described in detail from post-mortem specimens by Drennan and Sharrard (1971) and Specht (1975). There are differences in their findings indicating that the condition can be produced by variable muscle imbalance and, like idiopathic congenital vertical talus, present with variations in the degree of deformity and in the pathological anatomy at the mid-tarsal joint.

The characteristic deformity is equinus at the ankle, valgus at the subtalar joint, dorsiflexion, eversion and abduction at the mid-tarsal joint (*Figures 9.19, 9.20*). The navicular is dislocated from the head of the talus and lies on the dorsum of the neck of that bone. The deformity is rigid and cannot be corrected to the neutral position and the talonavicular dislocation cannot be reduced. Radiographs confirm the vertical position of a talus, the talonavicular dislocation and the valgus position of the heel.

Management of paralytic convex pes valgus
Since children with this condition are most frequently paralysed merely below the first sacral segment, their walking potential is generally good. The condition

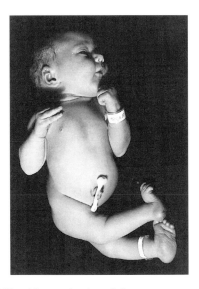

Figure 9.19 Vertical talus deformity in myelomeningocele. The ankles are in fixed equinus and the soles of the feet are convex to the head of the talus producing a palpable lump at the apex of the convexity. The subtaloid joint is in gross valgus.

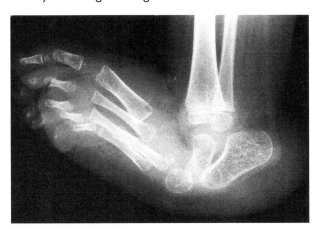

Figure 9.20 A lateral radiograph of the left foot of the child illustrated in *Figure 9.19*, showing the equinus position of the ankle and dislocation of the mid-tarsal joint.

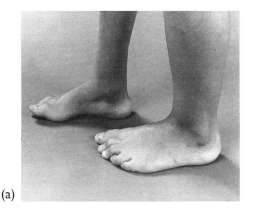

(a)

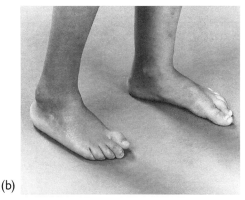

(b)

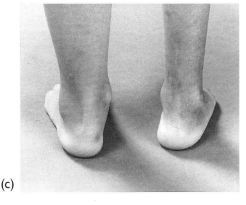

(c)

Figure 9.21 (a,b,c) Both feet of a girl aged 4 years and 6 months who had been born with a myelomeningocele affecting only the right leg and foot. At birth there was a right convex pes planus with rigid deformity of the ankle, subtalar and mid-tarsal joints. At the age of 8 months she was subjected to medial, lateral and posterior soft tissue releases and Grice subtalar arthrodesis. The result has been excellent.

demands surgical correction and this is best performed between the ages of 6 and 18 months. Sharrard and Grosfield (1968) report their experience in the operative treatment of 24 feet with vertical talus deformity; they note a high failure rate following a variety of procedures. Duckworth and Smith (1974) also highlight difficulties in the surgical management of this condition and provide a logical approach to the problem. Early release of any tight extensor tendons may be important in preventing the delayed form of the condition.

Soft tissue release with Grice inlay (Figure 9.21). This procedure is appropriate for the completely paralysed foot or the foot in which tendon transfers are deemed to be inadvisable. The subtalar and mid-tarsal joints are approached through medial and lateral incisions. All tendons on the dorsum of the foot are divided as are the ligaments of the subtalar and mid-tarsal joints. An elongation of a tendo achillis and posterior release of the ankle joint is performed through a separate posterior incision though some perform all the necessary surgery through a Cincinatti incision. Dislocation of the subtalar and mid-tarsal joints is reduced and the reduction maintained with two Kirschner wires. One is inserted between the first and second toes and passes proximally through the navicular and talus; the other passes vertically up through the calcaneum, talus and tibia. A Grice subtalar extra-articular arthrodesis is then carried out by the technique described earlier in this chapter. Some prefer to perform surgery for this condition in two stages. The foot is immobilized in plaster for 10 weeks. A polypropylene insert or a short double iron and inside T-strap is worn for a period of 12 months.

Soft tissue release and tendon transfer.   This is the treatment of choice when the appropriate motors are functioning strongly. The soft tissue release is performed by the technique already described above.

One of two tendon transfers may be performed. The peroneus brevis is detached from its insertion, led across the posterior aspect of the tibia and threaded into the tendon sheath of tibialis posterior to be inserted into the navicular; if the peroneus brevis is too short, then it is sutured to the tendon of tibialis posterior. Alternatively, the tibialis anterior may be detached at its insertion and reattached to the neck of the talus as recommended by Walker and Cheong-Leen (1973).

Excision of navicular combined with one of the procedures already described.   This operation would be logical for the older child in whom shortness of soft tissues prevented reduction of the talonavicular joint. We have no experience of the procedure. We have experience of one patient who had unusually rigid paralytic convex pes valgus and evidence of arthrogrypotic deformity elsewhere with knees stiff in extension, gross limitation of hip movement and generalized absence of skin creases on the flexor surface of joints (see *Figure 10.5*). Bilateral talectomy was performed. Twenty-four years later the feet remain trouble free.

Miscellaneous deformities of the foot and toes

Severe planus deformity has been noted but has not required specific treatment.

A calcaneus deformity plus supination–adduction deformity of the foot of sufficient degree to require surgery has occurred in three patients. A dorsal release of the capsules of the ankle and mid-tarsal joints and lengthening of the tendons of the dorsum of the foot has been performed. Some recur-

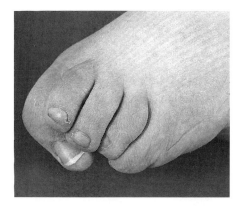

Figure 9.22   Flexion, pronation and valgus deformity at the interphalangeal joint of the hallux. The deformity is best treated by interphalangeal arthrodesis with correction of all elements of the deformity.

rence of the deformity has occurred after operation but has been sufficiently controlled by an AFO.

Claw toes of sufficient degree to require surgical correction may occur. If the deformity is mobile it is best treated by open flexor tenotomy in which the long flexor tendons are divided at the level of the proximal phalanx of each affected toe. If the deformity is fixed, in older children and adults, it has been satisfactorily corrected by filleting of half the proximal phalanx or by arthrodesis of the affected toes. Paralytic clawing of the hallux, if mobile, has been treated by tenodesis of the flexor hallucis longus (Sharrard and Smith, 1976). These authors report good results in 15 of 17 procedures performed up to the age of 11 years.

Hallux malleus may be associated with pronation and valgus deformity of the hallux (*Figure 9.22*) with recurrent trophic ulceration just medial to the great toe nail. Valgus deformity of the foot and external torsion of the tibia play a part in the production of this ulcer.

The ulcer will heal if all elements of the deformity are corrected by interphalangeal fusion. True ingrowing toe nails are encountered in adolescence and can be managed by wedge resection or radical excision.

Syndactylism was noted only twice in the feet (and once in the hands) yet this unimportant congenital anomaly has long been mentioned in association with myelomeningocele (Fuchs, 1909; quoted by De Vries, 1928). It was Fuchs who first coined the word 'myelodysplasia' and he mentions syndactylism of the second and third toes as one of the features of the condition.

Short legs have been noted in children with more marked paralysis on the side of shortening and in hemimyelomeningocele (*Figure 2.18a,b*) the discrepancy may be gross. Generally, if the leg length discrepancy is less than 3 cm conservative management is appropriate. For greater degrees of discrepancy, epiphyseal arrest of the longer leg provides the most appropriate

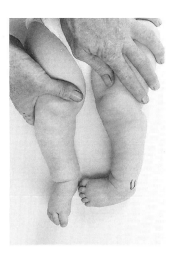

Figure 9.23 Internal tibial torsion on the left in a child of 20 months.

form of management in spina bifida. The place of limb lengthening is described on page 124.

Torsional Defects

Torsional defects in the lower limbs may occur at the hip, due to habitually assumed external rotation posture leading to contracture of the short external rotators, or at the femoral neck due to absence of normal femoral anteversion or in the tibia. Malalignment of the lower limbs is fully discussed by Dias *et al.* (1985) and by Fraser and Menelaus (1993).

Internal torsion of the intermalleolar axis relative to the axis of the knee is at first dynamic and may be found to be associated with strong medial hamstrings with weakness of the lateral hamstrings. Later internal tibial torsion develops (*Figure 9.23*) and this torsion may be present in the absence of any hamstring imbalance. Internal torsion generally manifests itself soon after the child is walking and is present in children who are ambulatory, generally in AFOs and with or without crutches. Its degree varies but most commonly it is gross and impedes walking.

If the rotational deformity is clearly impeding ambulation and the patient is tripping frequently, then twister cables may be used if the surgeon wishes to temporize. These will improve the gait while they are in use, but have no influence on the tibial torsion. If the condition is gross and impeding walking in a child who is clearly going to be a useful walker then osteoclasis of the tibia is applicable under the age of 2.5 years and has the advantage of low morbidity, rapid union and the absence of a surgical scar. The antero-medial bowing of the tibia which may be produced by this procedure remodels (Fraser and Menelaus, 1993). In older patients tibial osteotomy is the method of choice and

may be performed either at a mid-tibia level, with Knowles pins inserted above and below the osteotomy site and incorporated in the plaster, or at a supramalleolar level. Supramalleolar osteotomy is performed by a technique similar to that described in the management of external tibial torsion and valgus deformity of the ankle except that the rotation is made in an internal rather than an external direction at the time of surgery. The same complications may occur.

In the management of intoe gait, transfer of the medial hamstring muscles as described by Golski and Menelaus (1976) or the modification of this procedure described by Dias *et al.* (1985) has a small place in the management of selective patients with the appropriate muscle imbalance and good walking potential. Parents should be warned that tibial osteotomy may be necessary later or may be performed simultaneously with the tendon transfer, for a combination of fixed and mobile deformities.

External tibial torsion (*Figure 9.24*) generally appears over the age of 6 years and is part of a complex of deformities which may include contracture of the ilio tibial band, valgus deformity of the ankle joint with progressive shortening of the fibula at its distal end, and plano-abductor valgus deformity foot. These defects lead to an awkward gait, excessive shoe wear, difficulty with orthotic fitting and secondary trophic ulceration of the foot. Whilst the valgus deformity can be controlled by an orthosis it is generally best to ignore this complex of deformities. If orthotic control becomes impossible or the patient develops trophic ulceration, then tibial osteotomy to correct rotational deformity and associated valgus deformity is appropriate. Both deformities

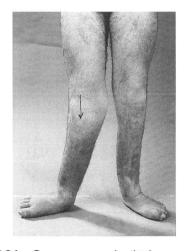

Figure 9.24 Gross external tibial torsion of the right tibia in a boy with an L5 lesion. Note the associated plano abducto valgus deformity of the right foot. The left foot had previously been similarly deformed and has been subjected to supra malleolar osteotomy.

can be corrected at a supramalleolar level by the technique described in the management of valgus deformity and carrying the same complications. The surgeon may elect, in the presence of gross subtalar valgus, to perform os calcis osteotomy, subtalar arthrodesis or subtalar and mid-tarsal arthrodesis (lateral inlay) in addition to supramalleolar osteotomy. The place of the Ilizarov method in management of torsional and angular defects is considered on page 125.

THE ILIZAROV METHOD IN THE MANAGEMENT OF THE LOWER LIMB IN MYELOMENINGOCELE
Shane A Barwood and H Kerr Graham

Introduction

The Ilizarov method has gained increasing acceptance throughout the world as a powerful tool for the management of congenital and acquired limb deformities. Correction is usually achieved by gradual distraction during which time new tissue may be formed including bone and soft tissues, following the law of tension–stress.

In the many reports that have been published describing the use of this technique, there are no published series dealing specifically with the Ilizarov method in the patient with spina bifida. Given the complexity of the deformities and the high risk of complications with conventional surgical techniques in this patient population, it is surprising that the Ilizarov method had not gained wider acceptance in corrective surgery of the lower limb in children with spina bifida. In recent major texts by both the Russian and Italian schools, spina bifida merits only a passing reference and no specific techniques or results are discussed (ASAMI Group, 1991; Ilizarov, 1992). Atar *et al.* in 1990 reported the correction of limb deformities in 10 patients with neuromuscular disease, including the correction of deformed feet in two patients with spina bifida (Atar *et al.*, 1990).

During the past 8 years, we have used the Ilizarov method in 19 children with spina bifida for a variety of indications including limb lengthening, rotational osteotomies of the tibia, correction of foot deformity and the early and late management of complications related to conventional reconstructive surgery.

Indications

Indications for the use of the Ilizarov method in reconstructive surgery of the lower limb in children with spina bifida are similar to those published by previous authors for neurologically intact children, but with a different emphasis. Pressure sores under casts and wound breakdown and infection are higher in the spina bifida population than in children with normal sensation and the recognition of such complications can be delayed, resulting in severe secondary morbidity. The use of an Ilizarov frame has the outstanding advantage of ease of inspection of surgical incisions as well as key pressure areas in the lower limb during the period of treatment.

In the management of complications associated with conventional reconstructive surgery, surgeons and parents may find it reassuring to be able to view the limb throughout the period of treatment, especially if there has been a previous history of pressure sores or wound breakdown.

One of the few advantages children with spina bifida enjoy is relative freedom from pain during Ilizarov procedures and they therefore tolerate the method extremely well.

Limb lengthening

The indications for limb lengthening in children with spina bifida are very limited (*Figure 9.25*). Minor degrees of limb length discrepancy are common in children with spina bifida, reflecting the asymmetry of the neurological lesion and associated deformities. In the majority of cases, given the dependency on orthotics, discrepancies are managed by shoe raises, orthotic modifications, or occasionally epiphysiodesis. However, in children with hemimyelomeningocele the discrepancy in limb length is usually in excess of 5 cm. These children are also highly functional because of their intact lower limb. The orthotic prescription, including a large shoe raise, can be very unwieldy for these functional children and we have therefore offered limb lengthening to four children for this indication. We have performed six tibial lengthenings in four children with hemi-myelomeningocele to correct shortening varying from 4 to 7 cm. Three lengthenings were in the proximal tibia and three were in the distal tibia. During lengthening, these children were largely free from pain and distraction was performed at the usual rate of 1 mm per day. Bone formation was neither unduly exuberant nor delayed. The frames were modified to include an above-knee orthosis to maintain knee extension during lengthening and also included a foot piece so that children could ambulate and weight bear throughout the period of treatment.

In two of three proximal tibial lengthenings, valgus bowing of the regenerate occurred during the early period after frame removal. One patient required a corrective osteotomy and the other reapplication of a

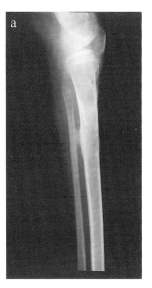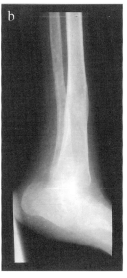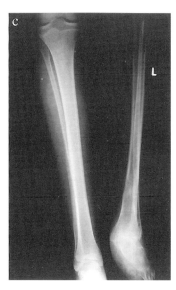

Figure 9.25(a,b,c)   Bifocal tibial lengthening in a patient with hemimyelomeningocele. Note the proximal and distal lengthening sites on the lateral view and the comparison with the neurologically intact limb on the antero-posterior view. Because of deformity of the foot and weakness on the affected side, it was decided to leave 1.5 cm of residual shortening.

frame. These children were analysed in the Gait Analysis Laboratory and the valgus deformity of the regenerate was clearly secondary to the internal varus moment across the knee during the stance phase of gait, which occurs in many children with mid-lumbar level spina bifida. By contrast, distal tibial lengthening was free from major complications, although in all patients the foot was included to prevent a secondary deformity.

A cast was applied in every patient after frame removal until the pin sites had healed and swelling had decreased. A new orthosis was prescribed with a reduced or absent raise.

Rotational and angular correction of the tibia

In children with spina bifida torsional deformity of the tibia in conjunction with angular deformity is very common. Corrective tibial osteotomy by an open supramalleolar technique is fraught with complications including wound infection, incomplete correction, loss of position, delayed union and non-union (unpublished data). These complications have been noted to be so frequent and severe that we have used Ilizarov techniques in four children for elective rotational and angular corrections of the distal tibia and in three other children as a salvage procedure after failed conventional surgery including two over corrections and one infected non-union (*Figure 9.26*). The advantages of an Ilizarov frame after supramalleolar osteotomy of the tibia are the ability to control the position of the small distal segment and foot and to make precise

adjustments until the appropriate position is achieved. Very small incisions are required for both the tibial and fibular osteotomies and the frames are easy to adjust in the outpatient department because of the diminished sensation exhibited by these children (*Figure 9.27*). We usually perform an acute correction of between 20 and 40° intraoperatively and complete the correction by progressive adjustments of the fixation frame. The rate-limiting step is the circulation distal to the osteotomy which can be compromised by too great an acute correction or by too fast a rate of postoperative correction.

In seven children who were managed by this technique, the surgical goals were achieved in all cases with the time to union being 6–10 weeks. In every case frame removal was followed by 6 weeks in a plaster cast and then prescription of an appropriate AFO.

Correction of foot deformity

Foot deformity in spina bifida is frequently severe in degree, rigid in nature and with a high tendency to relapse in recurrence. Equino-varus can be particularly recalcitrant and revision surgery is fraught with the complications of wound breakdown and cast sores. The Ilizarov method is ideal for most foot deformities apart from abducto valgus when stabilization with a bone graft to the subtalar or triple joint is preferred.

We have performed 12 foot corrections in eight children with spina bifida for either equino-varus, equino-cavovarus or equinus deformities. In eight feet some form of bony procedure or osteotomy was

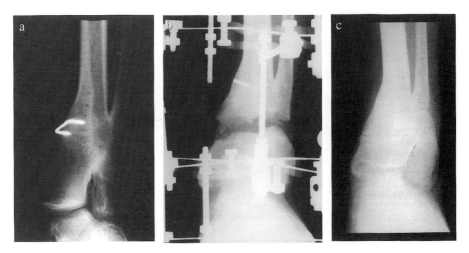

Figure 9.26(a,b,c)   Correction of a complex distal tibial deformity in a 15-year-old boy with a sacral level lesion and a previous distal tibial osteotomy complicated by deep infection, wound necrosis and synostosis formation (a). The lateral translation and valgus deformity led to a painful, unstable ankle with brace intolerance. A dome osteotomy was performed through medial and lateral incisions (b). Lengthening, medial translation, derotation and angular correction were performed and the final position shown in (c).

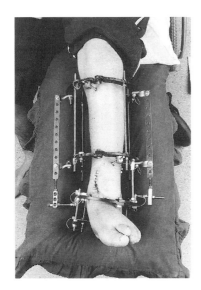

Figure 9.27   Ilizarov frame *in situ*, during translation phase.

performed and in four children distraction through the soft tissues was performed without a bony procedure. In comparison with similar procedures in children with relapsed congenital talipes equino-varus, children with spina bifida have been largely free from pain and have tolerated corrective procedures much better, including simultaneous bilateral corrections. In children with intact sensation the rate-limiting factor is usually pain during the distraction phase. In children with spina bifida we have been able to achieve correction with a mean time and frame of 7 weeks (range 5–12 weeks).

An essential part of the plan for reconstructive foot surgery using an Ilizarov frame includes efforts at muscle balancing if this has not already been achieved. This may involve lengthening or a resection of the tendo Achilles and tibialis posterior. Lateral transfer of tibialis anterior should also be considered at the conclusion of correction of the equino-varus foot if it is functioning and not spastic.

Following frame removal weightbearing in a plaster cast is used for a minimum of 6 weeks until the pin sites have healed and swelling has resolved. At the end of this period an AFO should be provided and long-term bracing continued.

In this small series of patients, complications have been minor and self limiting. There were no non-unions, malunions, neurovascular complications, deep infections or wound breakdowns. Superficial pin-site infections were common but were usually managed by pin-site care and oral antibiotics. It was not found necessary to admit patients to hospital for intravenous antibiotics nor to remove the wires or frames before the completion of treatment.

Conclusion

Application of the Ilizarov method to reconstructive surgery in the lower limb has been highly successful in a small number of children with spina bifida. In the majority of children in whom these techniques are indicated, diminished or absent sensation means that frames are well tolerated and correction can be performed more quickly than in children with intact sensation. Bone formation in lengthened segments or after osteotomy is not appreciably different to neurologically intact children. A particular hazard of proximal tibial lengthening is the varus moment across the knee which may procedure a valgus deformity in susceptible children. This can be predicted by preoperative gait analysis and avoided by overcorrection of the anatomic axis or opting for a distal lengthening.

We would consider the current indications for Ilizarov techniques in children with spina bifida to include limb lengthening in hemi-myelodysplasia, the fixation of complex multiplanar femoral and tibial osteotomies, the correction of relapsed foot deformity and the salvage of the limb when complications have occurred following conventional reconstructive surgery.

Chapter 10

The Knee

Malcolm B Menelaus

It is the presence of strong quadriceps muscles that largely determines whether the patient with myelomeningocele will be a useful walker as an adult. If two above-knee orthoses must be worn, then the patient's adult activities are severely curtailed and there is a tendency for obesity to develop. In these circumstances the demands made upon the hips, knees and feet are much less than those made by patients who do not require above-knee bracing. Thus the presence or absence of strong quadriceps muscles provides an index of the demands likely to be made on the lower limbs.

Flexion deformity at the knee implies weakness of the quadriceps muscle, with or without spasm in the hamstrings, and the likelihood is that there will be limited walking activity in adult life.

Schopler and Menelaus (1987) demonstrated that the assessment of power in the quadriceps muscles during the first few years of life generally gave an accurate prediction of quadriceps power at maturity. This is important; the surgeon is reluctant to perform sophisticated limb surgery unless the child is likely to remain walking into maturity and this is very dependent on quadriceps power. Schopler and Menelaus found that those with quadriceps power 4 or 5 as determined in the first 3 years are highly likely to have the same or increased power at maturity. Those with power 0, 1 or 2 are likely to have the same or reduced power at maturity. Ambulatory ability was closely related to quadriceps power.

If there is doubt as to quadriceps power, it may be wise to defer the management of dislocation and deformity at the hip joints as this management should be designed to meet the demands likely to be made on the hips; if long bracing is necessary, the hips will be largely restricted to hinge function.

The relatively small amount of knee surgery necessary plays an important role in enabling continued walking throughout childhood, in enabling the child with the knee that is rigid in extension to flex the knee and in preventing pressure sores that not infrequently occur in legs which have knee flexion or valgus deformity.

INCIDENCE OF KNEE DEFORMITY AND DISABILITY

Half of the children with thoracolumbar lesions have flexion or valgus deformity of the knee (70% of these have flexion deformity and 30% valgus deformity), 20% with lumbar lesions have flexion or extension deformity (80% flexion deformity, 20% extension deformity) and 15% of those with sacral lesions have a degree of flexion deformity (Parsch and Manner, 1976). Clearly, the incidence of deformity is related to the age of the children under study. The incidence of knee deformity reported by us in the first edition of this book (*Table 10.1*) was based on a study made in 1969 when the children attending our clinic had an average age of 6 years. The incidence of deformity has since increased.

Dupré and Walker (1972) found that 75% of a consecutive series of unselected spina bifida children had a knee problem; 60% had fixed flexion deformity, 5% were rigid (in extension or hyperextension) and 10% had limited flexion range. Birch (1976) reported that only 10% of his patients required knee surgery.

None of these figures record the incidence of weakness of the quadriceps muscles. In our experience, 43% of patients had weakness or paralysis of the quadriceps muscles at birth; because of deaths during the first 18 months of life, only 30% had such weakness or paralysis by the age at which walking occurred. These figures are based on an analysis published in 1971.

Table 10.1   Knee deformity in 91 knees of 60 patients (1971). (Four children had a different deformity in each knee; seven children had more that one deformity in the same knee)

Deformity	Extent of deformity	Number of knees	Number of patients
Fixed flexion	Varying from 10° to 70° of deformity	66	42
Limited flexion range	(a) Rigid in extension	8	5
	(b) Limitation of flexion, varying from 20° of limitation (relative to the normal knee) to a flexion range of only 10°	15	10
Recurvatum deformity	Varying from 15° to 60° of deformity (there was generally limited flexion also)	6	5
Valgus deformity	More than 13 cm of malleolar separation	3	2

KNEE ALIGNMENT AND VALGUS DEFORMITY

Work carried out at the Royal Children's Hospital, Melbourne, involving the review of about 434 patients from birth to 23 years of age (Wright *et al.*, 1992) indicates that children with spina bifida have neutral alignment at birth and gradually develop up to 6° of valgus – a pattern different from unaffected children. Valgus greater than 10° was observed in only 6% of patients and the degree of angular deformity was not affected by walking or by the use of an above-knee orthosis. Continued ambulation does not significantly contribute to lower limb extremity deformity. When valgus deformity occurs, it is usually in children with lower thoracic or upper lumbar lesions. It has been attributed to isolated activity in the tensor fascia latae and to spasticity in the biceps femoris, in which circumstance a portion of this tendon is excised. Inadequately treated fractures about the knee may also give rise to this deformity. Gross valgus deformity is seen in those children who develop renal rickets as a complication of spina bifida and may then be of an extremely severe degree. The life expectancy is too short for surgery to be warranted in these circumstances.

Sharrard and Webb (1974) mention the occasional occurrence of valgus deformity (and lateral tibial torsion) due to isolated reflex activity in the lateral hamstring muscles.

Management

Valgus deformity of moderate degree can generally be ignored or managed by appropriate modification to the orthosis necessary for that limb. More severe degrees of deformity require supracondylar osteotomy of the femur. Commonly, there is a combination of valgus and flexion deformity but this can be corrected satisfactorily by antero-medial impaction rather than by excising a wedge of bone. The former procedure leads to stability and a degree of rigidity without the use of internal fixation.

Stapling of the medial aspects of the lower femoral and upper tibial epiphyses is an attractive alternative to osteotomy as the child does not require any plaster immobilization or a significant period of debility.

THE NATURAL HISTORY OF KNEE CONTRACTURES IN MYELOMENINGOCELE

A multi-centre study of 850 patients, carried out in Melbourne and Seattle (Wright *et al.*, 1991) indicated that fixed flexion deformity contracture of 10° at birth decreased by the age of 9 months but increased thereafter if the patients level of lesion was higher than L3. In the thoracic and L1–L3 level patients the mean fixed flexion contracture was 18° if there was knee flexor spasticity and 17° without flexor spasticity. The range of knee flexion remained at 126° until the age of 3 years and decreased thereafter in patients with lesions higher than an L3 level. This study demonstrates that muscle imbalance and spasticity play a minimal role in the development of knee contractures. It is to be pointed out that normal neonates have a mean knee flexion contracture of 21.4° at birth, reducing to 10.7° at 3 months and 3.3° at 6 months (Broughton *et al.*, 1993b).

THE FLAIL UNDEFORMED KNEE

Flail knees and knees with minimal quadriceps control occur in any circumstance in which there is no function in the second, third or fourth lumbar segment. Above-knee bracing will be necessary. The range of flexion at the knee is commonly limited in those patients with high-level lesions. In two-thirds of the knees that are rigid in extension there is no useful power in the lower limbs (Birch, 1976).

THE UNDEFORMED KNEE WITH REDUCED QUADRICEPS POWER

This is common. It is helpful to use a floor reaction orthosis. If this is not adequate to enable ambulation, then it may be possible to use a long brace on one leg and a short brace on the other and to alternate braces on alternate days. The child does not tire as readily as when he or she is in short braces, but does not have the inconvenience of two long braces and either quadriceps muscle is exercised on alternate days. This is a short-term answer to the problem. The difficulty is that children in long braces, unless they can manage knee locks, cannot crawl which is likely to be quicker and less energy consuming than walking for these children.

Transfer of the hamstrings to the quadriceps mechanism has been reported as giving satisfactory results by Abraham *et al.* (1977), but we have no experience in this technique.

The production of a range of hyperextension at the knee by serial casting or posterior soft tissue release of the knee may facilitate brace-free walking in these patients.

FIXED FLEXION DEFORMITY

The natural history of fixed flexion deformity at the knee has been considered above (see the natural history of knee contractures in myelomeningocele). A flexion posture at the knee is imposed on the ambulant child if there is a fixed flexion deformity at the hip or calcaneus deformity at the ankle. If flexion deformity requires surgical correction, by posterior knee release, then it is wise to produce a range of hyperextension at the knee (*Figures 10.1–10.3*). It may not be possible to do this on the operating table because of tension on the wound, but serial casting postoperatively should be carried out to enable some hyperextension if the aim is to obtain an ambulant patient. On occasions, flexion deformity may require surgical management in the non-ambulant patient; such patients may find that gross flexion deformity makes transfer difficult.

Flexion deformity at the knee may develop following a period of cast immobilization or following juxta-epiphyseal fracture about the knee. The deformity has also been ascribed to the use of an abduction brace in the treatment of hip dysplasia.

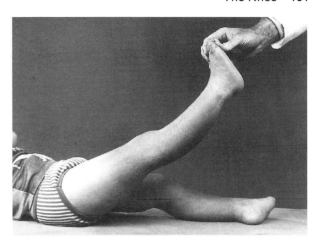

Figure 10.1 The right knee of a 5-year-old boy who, 6 months previously, had undergone a posterior knee release for 40° of fixed flexion deformity. Operation included division of semitendinosis, gracilis and the posterior capsule of the knee, and lengthening of semimembranosis and biceps femoris. Note that the knee now lies in 10° of recurvatum. If lesser degrees of correction are accepted then recurrent flexion deformity is inevitable.

Management

If the deformity is less than 10° and not increasing it can generally be ignored. For deformity a little greater than this then a series of well-padded plaster casts should be applied with great care. This is really specialized casting as the risk of pressure sores is high in unskilled hands. It is necessary to place generous felt pads over the tendoachilles and at the anterior aspect of the knee. The knee should be gradually extended by a series of casts with frequent removal of the casts for inspection for pressure sores. Norton and Foley (1959) emphasize the risks of passive stretching in the correction of flexion deformity at the knee.

Indications for Surgery

The indications for surgery differ according to the walking ability of the patient. In patients who can walk, surgery is offered if there is a fixed flexion contracture which restricts ambulation, has been increasing over a period of observation and is in excess of 30°. Surgical release is also offered to those patients with less fixed flexion contracture associated with quadriceps weakness. Such children tend to develop further knee flexion when walking, especially when tired, and release of the hamstrings allows more effective action of the quadriceps.

(a)

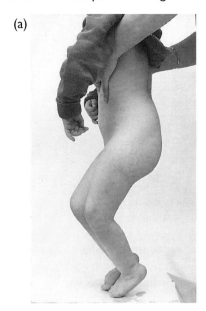

(b)

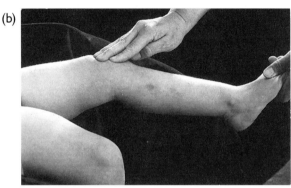

Figure 10.2(a,b)   Child aged 2 years and 6 months with bilateral fixed flexion deformities of the knees (see also *Figure 10.3*).

In non-walkers surgical release is indicated when flexion contracture is impeding, or likely to progress to a degree that would impede sitting balance, standing to transfer, or transfer from chair to bed. In the last category, we have found that, in patients with flail legs, transfer from chair to bed may be difficult if there is gross knee flexion contracture.

Surgery

In the past we used to perform a transfer of the hamstrings to the lower end of the femur (Eggers, 1952). We found that such a transfer is not effective in producing hip extension power and prefer a combination of division and lengthening of the hamstrings as indicated in *Figure 10.4*. If the deformity cannot be corrected by hamstring release alone, then posterior capsulotomy is performed in addition, and in these

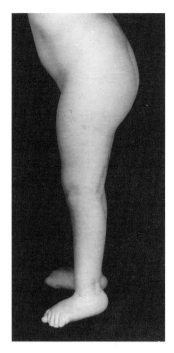

Figure 10.3   The same child 4 months later following bilateral lengthening of the hamstring muscles.

circumstances all the hamstring tendons are divided together with the tendon of gracilis and the ilio-tibial band. It should be possible to place the knee in 10° of hyperextension on the operating table and this may require division of the cruciate ligaments and the posterior fibres of the medial and lateral ligaments at the knee as well as a complete posterior capsulotomy. That division of all the hamstring tendons may produce a recurvatum deformity need not be feared in the spina bifida patient unless such surgery were performed in the absence of a significant flexion deformity and in a child under the age of 6 years.

We prefer to perform the operation through a vertical posterior mid-limb incision down to the flexion crease at the knee. Through this incision the hamstring tendons can be divided or ring barked (as indicated in *Figure 10.4*) and by retracting the neurovascular bundle medially and then laterally the whole of the posterior capsule, the posterior fibres of medial and lateral ligament and the posterior cruciate ligament can be divided under clear vision.

Postoperatively the knee is immobilized in a well-padded cast as has already been described for the conservative management of flexion contracture. The initial plaster cylinder immobilizes the knee in some flexion. A week later the cast is wedged into a position of 10° of hyperextension and if this position cannot be achieved then the cast is changed as often as necessary to achieve that degree of recurvatum.

There is a high incidence of incomplete correction

(a) Minimum Procedure

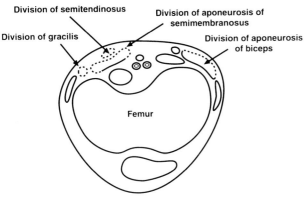

(b) Additional Optional Procedures Above Joint Level

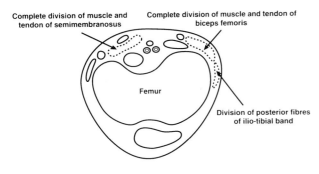

(c) Additional Optional Procedures at Joint Level

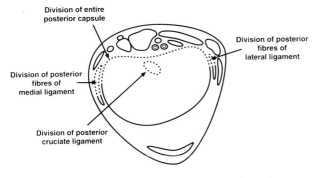

Figure 10.4(a,b,c) Surgery necessary for the correction of knee flexion deformity.

of flexion deformity at the knee. Birch (1976) found that 50% of his patients had incomplete correction after a radical posterior release and a higher percentage were incompletely corrected by a partial posterior soft tissue release. A prospective long-term follow-up of the author's posterior release procedures, combined with detailed advice as to the nature of the surgery to be performed is to be found in the article by Marshall *et al.* (1996); the mean knee flexion contracture before surgery was 39° which improved to 5° at maximum correction and 13° at follow-up at a mean period of 13 years after surgery.

The results of surgical correction of knee flexion deformity have also been published by Dupré and Walker (1972), Birch (1976), Dias (1982) and by Jrujic and Frecaparisi (1982).

We have not been impressed by the results of passive stretching in the management of flexion deformity at the knee (or at the hip) whereas this method of treatment is stressed by others.

If flexion deformity recurs after soft tissue release, then we prefer to repeat a soft tissue release rather than to perform osteotomy which, itself, may require repeating. In the older child supracondylar osteotomy of the femur may be necessary to correct gross flexion deformity. It is advisable to divide hamstring tendons, in addition, lest activity in these tendons, though slight, produces recurrent deformity. Supracondylar osteotomy is reserved for patients as close to skeletal maturity as is possible; if performed on the immature child, the femur will re-deform. For gross deformity both soft tissue release and extension osteotomy may be necessary, otherwise the articular surface of the lower femur may finish up in a vertical position. Supracondylar osteotomy may be performed by a variety of techniques. We divide the bone transversely and encourage anterior impaction as the leg is extended at the osteotomy site. Rarely, an anteriorly based wedge is excised, for gross deformity. Sharrard and Webb (1974), removes an anterior wedge, retains the posterior cortex and then corrects the deformity by bending this posterior cortex. For the immature patient we prefer to internally fix the osteotomy with crossed K-wires and employ a cylinder cast on the limb. After maturity an AO blade plate is preferred. Zimmerman *et al.* (1982) report experience with supracondylar osteotomies and point out that, for those with gross flexion deformity, femoral shortening is the key to success. They also point out that there is a significant complication rate including fracture, infection and recurrent deformity. Carstens *et al.* (1992) report their considerable experience with soft tissue and bony procedures, alone and in combination.

LIMITED FLEXION RANGE AND RECURVATUM DEFORMITY

Two-thirds of the legs which have a knee that is rigid in extension have no useful muscle power in that limb; one-third of such legs have significantly greater power of extension than of flexion. Birch (1976) provides these and other interesting statistics relating to knee deformity.

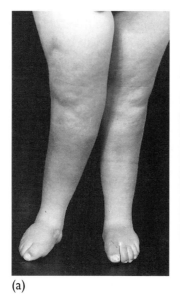 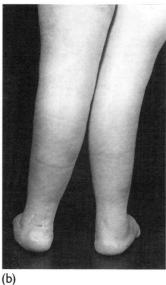

(a)   (b)

Figure 10.5(a,b)   Fixed recurvatum deformity of both knees. Note the featureless appearance and absence of skin creases on the flexor surface of the joints. This patient had surgery for the correction of bilateral vertical talus deformity 10 years previously.

The knee may be rigid in extension and have a featureless appearance as is seen in arthrogryposis multiplex congenita (*Figure 10.5a,b*).

Lindseth (1976) describes experience with 16 patients with extension contracture of the knee of whom only three where ambulatory; 13 of these patients had a neurosegmental level of lesion of L3. We have reported our experiences with this condition (Sandhu *et al.*, 1995) in 15 knees from a data base of 297 children with spina bifida. This condition may be present at birth or develop insidiously.

Management

In the first 6 months of life carefully applied serial casting may enable the knee to be flexed to 90°. Care must be taken to ensure that the casting is resulting in flexion at the joint, as confirmed by serial radiographs. Care also must be taken to avoid any pressure affects from casting. If casting is ineffective and the child's general condition and neurosegmental level suggest that walking is likely then formal lengthening of the quadriceps mechanism should be carried out. Rarely is this procedure indicated at a later age, in children with good walking ability yet with fixed recurvatum deformity.

Knees that are rigid in extension in children who have no useful muscle power in the legs are best subjected to subcutaneous tenotomy of the ligamentum patellae and any other tight anterior structures. This is a small procedure which carries great benefits (Sandhu *et al.*, 1995) and is performed at an age when the child is old enough to manage knee-locks without assistance. At this age legs are becoming long and protrude far when the child is seated which presents difficulties in the classroom and in transport. A removable plaster cast with the knee at 90° is worn as a postoperative night splint. Walking can be recommenced within 2 weeks of surgery.

Rarely is supracondylar flexion osteotomy of the lower femur indicated for this deformity; we have performed the procedure twice with satisfactory results.

LATE KNEE PROBLEMS IN MYELOMENINGOCELE

We carried out a study of 72 community ambulating adult patients (Williams *et al.*, 1993). Of these patients 24% had significant knee symptoms. These had low lumbar lesions and hip abductor and calf muscle weakness. There was an abductor lurch with the knee deforming into valgus and flexion during the stance phase followed by a swivel push-off on a fixed pronated foot. This characteristic gait placed abnormal stress on the knee leading to medial and antero-medial rotary instability and eventual degenerative change. It is likely that disability from knee symptoms will be a factor precluding continued ambulation in these patients. We do not have an answer to this problem.

Chapter II

The Hip

Nigel S Broughton

INTRODUCTION

Many children with spina bifida develop hip deformity and dislocation. In the past much unnecessary surgery has been carried out, in our hands and generally, in the management of these conditions.

It has previously been assumed that (i) all spina bifida children should walk for their general well-being; (ii) in order to give them the best chance of walking, they should not have hip deformity or dislocation; and (iii) muscle imbalance around the hip leads to hip deformity and dislocation and can be prevented by early prophylactic surgery. Unfortunately, all these considerations are probably incorrect.

We now appreciate that it is not desirable for all children with spina bifida to walk in the long term. They can lead useful lives using a wheelchair for mobility. The physical effort and enthusiasm used in attempting cumbersome walking is best spent in other intellectual pursuits and socializing with other children. We recognize that most of these children attempt to put themselves into an upright position and in their early years splintage should be provided for them to achieve this. However, after the age of 10 years most of the children with high-level spina bifida find that mobilization is easier in a wheelchair and this should not be discouraged or seen as a failure.

Hip dislocation has little effect on the child's ability to walk. Most of the problems around the hip associated with poor walking are due to a fixed flexion deformity giving excessive lumbar lordosis.

The natural history of hip deformity and dislocation around the hip is now better appreciated, particularly following a study of children treated at the Royal Children's Hospital, Melbourne and Children's Hospital, Seattle. Many of the children with muscle imbalance around the hip do not develop dislocation and the progression of hip flexion deformity is unpredictable.

The management of hip deformities around the hip has therefore changed substantially since the last edition of this book, and most authorities on the subject have changed their approach to operative management in this area over the past 10 years. Surgeons should constantly remind themselves that when they operate on the spina bifida hip they are playing with fire; if the operation does not make the patient better it is likely to make him or her worse.

NATURAL HISTORY OF HIP DEFORMITY IN MYELOMENINGOCELE

A group of 1061 children with spina bifida has been studied in Seattle and Melbourne from 1971 to 1988 (Broughton *et al.*, 1993b). At their first attendance a specially trained physiotherapist recorded the range of movement in each direction at the hip together with strength of the muscles around the hip, walking ability and any orthopaedic operations performed. The neurosegmental level in each case was assessed by a modification of Sharrard's classification. An overall neurosegmental level for each child was determined from all available assessments in the knowledge that muscle strength assessment becomes more reliable after the age of 5 years. In addition 3184 radiographs of 802 patients were assessed for dislocation.

Hip Dislocation

The results of the rate of dislocation are presented in *Figure 11.1*. When operations are performed it is impossible to determine whether the hips would have dislocated without surgery. Accordingly, we gave two curves for each neurosegmental level: one is for the

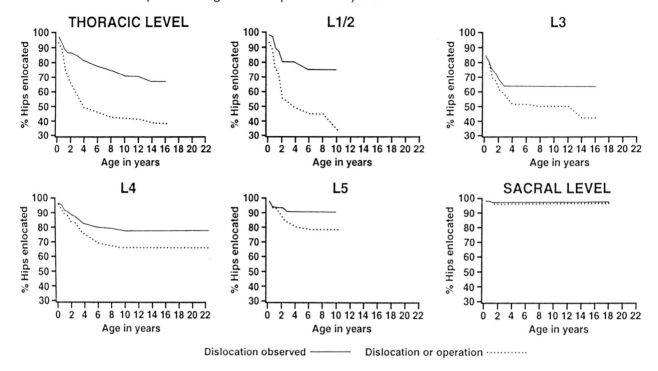

Figure 11.1 Hip dislocation rates in children with myelomeningocele. Results are for different neurosegmental levels and expressed as percentages of hips not dislocated at the various ages.

observed dislocation rate, the other includes dislocations and hips on which an operation had been performed. The natural dislocation rate without any operation must lie between these two curves. The graphs show that there is no significant difference in the dislocation rate between thoracic, L1/2 and L3 levels. In each of these neurosegmental levels there were around 47% of children who neither dislocated nor had operations performed on their hips.

In the children with L1/2 level only 30% had dislocated hips by the age of 11 years and 45% had been operated upon usually for progressive flexion deformity. This means that 25% had neither dislocated nor been operated upon.

In the children with L3 level only 36% of hips had dislocated by the age of 5 years and this number did not increase in later life. In all, 42% of the hips of children with L3 level neither dislocated nor had operations.

Maximum muscle imbalance at the hip is seen in children with L4 neurosegmental level. However, the rate of dislocation in these children was less than in the upper level lesions so that 67% of hips with L4 level had neither dislocated nor had operations performed upon them and 80% of children with L5 neurosegmental level had neither dislocated nor had operations performed on their hips. This rate of dislocation is much less than that which had previously been described by Sharrard (1964c).

Within each neurosegmental level we could not identify factors making hip dislocation more likely. We therefore concluded that hip dislocation was not inevitable in any of these children and within each neurosegmental level was unpredictable. Dislocation was less in those children with maximum muscle imbalance across the hip.

Hip Flexion Contracture

Hip flexion contracture is common in normal neonates (Broughton *et al.*, 1993a) and in children with myelomeningocele (Shurtleff *et al.*, 1986) but by the age of 9–15 months the children with thoracic-level lesions had not resolved whereas those with sacral and no loss lesions had largely resolved (see *Tables 11.1, 11.2*) (Broughton *et al.*, 1993b).

Hip flexion contracture of the hip is common in patients with high-level lesions; by the age of 11 years in thoracic-level patients the average hip flexion contracture was 22°. Children with adduction and flexion power with L1 or L2 levels at the same age had an average hip flexion contracture of 33° but this was not statistically different from the thoracic levels (*Table 11.3*).

The average hip flexion contracture in the L4

Table 11.1 Average hip flexion contracture in children with myelomeningocele from birth to age 3 months

| Level | Hip flexion contracture (degrees) | | |
	No. of hips	Mean	SD
Thoracic	128	21.31	20.57
L1/2	54	26.43	17.14
L3	39	32.21	16.49
L4	205	28.51	15.66
L5	82	27.5	11.53
Sacral	118	18.25	13.17
No loss	28	6.0	16.6

Table 11.2 Average hip flexion contracture in children with myelomeningocele from 9 to 15 months of age

| Level | Hip flexion contracture (degrees) | | |
	No. of hips	Mean	SD
Thoracic	87	11.44	16.63
L1/2	36	9.64	14.63
L3	31	7.74	13.65
L4	184	4.92	9.88
L5	82	5.98	12.30
Sacral	118	1.15	7.36
No loss	38	0.0	6.97

Table 11.3 Average hip flexion contracture in children with myelomeningocele from 9 to 11 years of age

| Level | Hip flexion contracture (degrees) | | |
	No. of hips	Mean	SD
Thoracic	61	22.16	21.44
L1/2	12	32.91	10.54
L3	13	11.23	15.59
L4	49	9.48	17.47
L5	39	5.38	10.22
Sacral	100	3.53	8.76
No loss	24	− 1.25	7.10

group, aged 8–11 years, was significantly less than that in children with flail hips, as it was in the L5 group.

Hip deformity and dislocation is therefore not as common as was first assumed and the development of these abnormalities cannot be predicted on the basis of the level of the lesion. The concept that muscle imbalance is responsible for deformity and dislocation is no longer tenable. There is therefore no rationale for early or prophylactic management to correct muscle imbalance at the hip in the expectation of preventing deformity and dislocation.

Abduction External Rotation Deformity

Many of the children with extensive paralysis lie with the hips in a position of abduction and external rotation. These deformities may become fixed.

Although there is uncertainty as to the effectiveness of the measure, we discourage the posture by suggesting that the hips be placed for much of the time in a sleeve that holds the hips in adduction and internal rotation.

If there is contracture of the tensor fascia lata there may be associated flexion and external rotation contractures at the hip. A release of tensor fascia lata at its origin, together with any other tight bands on the lateral or anterior aspect of the hip, plus division of the ilio-tibial band distally, will then be necessary.

Limitation of Abduction

In children with high-level lesions there may be a limitation of abduction or in severe cases an adduction contracture. This may be due to spastic adductors and psoas or their unopposed action. This makes toileting difficult, intertrigo common, and may lead on to pelvic obliquity and pressure sores.

This should be treated, particularly in those with a tendency to hip subluxation, by a soft tissue release of the psoas and adductors. This often results in improved balance whilst sitting.

HIP DISLOCATION

It has previously been assumed that dislocated hips in these children should be reduced to improve function and prevent complications. Over the past 20 years this approach has been increasingly questioned and it has been noted that some children are worse after hip surgery.

The gait of these children is defective because of a complex of factors including muscle weakness and fixed flexion deformity; dislocation may be less relevant than these other factors. We have studied groups of children with unilateral and bilateral hip dislocation to identify the place of surgery in these children.

Unilateral Hip Dislocation

Unilateral hip dislocation produces a variable leg length discrepancy. In some patients it may produce pelvic obliquity and ischial ulcers from prolonged sitting with a hip asymmetry. In our recent long-term study on 16 patients with unilateral dislocation of the hip we found that there were few problems in the children with high-level dislocation. Of the nine children with high-level dislocations, only one was a walker. In two of these children surgery to reduce the dislocation had been unsuccessful, both had a 5 cm leg length discrepancy and one had a scoliosis and ischial pressure sore on the left buttock. In the five children who had no surgery, all had scoliosis and one had an ischial pressure sore. In the three children who had successful surgery, one had scoliosis with pelvic obliquity and then developed dislocation of the other hip, and another, although a walker, had a 2-cm leg length discrepancy (Fraser *et al.*, 1995).

As a result of this and other studies (Feiwell *et al.*, 1978; Crandall *et al.*, 1989) we conclude that unilateral dislocation of the hip in high-level lesions produces few fuctional problems and there is a significant failure rate of attempted reduction of the hip. As the vast majority of these children are non-walkers in the long-term, we feel that surgery to reduce a unilateral dislocation in a high-level lesion should seldom be performed.

In the same study there were seven children with unilateral hip dislocation and a low lesion between L4 and sacral. All these children were walkers. Surgery had been attempted and was successful in six of these children, but one had a scoliosis and two had significant leg length discrepancies. The other child had no surgery performed, was a walker but had 4-cm leg length discrepany and an ischial pressure sore on the right buttock.

As a result of this and other studies we feel that in the low-level lesion with unilateral dislocation surgery is usually successful and should be attempted to reduce the functional problems, but there is still an incidence of leg length discrepancy and scoliosis.

Bilateral Hip Dislocation

Children with bilateral hip dislocation may have a poor gait because of the dislocation or an associated fixed flexion deformity and sometimes pressure sores from the prominent upper femur.

Our study identified 19 patients with a minimum follow up of 10 years. Some of these children had been treated with attempts to reduce the hip, some with attempts to reduce the fixed flexion deformity and some not at all. In the upper-level lesions the only

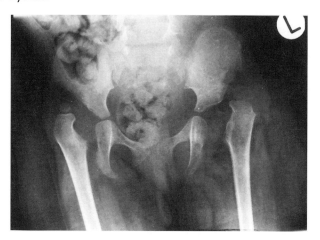

Figure II.2 Gross dislocation of the hips in a 2-year-old child with an LI lesion. These hips are best left untreated. If fixed flexion deformities develop at a later stage they should be managed with a soft tissue anterior hip release.

three children who were walking all continue to have bilateral hip dislocations. In the low-level lesions all eight patients were walkers, five had enlocated hips and three had bilaterally dislocated hips. Only one child in the series developed occasional pain in one hip and none of these children developed pressure sores.

We concluded that reduction of the hips did not improve function in these children. Our aim with surgery in the upper-level lesions is to achieve a stable upright posture with correction of the flexion deformity of the hip (*Figures 11.2–11.4*). This allows the use of a reciprocating gait orthosis. We advocate a similar approach for the lower-level lesions with management aimed at preventing the occurrence of fixed flexion deformity of the hip.

This view has been borne out by the recent study from Toronto on the function of dislocated hips in children with lower level spina bifida. Alman *et al.* (1996) identified 52 children with dislocated hips and neurosegmental levels of L3 and L4. Thirty had been treated by attempts at reduction surgically and 22 conservatively. Of the 30 treated by surgery, 10 had failed. The results in those with failed surgery were significantly worse than those with successful surgery. However, the results in those with failed surgery were worse than in those who had not had surgery. The results in those with successful surgery were better than those treated conservatively, but not statistically significant. They concluded that the benefit of surgical relocation of the dislocated hip was marginal. Other authors have reported similar conclusions (Feiwell *et al.*, 1978; Bazih and Gross, 1981; Crandall *et al.*, 1989). We have also noted a high incidence of postoperative pathological fractures and heterotopic ossification and

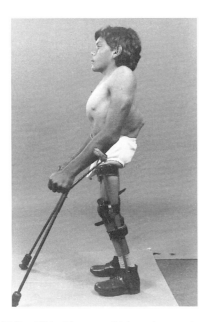

Figure II.3   This 17-year-old boy has a thoracic-level lesion but remains a household ambulator because of his satisfactory extension posture. Both hips are dislocated and have never been treated.

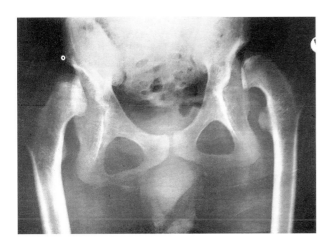

Figure II.4   The radiograph of the boy in *Figure II.3* shows that the dislocated hips have formed false acetabula.

stiffness if high-level lesions have surgery for dislocation.

Furthermore, Barden *et al.* (1975), in a review of adult myelomeningocele patients, found that walking ability did not correlate with the dislocated state of the hip. All patients with a deficit below L3 and dislocation were walking and pain free.

THE AIMS OF MANAGEMENT AND GENERAL CONSIDERATIONS

The aim of management in these children should be to fulfil their greatest potential. The child should be comfortable, pain free and able to mobilize and socialize to the best of their ability. This does not necessarily mean that they should ambulate. Some children are most mobile in a wheelchair.

High-level Lesions

Children with high-level lesions and no quadriceps are unlikely to continue to be long-term walkers. They will strive to adopt an upright posture and this should be encouraged with braces and splintage. Within these aids they will attempt walking and this should be encouraged. However, as they approach adolescence they will often find mobilization easier in a wheelchair. Intervention and surgery should therefore be directed to allowing walking in a brace in the first 10 years of life, but bearing in mind that the child will probably adopt a wheelchair existence later in life. Surgery should be simple to reduce the effects of deformity and allow brace fitting but to keep mobility so the child can sit in later life. We generally find that extensive osteotomies to realign the bony architecture, such as acetabuloplasty or upper femoral osteotomies, are unnecessary and that simple tendon releases are as effective. However, even after simple tendon releases there is still a risk of heterotopic ossification and stiffness in these children.

Low-level Lesions

Those children with strong quadriceps will probably continue walking into adult life using short orthoses. Surgery should therefore be directed with a long-term view in mind and often surgery both to minimize flexion deformity and to reduce hip dislocation is appropriate.

PRINCIPLES OF MANAGEMENT

Orthopaedic surgeons should understand the natural history of the condition that they are dealing with so that they set realistic goals for children subjected to their surgical endeavours. Their management should be condensed so that all orthopaedic procedures are performed at the same time with single event multilevel

Table 11.4   The indications for reduction of hip dislocation in spina bifida

	Unilateral	Bilateral
High-level lesion No quads, unlikely to be long-term walkers	Occasionally reduce if the other leg has a low lesion, or surgery is required in any case for flexion deformity	Never reduce
Low-level lesion Strong quads Usually walkers in ankle–foot orthosis (AFOs)	Usually reduce	Occasionally reduce if surgery is required in any case for flexion deformity

surgery. Surgery should be performed to minimize the period of immobilization postoperatively.

The natural history of deformity and dislocation cannot be assumed from the neurosegmental level. Treatment should be directed at the deformity as it arises rather than prophylactically to try and prevent the development of deformity.

Reduction of hip dislocation is usually unnecessary (see *Table 11.4*). Most cases of unilateral hip dislocation in the low-level lesion should be reduced to prevent leg length discrepancy, pelvic obliquity and scoliosis. However, there are few indications for reducing the hip in a unilateral dislocation in a high-level lesion and in a bilateral dislocation in a low-level lesion.

Most children walk better without a fixed flexion deformity of the hip. Although a hip flexion contracture of up to 30° can be accommodated in the reciprocating gait orthoses, most of the surgery of hip deformity should be directed at establishing a stable upright posture without fixed flexion deformity of the hip (*Figures 11.5–11.7*).

Much has been written in the past about providing extension and abduction power to the hip to prevent the Trendelenberg gait and produce a more stable gait. Sharrard (1964c) advocated the use of a posterior ilio-psoas transfer. Unfortunately, when EMGs have been taken of the transferred muscle there has been no activity recorded in stance so its effect seems to have been more as a tenodesis (Buisson and Hamblen, 1972). Gait analysis studies have also failed

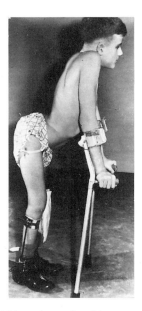

Figure 11.5   We are usually able to correct deformity with an extensive soft tissue anterior hip release but on this occasion because of the severity extension femoral osteotomies have been performed. No attempt was made to reduce the left hip; he remains a community ambulator.

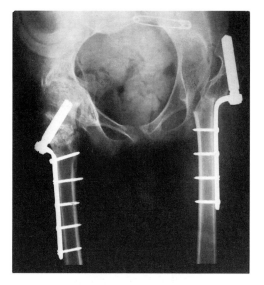

Figure 11.6   Undesirable flexion posture in a boy with L4 lesion. He has strong psoas and quadriceps but gluteal weakness and has developed fixed flexion deformity of both hips. Note the gross lumbar lordosis and that his centre of gravity is in front of rather than directly over his feet.

to show more efficient walking after the transfer (Duffy *et al.*, 1996c); indeed, the procedure leads to undesirable gait characteristics as described in Chapter 8. For those reasons we no longer perform this or other tendon transfers in the management of hip deformity or dislocation. Any improvement in gait that occurred after these transfers, and we performed over 120 of these procedures over 30 years, was equalled by the improvement in gait of patients undergoing correction of flexion deformity with or without reduction of dislocation. Some improvement in gait, following any surgery at the hip, can be explained on the basis of maturation of the child in the year or two between surgery and assessment. Gait analysis (see Chapter 8) offers an opportunity to confirm or deny these propositions.

The triple transfer as recommended by Yngve and Lindseth (1982) consists of external oblique transfer of the greater trochanter, transfer of the adductor origin posteriorly, and posterior transfer of the origin of tensor fascia lata. It is often used in combination with a varus femoral osteotomy to improve gait and reduce the risk of dislocation. Phillips and Lindseth (1992) has reported improved gait following these procedures in 47 patients. This type of approach is recommended by some surgeons in an attempt not only to reduce the risk of dislocation but also to produce a more stable, energy efficient gait (Weisl *et al.*, 1988). We have not performed this type of surgery and remain unconvinced about its value in the management of these children.

Transfer of the ilio-psoas to the anterior greater trochanter has been described by Mustard (1952, 1959).

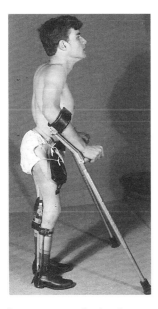

Figure 11.7 Postoperatively he has a much better extension posture, although some of his lumbar lordosis is fixed.

Our experience has been that fixed flexion deformity of the hip following the procedure is common.

Management

Up to the age of 3–4 years, we observe the child, recording the fixed deformity and strength of muscles around the hip. As the child grows and becomes more co-operative the assessment of the neurosegmental level is more consistent. The development of fixed deformity is monitored. During this time appropriate positioning helps in the prevention of external rotation, abduction deformity and may help in the slowing of hip flexion deformity. However, we would not recommend the use of soft tissue stretching or manipulation by a physiotherapist. Any dislocation or subluxation is monitored but abduction bracing is not used. If there is limitation of abduction and subluxation a psoas and adductor release should be performed.

Fixed flexion deformity of the hip of more than 30° usually causes problems with walking and the fitting of an orthosis and it is at the age of 3–4 years that this may be first addressed by a soft tissue anterior hip release. Fixed flexion deformity of the hip may develop later and if it is causing a problem can be managed by anterior hip release. This is now our most common intervention at the hip in these children. In a case of bilateral dislocation of the hip with fixed flexion deformity we would usually ignore the dislocation and correct the fixed flexion deformity by soft tissue release.

Hips that become stiff after surgery are very difficult to manage. Taylor (1986) described poor results after excision of the upper end of the femur in eight patients due to extensive new bone formation.

Author's Current Surgical Management for Hip Dislocation

If, based on the foregoing considerations, reduction of the hip dislocation is indicated then we perform at least the first two of the following five procedures. The need for the remainder of these procedures is apparent at surgery. All the necessary surgery is carried out at one stage, enabling a minimum period of immobilization of the child. The surgery necessary is performed over the age of 3 years, as the need for hip reduction is unclear until that age, and before the age of 6 years as after this there is an increased likelihood of redislocation.

1 *Open reduction of the hip.* Open or closed adductor tenotomy is performed as a preliminary if there is a limited range of abduction of the hip. An anterior Smith–Petersen approach through a Salter skin

incision, is employed. Whilst the hip may clinically appear to reduce by closed means we prefer open reduction because (i) the head will seat better after removal of acetabular fat and division of the transverse ligament of the acetabulum; and (ii) there is invariably redundant anterior capsule which can be efficiently plicated at the conclusion of the procedure, hence further stabilizing the hip.

2 *Psoas recession*. The psoas tendon alone is divided unless there be fixed flexion deformity necessitating complete division of iliopsoas.

3 *Anterior hip release*. This is performed by the technique described below if there is fixed flexion deformity.

4 *Pemberton osteotomy* (Pemberton, 1965). This gives great stability to the hip so that only a short period of postoperative immobilization is necessary. Displace-

ment of the osteotomy can be varied in direction and extent depending on the stability of the hip following open reduction. If the inserted graft is not completely stable in all positions of the hip, then it is stabilized with a K-wire (*Figures 11.8, 11.9*).

5 *Intertochanteric varus derotation osteotomy*. If the hip still dislocates, after the above procedures have been completed, then this procedure is performed with displacement as necessary to produce complete stability. Internal fixation is with an AO or Altdorf blade plate. It is generally preferable to defer capsular reefing until the femoral osteotomy has been secured. A hip spica is applied with the hip in full extension, neutral rotation and 20–30° of abduction and maintained for 6–10 weeks. The patient is admitted to hospital for a few days when removed, for gentle mobilization (*Figures 11.10, 11.11*).

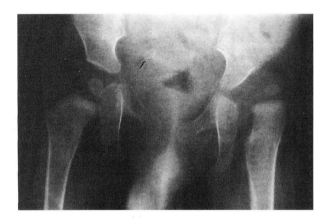

Figure 11.8   Unilateral hip dislocation in a child with an L4 lesion.

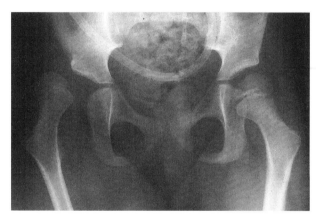

Figure 11.10   Unilateral hip dislocation in a 3-year-old with an L4 lesion.

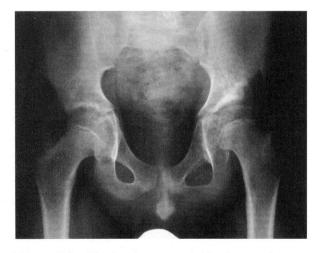

Figure 11.9   This has been treated by open reduction, psoas lengthening and a Pemberton osteotomy. Follow-up film after 10 years shows that the hip has remained reduced.

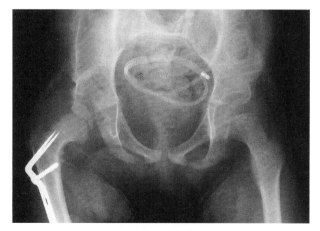

Figure 11.11   This has been treated with open reduction, psoas lengthening, Pemberton osteotomy and on this occasion a varus derotation osteotomy of the upper femur to maintain a reduction.

Other Surgical Procedures

Anterior hip release

The patient is placed supine with a folded towel under the buttocks. A steri-drape is used to cover the genitalia and perineum and this and the skin are painted with iodine from the waist to below the knee on both legs, even for a unilateral procedure, so the Thomas test can be performed during the operation to check on complete correction of the deformity. Bilateral operations when necessary are performed at one session since this greatly simplifies postoperative management.

The iliac apophysis is split and each half is detached with the periosteum of the inner and outer surfaces of the ileum posteriorly to the level of the midpoint of the hip. In patients with high-level lesions, the gluteii, tensor fascia lata and iliacus muscles are often represented by fibro-fatty tissue. Sartorius is displaced medially and dissection continues down the anterior ilium to the anterior–inferior iliac spine; both heads of rectus femoris are detached and retracted distally. The psoas tendon is pulled from its sheath and 1 cm of the tendon is excised. The anterior capsule of the hip is exposed and divided transversely from as far postero-laterally to as far postero-medially as can be reached. The operation site is then carefully palpated whilst the Thomas test is performed by flexing the opposite thigh. Any additional tight bands are divided.

At the end of the operation the only tight structures crossing the anterior aspect of the hip are the femoral nerves and vessels. At this stage the anterior superior iliac spine and the adjacent part of the iliac wing protrude forwards in front of the periosteum and muscles which lie posteriorly and inferiorly. This protruding part of the iliac wing is excised and the deep fascia is closed as are the fat and the skin over a suction drain. Postoperatively, the patient is placed on a Bradford frame and nursed in a prone position for as long as can be tolerated each day. This or a supine position with the hips in full extension is continued for 6 weeks. In the last 4 weeks of this period patients are allowed to stand for up to 1 hour a day using a gait orthosis which allows the hips to be locked in full extension.

We have recently reported good results from this surgery (Frawley et al., 1996). Of 57 hips, 43 had had good correction maintaining less than 30° of fixed flexion deformity. Ten had recurred and four had initially been good but then relapsed late over 3 years after surgery.

Extension femoral osteotomy

In older patients with severe fixed flexion deformities an anterior hip release may not fully correct the fixed flexion deformity of the hip (*Figures 11.5–11.7*). This can be corrected by an intertrochanteric osteotomy performed either as a posterior closing wedge or an anterior opening wedge. We would normally use rigid internal fixation following this. Some surgeons perform the procedure and use external fixation to maintain position.

Pelvic osteotomies

Whilst the Pemberton osteotomy, discussed above, can be performed up to the age of 7–8 years, there are occasions when the late presenting patient with unilateral dislocation and a low lesion requires acetabulo-

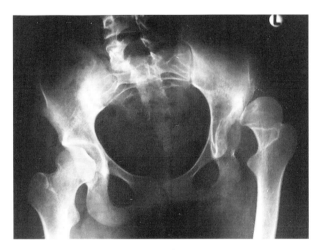

Figure 11.12   The radiograph of a 16 year old with an L5 lesion. He had developed pain in the subluxed hip, an unusual complication as such hips are rarely painful.

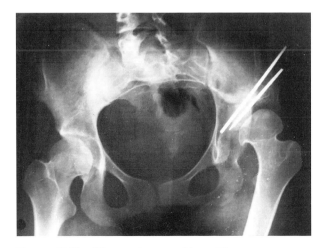

Figure 11.13   This was treated by a Chiari osteotomy, which has been most successful in relief of his pain over the last 14 years.

plasty. If lateral cover is required then it may be elected to perform a Salter osteotomy. If the prerequisites for a Salter osteotomy are not met then rarely Chiari osteotomy (Chiari, 1974) is indicated for the older patient, and in those very rare circumstances where the hip is painful (*Figures 11.12, 11.13*).

Chapter 12

The Spine

Ian P Torode and D Robert V Dickens

With improvements in understanding of the genetic implications for neural tube defects and with improvements of prenatal ultrasound examination, amniotic fluid examination and chorionic villous sampling, there has been a reduction in the incidence of children born with myelomeningocele. Despite improvements in cerebrospinal fluid (CSF) shunting techniques the relative frequency of spinal deformities in these children has not significantly altered. The management of spinal deformity in many of these children is a major component of their care. Without this, improvements in daily living, that might be expected by treatment of other associated problems may not be realized.

Spinal deformity not only impedes effective walking, it may also make sitting difficult. If the child has poor sitting balance because of a spinal deformity and has to use their hands to maintain the upright posture then the spinal deformity results in a crippling impairment of function. Because of subtle neurological disturbances in the upper limbs, spina bifida patients commonly need to use both hands for functions that unaffected people can carry out with one hand.

At the time of writing the second edition of this text the implants that were in use for spinal instrumentation were the Harrington and Dwyer systems. Since then there has been a vast development of both implants and surgical techniques for the management of spinal deformity. The use of these new techniques and implants in the management of deformities of the spine associated with myelomeningocele are described. Detailed descriptions of the posterior and anterior approaches to the spine are well described and do not need to be reiterated, although the lessons learned from our previous experience need to be examined and put into practice (Mazur *et al.*, 1986a). The importance of segmental fixation, either by pedicle screws or sublaminar wire, has been widely recognized and where possible the principal of segmental fixation is particularly relevant to instrumentation of the spine in meningomyelocele patients.

Despite these advances in implant design and infection control, spinal surgery for deformity in myelomeningocele is still bedevilled by complications. Hull *et al.* (1974) reported a 43% incidence of major infection and a 76% pseudarthrosis rate. A review of patients undergoing surgery for scoliosis in myelomeningocele at our institution also revealed a decreased but significant incidence of complications in these patients. However, examination of these earlier papers does reveal that the best results in the management of these children is by the combination of both an anterior and posterior approach to the spine with segmental instrumentation where possible. This has resulted in an improvement in terms of radiographic outcomes and also an improvement in the patients functional status. The use of these techniques and improved fixation has enabled earlier mobilization of the patients which in turn has reduced the degree of disuse osteopenia and hence secondary fractures, reduced the incidence of genitourinary complications and enabled discharge of the patients with a significantly shorter hospital stay.

CLASSIFICATION OF SPINAL DEFORMITY

In the context of spinal deformity in myelomeningocoele patients the terms *developmental* and *paralytic* should be considered as synonymous; the term congenital means 'associated with congenital anomalies' of the spine rather than the more limited 'present at birth'. The incidence of congenital vertebral anomalies in children with myelomeningocele is between 15 and 20% (Samuelsson and Eklof, 1988).

The congenital vertebral abnormalities in myelomeningocele are:

- Defects of the neural arch and wide separation of the pedicles at the level of the meningocele lesion. These defects range from minor degrees of spina bifida, which are difficult to demonstrate radiologically, to complete absence of the neural arch and hypoplasia of the pedicles.
- The full range of vertebral body anomalies seen in congenital scoliosis and occur either at the level of spina bifida or at any other site in the spine. These anomalies include:
  1. Defects of segmentation. Including defects in disc development, unilateral unsegmented bar (anterior and posterior), and total defects of segmentation with shortness of the affected portion of the spine but often without curvature.
  2. Defects of formation: (i) pure anterior defect with partial or complete absence of one or more vertebral bodies; (ii) antero-lateral defect with absence of half of the anterior portion of one side of the vertebral body and complete absence of the other side; and (iii) lateral defect leading to a hemivertebra (*Figure 12.1*). Hemivertebrae may be single or multiple and may be associated with a contralateral defect of segmentation.
  3. Mixed defects (*Figure 12.2*). Any of the anomalies may be seen together at the same or another level of the spine. In myelomeningocele, it is the lumbar spine which is the most common site for these congenital anomalies (*Figure 12.3*). Almost invariably there are multiple anomalies of mixed type. The above classification is based on that suggested by Moe *et al.* (1978).

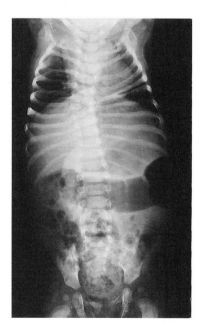

Figure 12.1 Hemivertebra and thoracic scoliosis with lumbar spina bifida.

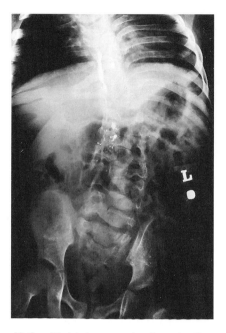

Figure 12.2 Multiple vertebral and rib anomalies with lumbar spina bifida and myelomeningocele.

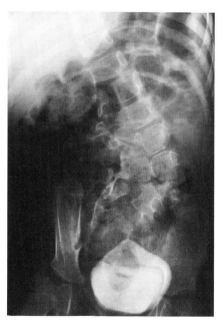

Figure 12.3 Congenital scoliosis at the level of the spina bifida.

- Diastematomyelia (*Figure 12.4a,b*).
- Spondylolisthesis.
- Absence of the sacrum – either partial or complete (*Figure 12.5a,b*; also *Figures 2.13, 2.14*).
- Kyphosis. Paralytic and congenital forms occur. Muscle imbalance is a major factor leading to progression.
- Lordosis. The commonest form of lordosis is not structural but secondary to fixed flexion deformity of

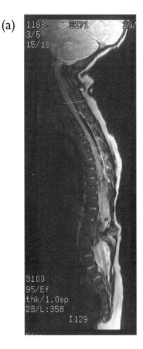

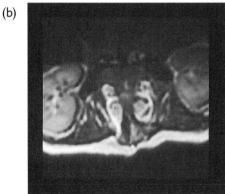

Figure 12.4(a,b) Diastematomyelia in association with myelomeningocele. The spine of a girl aged 2 years and 3 months who was born with myelomeningocele which was closed at birth. She had presented with spasticity in both legs. The bony spur associated with diastematomyelia can be seen just below the defect of segmentation at the thoracolumbar junction. Surgical release corrected the neurological deficit.

the hip. The curve may become fixed and there may be paralytic elements. Seldom is the curve congenital.
• Scoliosis. Paralytic scoliosis is the most common form of scoliosis occurring in myelomeningocele. This is true for approximately 90% of curves and a higher percentage of those that require surgical treatment are paralytic in nature. Congenital and mixed congenital and paralytic curves also occur. The curve may be a lordoscoliosis or a kyphoscoliosis.

GENETICS

Anencephaly and spina bifida cystica have a genetic relationship to those conditions that are characterized by multiple anomalies of the vertebral bodies without spina bifida cystica (Wynne-Davies, 1975). This implies that there is an increased risk of spina bifida cystica in the siblings of children who present with congenital scoliosis. Should the mother of a child with congenital scoliosis become pregnant, then she should be advised to undergo ultrasound examination, amniocentesis and serum examination. Isolated single anomalies of vertebral body development are not familial and carry an extremely low risk to subsequent siblings.

Laurence *et al.* (1968a) and Laurence (1970) have described the vertebral and other abnormalities occurring in parents and siblings of cases of spina bifida and of anencephaly.

KYPHOSIS

A major kyphotic deformity of the spine associated with myelomeningocele is present in approximately 10% of patients (Hoppenfeld, 1967; Banta and Hamada, 1976). This deformity is often termed congenital because it is present at birth and is due at least in part to the congenital deficiency of the posterior elements of the spine at the level of the kyphosis.

The deformity usually progresses with time. This progression is due to the unopposed action of the psoas muscles anteriorly The erector spinae muscles sublux laterally and act as spinal flexors and the effect of gravity on this unsupported spine adds to the deforming forces. With progression of the deformity, particularly with the patient sitting, there is frequently skin ulceration over the gibbus, a crowding of the abdominal contents and respiratory embarrassment. For sleeping, the patient must lie on their side as lying on the back is either physically difficult or alternatively results in pressure ulceration and further skin breakdown. In the sitting position the patients often need to use their hands for support and this significantly compromises their functional capabilities (*Figure 12.6*).

Incidence

Hoppenfeld (1967) reported an incidence of kyphosis at birth of 1 in 8 babies born with myelomeningocele.

Shurtleff *et al.* (1976) demonstrated the relationship between kyphosis, the level of the lesion (clinically and radiologically) and the age of onset of the deformity. Those children with thoracic lesions had an incidence of kyphosis of approximately 1 in 10 at

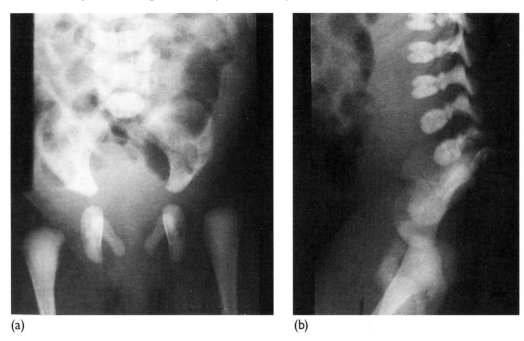

(a)   (b)

Figure 12.5(a,b)   Kyphosis with gross anomalies of vertebral bodies. Radiographs on the first day of life demonstrate multiple vertebral and rib anomalies including absence of vertebral bodies at the apex of the kyphosis and almost complete absence of the sacrum; only the right half of the first sacral vertebra is present.

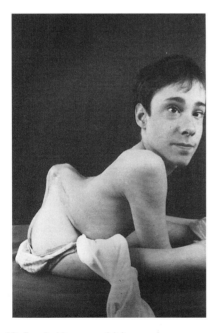

Figure 12.6   A 16-year-old boy who presented with this gross kyphosis. The deformity had progressed throughout childhood and there was a history of frequent ulceration.

birth: by early adolescence just over one-third have kyphotic curves over 65°. Children with lumbar lesions did not have kyphosis at birth but there was a 3% incidence in children with asymmetrical lesions. Minimal increases, with advancing age, in the occur-

rence of kyphosis amongst the sacral and asymmetrical groups of patients suggest that their risk of acquiring kyphosis is approximately 1 in 7 to 1 in 10. The risk to children with lower lumbar paralysis developing a kyphosis is less than 1 in 20. Twenty-six of 42 patients with kyphosis had developed the deformity before the age of 6 years. It is thus clear that there are both congenital and paralytic forms of kyphosis.

Pathology

This has been well described by Hoppenfeld (1967) and by Sharrard and Drennan (1972). The vertebral bodies may show congenital division with two centres of ossification. At occasional levels the articular facets are fused forming a continuous lateral cartilaginous linkage. In addition, the widely separated pedicles are associated with lateral and anterior displacement of the extensor muscles of the spine, which are poorly developed. The psoas muscles lie anterior to the kyphosis. These muscular displacements (particularly the displacement of the long spinal muscles – the psoas is seldom completely innervated) are regarded as being major factors responsible for progress of the deformity.

   Not only are the pedicles widely separated but their posterior ends are more laterally placed than the anterior ends, which are attached laterally to the vertebrae. The facets in the kyphotic lumbar area articulate with each other in the coronal plane instead

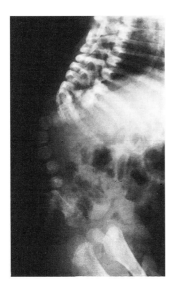

Figure 12.7 Radiograph of the typical kyphotic deformity in a young spina bifida patient.

of the normal sagittal plane; this is because the articular process and facets maintain their normal relationship to the pedicles, the pedicles themselves being directed and rotated laterally.

Disc spaces are narrowed, more so anteriorly. The nucleus pulposis is located posteriorly at the apex of the deformity. The anterior longitudinal ligament is shortened and may be thickened. The transverse processes are present and separate the psoas muscle from the laterally displaced paraspinal muscles. The rudimentary laminae are angulated laterally, so that their original anterior surface faces posteriorly (*Figure 12.7*).

There is generally a fixed lordosis above the kyphosis and sometimes a fixed lordosis below it (Lindseth and Seltzer, 1979). Donaldson (1974) noted that the great vessels do not follow the kyphosis and thus could create significant problems in treatment; however, this has not been our experience. Park and Watt (1975) confirmed displacement of the aorta by aortography. Portions of the erector spinae muscles lie anterior to the axis of flexion and thus become flexors of the spine. The quadratus lumborum is also displaced so that the majority of its fibres are anterior to the axis of flexion.

Those children who are born with a lumbar kyphosis generally have complete paralysis of the leg muscles. In a series of 11 patients undergoing surgical correction (Lowe and Menelaus, 1978) only one child had activity in the psoas and quadriceps muscles, and this activity was preserved.

Kyphosis may be associated with multiple anomalies at multiple levels of the spine. Children who are born with a kyphosis generally have hydrocephalus and are among the most severely affected children. Hence, decisions on management require very careful consideration. Children who survive the first few weeks and then develop hydrocephalus will require a shunt procedure and subsequently excision of the sac. Some parents may demand initial vigorous and active treatment of all conditions, others may not. Some children, initially without spinal deformity, later develop a kyphosis. We must then be prepared to treat this difficult and disabling condition.

Management

Non-operative management

The non-operative management of these children involves care of the associated problems rather than treating the deformity *per se*. Spinal orthoses usually do not control this deformity and are not recommended.

In the very young child, care must be given to seating and the way the child lies. The attenuated skin over the apex of the deformity must be protected from prolonged pressure and this area must be inspected regularly. As the child grows and graduates to a wheelchair, a cavity needs to be created in the upright cushion of the wheelchair to accommodate the protruberant gibbus and prevent ulceration of the skin. Side supports often are helpful in the wheelchairs of these children, not so much for lateral control of any spinal deformity, but simply for support of the child to allow more free use of the hands. Many children find themselves trapped, placing their hands on the arms of the chair for support and thus are significantly compromized with regard to function.

In children who have undergone urinary diversion, the progression of the kyphosis often compromises access to an abdominal stoma. In these children consideration should be given to rediversion of the urinary tract with sphincter implant or catheterization.

Historical review

With regard to surgical treatment, Kilfoyle *et al.* (1965) reported good results in two of three interbody fusions for kyphosis with paraplegia from varying causes. Sharrard (1968) described osteotomy resection of the spine in the newborn, and in older children transverse osteotomy with overlapping of the fragments and fixation by four screws. For the less severe kyphosis in which there was a liability to ulceration of the skin on either side of the midline, he described excision of the laterally directed pedicles and laminae.

Sharrard and Drennan (1972) later reported the results of osteotomy excision of the lumbar spine in 18 children aged 3–12 years. Fusion was limited to the area of bone excision, where Blount staples and crossed oblique pins were used for internal fixation; compensatory curves were not corrected. The results of osteotomy excision have also been described by Eyring *et al.* (1972) and by Cotta *et al.* (1971). The duration of follow-up in these series is short.

Sriram *et al.* (1972) described a case effectively treated by excision of the vertebral body and fusion using Harrington compression apparatus inserted into the vertebral foraminae. Eckstein and Vora (1972) reported the results of spinal osteotomy in 16 children under the age of 8 years; they preferred not to use internal fixation. Five of the 16 children died after the operation.

Poitras and Hall (1974) report six cases operated upon by a posterior approach with excision of the sac, excision of the bony elements and fixation of the osteotomy with compression rods.

McKay *et al.* (1976) described a method of correction that did not involve excision of bone. The fact that the child regained normal height after this procedure could prove a disadvantage as a shorter child has a lower centre of gravity and therefore greater stability. This method was reported by Duncan *et al.* (1976). Moe *et al.* (1978) suggest, for the child under the age of 3 years, direct anterior fusion with excision of the anterior longitudinal ligament, annulus and discs, and a strut graft fusion.

Lowe and Menelaus (1978) describe the results of management in which a long length of the spine is corrected and fused using longitudinal heavy threaded wires as internal fixation. This method of treatment finds its best application between the age of 3 and 6 years.

Indications for operation

The principal indication for surgery is chronic or recurrent skin ulceration. However, correction also gives subsidiary benefits. Without the kyphos a brace is more easily fitted and pressure over the unstable skin avoided. With a stable and erect spine the child is able to sit in greater comfort, use their hands for independent activities and there is improved access to the abdomen.

The mortality rate of operation is too high for the last three factors to be regarded as indications unless there is also chronic or recurrent ulceration. Unlike Sharrard and Drennan (1972), we have not operated to improve neurological deterioration, painful kyphosis or gross deformity alone. In our experience neurological deterioration has not been an issue as these children have no useful neurological function distal to the kyphosis and pain from the kyphotic deformity has not been a common finding. Whilst the deformity always progresses with frequent skin ulceration over the gibbus, these children are generally unwell and may

not survive long. In general, children with gross kyphosis are paraplegic or have so little muscle power in the legs that there need be no concern regarding further loss of neurological activity due to progress of the deformity. If there is activity in certain muscles the surgeon may spare the appropriate nerve roots but cannot guarantee that useful muscle function will be preserved. Nevertheless, surgery should be undertaken in these circumstances as the progressive kyphosis will itself prevent walking using a Reciprocating Gait Orthosis (RGO) if it is not corrected.

Preoperative management

Vigorous endeavours are made to heal ulceration over the kyphosis. This usually means discarding all bracing for some weeks, the use of protective pads and prone lying; it may be necessary to carry out this management in hospital for several weeks before operation.

Urine cultures and tests for the antibiotic sensitivity of any organisms present are performed. A course of the appropriate antibiotic is commenced 24 hours before operation and continued until the wound has healed. If the urine is sterile and there are no other foci of infection a broad-spectrum antibiotic is used. The volume of blood cross-matched before operation should exceed the patient's blood volume as the loss may range from 500 to 1500 ml. CSF pressure and shunt valve function must be checked preoperatively.

Principles of surgical correction

It is generally agreed that correction of severe kyphosis can only be achieved with reliability by excision of bone and that maintenance of correction can only be obtained by solid fusion in front of, between and behind the vertebral bodies over the entire length of the deformity. McKay *et al.* (1976) has shown that it is technically possible to correct kyphosis without excision of the bony elements but his method is only applicable to paralytic deformity over the age of 6 years. The authors have no experience of the procedure.

Recommended surgical techniques

The choice of the form of surgery for the correction of kyphosis must depend on the previous experience and preference of the individual surgeon. There are few long-term follow-up studies in the literature and a paucity of hard facts on which to base firm recommendations. It is wisest at the time of surgery to maintain a versatile approach that allows variations in the technique of fusion and of internal fixation according to circumstances. Whilst Hall (1964) has employed the Harrington compression apparatus with success at as

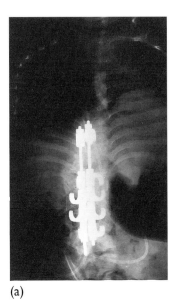
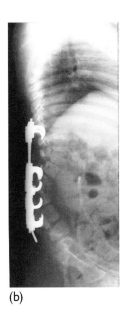

(a)   (b)

Figure 12.8(a,b) Radiographs of the spine of a child who had surgery at 2 years of age. The spine was exposed up to the seventh thoracic vertebra which meant that there were three intact laminae above the defect. The functionless lower end of the cord was excised and the dura closed. The whole of the bodies of the first and second lumbar vertebrae and part of the body of the 12th thoracic vertebra were excised. A Harrington double compression system was then employed using: (i) the transverse processes for the hooks close to the apex of the curve; (ii) the laminae for the most proximal anchoring hooks; and (iii) the intervertebral foraminae for the lowermost hooks Fourteen months later, her spine was re-explored and the internal fixation removed at the lower ends of the rods were tenting the skin. The fusion was solid. (Radiographs kindly proved by Dr John Hall of Boston. He and Dr Kenneth Winston carried out the surgery on this patient and acknowledgment is made to them.)

early an age as 3 years, we have been concerned that the bulky apparatus might be exposed by wound breakdown, notably in small children with very scarred and unstable skin (*Figure 12.8a,b*). This leads us to prefer intramedullary wire fixation in these circumstances. A strut graft is also appropriate for young children with scarred skin but carries the disadvantages that further surgery is inevitable as the deformity is never totally corrected by this technique and there will be a recurrence of the deformity.

In the present state of our knowledge the most appropriate surgery would be as follows.

Correction in infancy
Lindseth technique. This technique involves resection of the appropriate posterior elements and the apical ver-

tebra at the time of closure of the meningocele. A crucial part of the operation is the re-approximation of the erector spinae muscles to the midline so that they may act as spinal extensors and resist recurrence of the kyphosis (Lindseth, 1995).

'Bloodless kyphectomy'. In this technique the apical vertebra is excised through the adjacent discs. The anterior longitudinal ligament is divided but the posterior longitudinal ligament is preserved. Sutures are passed around the pedicles to approximate the vertebral remnants (Cherny *et al.*, 1995).

Operation for children 1–3 years of age
Anterior strut graft. This method is described by Moe *et al.* (1978) and is suggested for use in the child under the age of 3 years with a rapidly progressive deformity. It involves direct anterior fusion with excision of the anterior longitudinal ligament, annulus and discs, and strut graft fusion. The authors illustrate the method by radiography and photographs of a patient who underwent this surgery at the age of 1 year and 7 months. There was only 3° loss of correction 4.5 years later. The curve had extended and would require further fusion but progression of the curve had clearly been delayed.

Operation for children 3–7 years of age
Kyphos excision, extension fusion and longitudinal wire fixation (Lowe and Menelaus, 1978). In this age group most children can be managed by attention to seating and vigilance of the soft tissues over the apex. If persistent skin breakdown precipitates surgery the technique advocate is that described by Lowe and Menelaus (1978) (*Figures 12.9, 12.10*).

In this procedure the patient is placed prone and

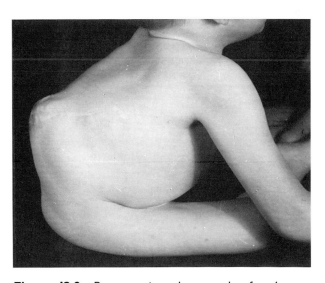

Figure 12.9 Preoperative photograph of a 4-year-old boy with a kyphosis of the upper lumbar spine.

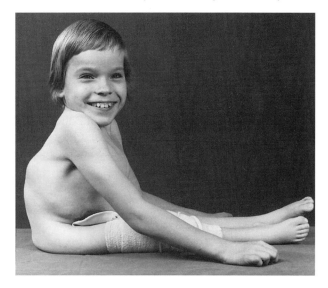

Figure 12.10 The appearance 4 years after kyphosis excision, extensive fusion and heavy threaded wire fixation. The wires were removed 6 months after operation.

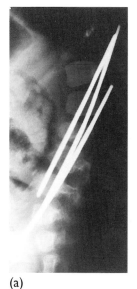
(a)

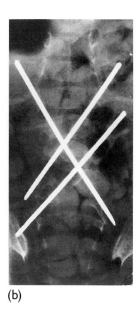
(b)

Figure 12.11(a,b) AP and lateral radiographs taken after operation showing the heavy threaded Kirschner wires that are preferred for internal fixation with the Menelaus technique.

the kyphotic segment of the spine is exposed subperiosteally. The dura is dissected free from the vertebral bodies and transected and folded upwards. Care must be taken to leave open the lower end of the cord so that spinal fluid can escape from the central canal of the cord to the arachnoid. The dura is oversewn to prevent CSF leakage. Acute elevation of intracranial pressure following transection of the non-functioning spinal cord may otherwise occur (Winston *et al.*, 1977). Care is taken to avoid damage to nerve roots.

At least one vertebra is removed from the apex of the kyphos and then the discs above and below are removed. The anterior longitudinal ligament is preserved. The intervertebral discs are then excised from between any vertebrae which form part of the residual kyphosis or part of a fixed lordosis above or below it. The upper and lower segments of the spine are then brought end to end. The resected vertebral bodies are used as bone graft. Three or four heavy threaded Kirschner wires (gauge 7/64 in or 2.75 mm) have then to be passed along the length of spine to be fused (*Figure 12.11a,b*). The wires that have been inserted proximally are then passed distally into the caudal segment of spine. If possible they are driven into the iliac crests. In some circumstances it may be easier to pass the wires in a cephalic direction.

Hall and Poitras (1977) suggests that fusion should not necessarily be carried down to the sacrum, unless the apex of the kyphosis is mid-lumbar or lower. The preservation of some mobility at the lumbosacral junction is more likely to lead to successful fusion at the apex of the curve. Furthermore, mobility at this joint

may protect against ischial pressure sores. Postoperative immobilization is carried out in a bivalved soft-lined polypropylene jacket with thigh extension. Fusion is usually solid enough at 3 months to remove the thigh extensions and allow sitting in the brace. Spinal support is continued for an additional 6–9 months.

The older child
In the children over 8 years of age usually the vertebral bodies are of reasonable size that will accept internal fixation of sufficient dimension to impart stability to the corrected spine.

The approach in the older children is similar to that described previously for the younger child. In the older child, however, the spine needs to be mobilized to a slightly greater extent and this usually involves excision of the anterior longitudinal ligament and excision of more than one vertebral segment.

The incision is made in the midline extending distally from approximately T3 down to the upper aspect of the sacrum. The subperiosteal dissection is begun in the proximal region as these levels are usually intact and anatomy more normal. This allows one to carefully follow the bony elements distally until the defect in the bifid lamina is encountered and the dural elements dissected free.

The bony dissection is carried distally around the bifid segment and along the tips of the out-turned bifid laminae on each side of the spine. The subperiosteal dissection is carried anteriorly along the line of the pedicles at the apex of the kyphosis and around the

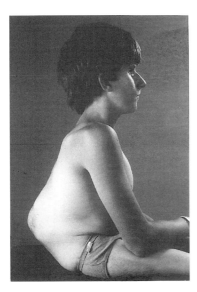

Figure 12.12   Clinical appearance of a 13-year-old boy with a spina bifida kyphosis prior to surgical correction of the deformity by resection and intramedullary rods.

vertebral bodies until the vertebral column is free of soft tissue attachments at the apex and over a level of approximately 3–4 vertebrae.

Great care is taken to stay close to the vertebral bodies and avoid injury to the intra-abdominal contents, particularly the great vessels. Authors have raised concerns regarding the great vessel anatomy (Donaldson, 1974; Loder *et al.*, 1991). Park and Watt (1975) also confirm the great vessel anatomical course by aortography. The vertebrae resected usually include the apical vertebra and one or two of the more proximal

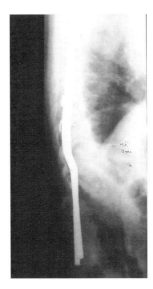

Figure 12.14   Postoperative lateral radiograph of the spine of the boy shown.

vertebrae of the kyphos. Once these vertebrae are resected the spine can then be readily realigned. The preferred technique is to use the Luque rod as an intramedullary rod and the tails of the 'U'-shaped Luque rod are passed into drill holes made in the vertebral bodies in the lumbar spine (Torode and Godette, 1995) (*Figures 12.12–12.15*).

The spine is instrumented by passing the Luque rod into the holes drilled in the lumbar vertebra and extending into the upper portions of the sacrum. The

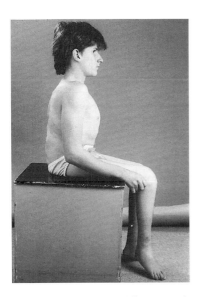

Figure 12.13   Postoperative photograph illustrating the correction obtained by the technique described.

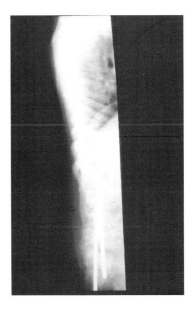

Figure 12.15   Postoperative lateral radiograph of a different child showing the implantation of the Luque rods into the bodies of the distal vertebrae, with sublaminar wiring of the thoracic vertebrae.

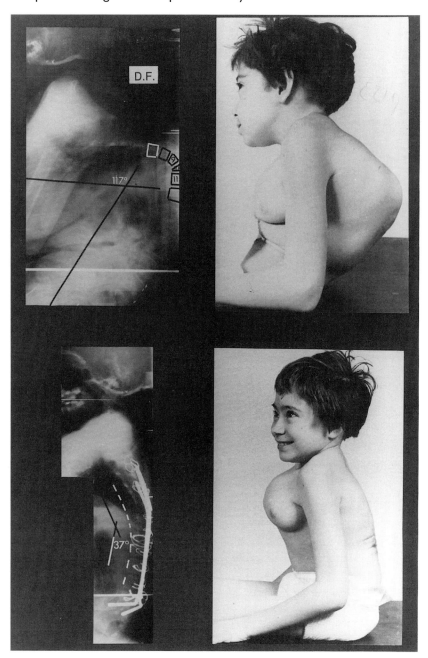

Figure 12.16   Pre- and postoperative photographs and radiographs of a spina bifida kyphosis patient who underwent correction utilizing the vertebrectomy and fixation with Luque rods and Galveston technique (courtesy of Dr Robert Gillespie).

rod is then bent so that it lies in a satisfactory plane along the posterior aspect of the thoracic spine and fixed to that segment of the spine by sublaminar wires. Even if there has been skin ulcers present and poor tissue over the apex, this can usually be excised and the skin and subcutaneous layers mobilized on both sides of the trunk around the abdomen to allow apposition of the margins of the wound without tension and avoidance of any skin flaps.

Other techniques of fixation of the Luque rod to the pelvis have been described with satisfactory results. These include:

- Fixation into the posterior iliac wings using the Galveston technique (Allen and Ferguson, 1979). Unfortunately, many of these children have a hypoplastic pelvis because of the lack of normal muscle activity and hence the posterior iliac wings are underdeveloped (Heydemann and Gillespie, 1987) (*Figure 12.16*).

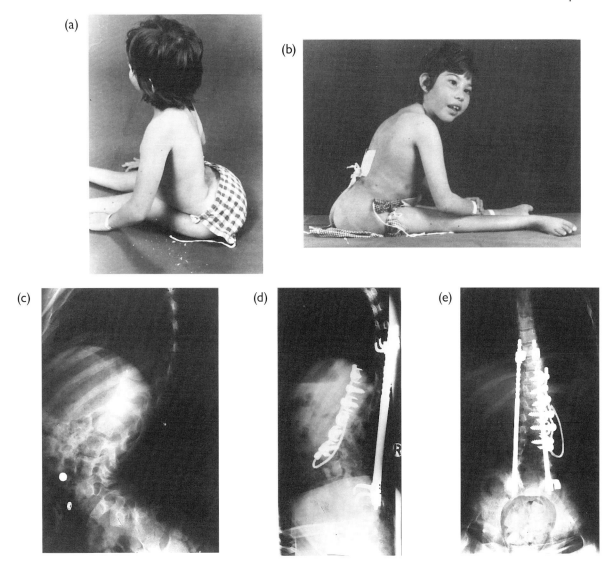

Figure 12.17 (a–e)   The clinical and radiological appearance of a 9-year-old girl before and after surgery to correct lordosis. The surgery involved bilateral anterior hip releases followed later by anterior and posterior spinal surgery with instrumentation. (a) Preoperative clinical photograph. (b) Postoperative clinical photograph. (c) Preoperative lateral radiography. (d) & (e) Postoperative radiographs.

• Fixation of the Luque rods over the alar of the sacrum with circumferential vertebral wiring (Loder *et al.*, 1991).

• Fixation of the Luque rod to the vertebral bodies by segmental AO cancellous screws and wires. In this technique the standard sublaminar wiring is performed proximally whereas in the distal segment points of fixation are made by inserting AO cancellous screws into the hypoplastic pedicles and vertebral bodies of the lower lumbar vertebrae. Stainless wires are then placed around these AO screws and then fixed to the Luque rods (Holt, 1996).

Complications

This form of surgery represents a major insult to these children and hence complications can and will ensue. These are outlined later in the chapter.

LORDOSIS

A particularly malignant form of lumbar hyperlordosis has been noted in children who have undergone lumboperitoneal shunting for hydrocephalus. It is possible that the deformity that arose in these children is due to arachnoiditis associated with the physical properties of the tubing used rather than the shunting procedure itself. This particular deformity is rarely seen now.

We are here concerned with excessive lumbar

lordosis. Lordoscoliosis will be discussed under the heading 'Scoliosis'.

Deformity severe enough to warrant surgery is now seldom seen, which probably correlates with the cessation of lumbo-peritoneal shunt procedures. It must be recognized that a modest degree of hyperlordosis is acceptable in a wheelchair-bound patient as it allows a broader weightbearing area for seating on the posterior aspect of the thighs without compromising function.

Major methods of treatment utilized for this deformity include:

- *Posterior approach and Harrington instrumentation.* The surgical approach as reported by Hall (1964), Jackson (1966) and King and Hall (1970). It must be recognized, however, that in patients in whom the deformity is due to lumbo-peritoneal shunting, the associated arachnoiditis and neural tethering means that the neurological structures are at risk if distraction instrumentation is utilized.
- *Anterior approach with Dwyer instrumentation.* This technique was employed in an effort to shorten the spinal column and reduce the distraction of the scarred neural elements as mentioned above (Dwyer *et al.*, 1969).
- *Combined anterior–posterior approach.* As in other areas of spinal deformity in the spina bifida children, the combination of an anterior and posterior approach often gives the best combination of fusion area and mobilization of the spine. The anterior approach in the hyperlordosis allows for disc excision and approximation of the involved vertebral segment. This approximation can be made by the use of the Dwyer instrumentation or Zielke instrumentation. If there are sufficient laminae posteriorly to obtain segmental instrumentation, then the use of anterior instrumentation can be avoided, stability being obtained via posterior means alone. It is possible to avoid the use of distraction methods by using a Luque rod with sublaminar wires. The sublaminar wires are used to draw the vertebral column to the rods to reduce the lordosis (*Figure 12.17a–e*).
- *Anterior wedge resection and skeletal suspension (Hall procedure).* Hall and Bobechko (1973) provide details of this technique for the correction of extreme lordosis. They point out that when hyperlordosis is present, the vertebral bodies can be palpated under the anterior abdominal wall. In these circumstances, the simplest approach is directly to the front of the spine across the peritoneal cavity. Because of the scarred and tethered cauda equina and dura, lengthening of the spinal column is to be avoided. This method involves resection of vertebral bodies to allow straightening without traction on the neural elements.

The authors point out that children with extreme lordosis have disturbed anatomy. The aorta and vena cava are displaced laterally. The renal pedicle is displaced proximally and the bifurcation of the great vessels displaced distally. This altered anatomy aids the surgeon to obtain a direct approach to two vertebral bodies at the apex of the lordosis. One disc plus one half of each of the two adjacent vertebrae are removed together with the involved pedicles. The deformity is not corrected on the operating table but is gained slowly in the postoperative period by means of skeletal suspension. Pins are placed through the lower ends of the femora and vertical traction is applied with the child lying supine and with the hips and knees flexed to 90°. If the spine does not commence to straighten within the first few days of suspension, then a second-stage posterior release is performed and the child replaced in suspension. Correction is usually complete at the end of the 2 weeks when a plaster cast is applied and retained until bony union has been secured.

This method is only applicable when there is a severe degree of lordosis as only in those circumstances have the vertebral bodies dissected through the posterior vascular structures. For lesser degrees of lordosis, Hall recommends the Dwyer procedure.

Steele and Adams (1972) and Moe *et al.* (1978) report experience with similar techniques of correction of extreme lumbar lordosis. As early as 1968, Simmons had described a method of correction of lumbar lordosis by wedge resection of bone from the apex of the lordosis, sometimes followed by posterior spinal instrumentation

SCOLIOSIS

This section deals with scoliotic deformities of the spine in contra-distinction to deformities in the sagittal plane. However, it is not uncommon for patients with spina bifida to have significant deformities in the sagittal plane in association with a major scoliotic deformity of the spine. The commonest form of scoliosis in myelomeningocele is a paralytic curve. This typically is a long lumbar or thoraco-lumbar curve associated with pelvic obliquity. Whereas kyphotic deformity of the spine result in soft tissue ulceration over the apex of the kyphosis, patients with scoliosis and pelvic obliquity are at major risk from soft tissue breakdown under the buttocks due to poor pressure distribution across the ischial tuberosities. The lower ischial tuberosity, which is on the convex side, is usually the site of ulceration as that side takes the bulk of the body weight. Furthermore, the presence of the spinal deformity and the pelvic obliquity results in poor sitting balance, which also compromises the function of the patient in a

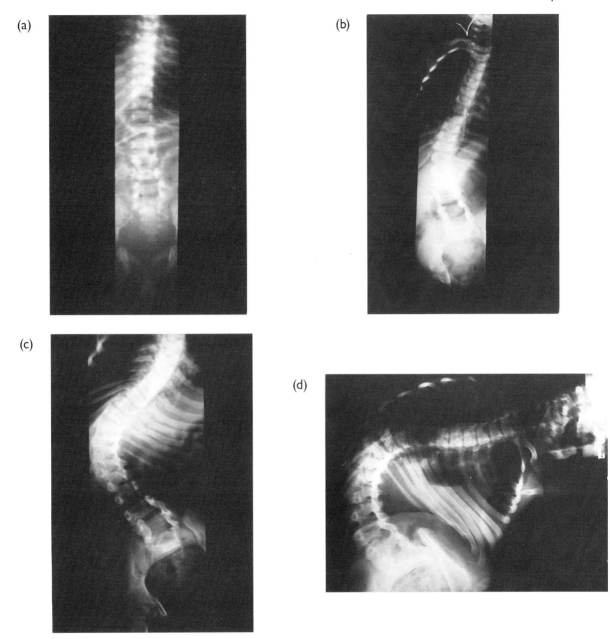

Figure 12.18(a–d)   Radiographs of the spine of a girl from infancy through to 15 years of age. These demonstrate the marked progression of the deformity and that intervention early in the development of the deformity should have been employed.

wheelchair as they need to use their hands for support (*Figure 12.18a–d*).

In ambulant children the pelvic obliquity results in an apparent leg length discrepancy and uncovering of the femoral head on the high side. Continued subluxation of the hip may follow and further compromise both the ability to stand and sit.

Curves in the thoracic region occur either alone or in association with a lumbar curve and these may also be related to paralysis but the curve may be attributed to abnormalities of the spinal cord rather than pure paralysis. These abnormalities include Chiari malformations types I and II, syringomyelia, intracanal and spinal lipomata or diastematomyelia. These abnormalities have been noted in the past at surgery and with myelography but with the advent of the MRI, the brain, brainstem and spinal cord can be examined non-invasively. Virtually all children with spina bifida have some degree of spinal cord tethering.

The third significant component in deformities of the spinal column in spina bifida is the presence of congenital vertebral anomalies as distinct from the presence of the bifid lumbar spine. Fifteen to 20% of children who have myelomeningocele also have other congenital vertebral abnormalities (Samuelsson and Eklof, 1988). These anomalies can also produce deformities depending on their extent, location, and growth capacity. From a clinical standpoint deformities due to congenital anomalies are more rigid than those due to paralysis and continued growth may result in progression of those curves. The site of these deformities may be distant from the bifid part of the spine and hence surgery to correct or prevent progression of those deformities may involve operating on a segment of the spine that is neurologically intact. Care must be taken to protect those intact spinal levels. It is recognized that some children have spinal deformities in which there are more than one of the aforementioned components involved in the progression of the deformity. Careful examination and work-up of these patients is therefore necessary to obtain a good surgical outcome.

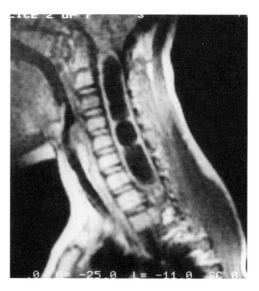

Figure 12.19   MRI scan of a boy with a scoliotic deformity of the spine demonstrating a large syrinx of the cervical cord.

Hydrosyringomyelia as a Cause of Scoliosis

Patients may develop progressive scoliosis due to hydrosyringomyelia (Sharrard and Drennan, 1972; Hall *et al.*, 1975, 1976; Hight *et al.*, 1976). These workers have demonstrated that myelomeningocele patients with spontaneously arrested hydrocephalus commonly have associated hydrosyringomyelia. They feel that the hydrosyringomyelia in these circumstances is probably acting as a decompressive vent for the associated hydrocephalus. Most of their patients affected by this lesion presented with either progressive scoliosis alone or with both paralytic scoliosis and progressive neurological deficit. Three of their 17 patients presented with progressive paralysis alone. These problems often began at the age of 5–10 years. The gradually increasing scoliosis was usually thoracolumbar but at times was purely thoracic. Parents had sometimes complained that these children were increasingly lazy and had stopped using their braces. Clinical examination of the extremities might reveal increased weakness both in arms and in legs. Ventricular size and shunt function should be studied in these circumstances.

    These authors report that early scoliosis may be arrested, and even reversed by shunting, but that curves of 50° or more may progress despite adequate treatment. This concept suggests that shunting may be of benefit in preventing the onset of scoliosis. The frequency of hydrosyringomelia as a cause of scoliosis in myelomeningocele remains uncertain (*Figures 12.19–12.21*).

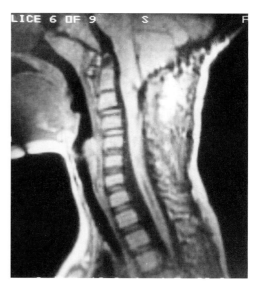

Figure 12.20   MRI scan of the same patient following surgery for the syrinx.

Incidence

Shurtleff *et al.* (1976) have investigated the incidence of scoliosis and related it to the clinical and radiological level of the lesion and the age of development of the curvature. Their findings are shown below.

Thoracic lesions

One per cent of those with paralysis in the thoracic area had scoliosis greater than 30° during the first month of

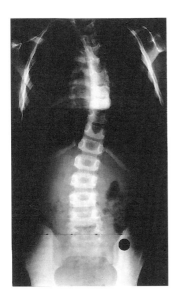

Figure 12.21 AP radiograph of the spine of this patient.

life. By the age of 4 years 17%, by the age of 10 years 33%, by the age of 15 years 81% and by the age of 20 years 88% had curves of this magnitude.

High lumbar lesions

A smaller group of patients were studied. None was reported as having scoliosis under the age of 2 years when 4% had scoliotic curves. By the age of 4 years 14%, by the age of 10 years 22% and by the age of 15 years 44% were so affected. Over the age of 20 years, 81% were affected.

Lower lumbar lesions

None was affected in the first month of life, 3% were affected by the age of 4 years, 18% by the age of 10 years, 23% by the age of 15 years and the same proportion of patients over the age of 20 years had this deformity.

Sacral lesions

Under the age of 14 months, no patients were affected; at that age, 3% were affected. The incidence remained at 3% until the age of 15 years after which 9% had scoliotic deformity.

Asymmetrical lesions

At the age of 4 years 6%, at the age of 10 years 25% and at the age of 15 years 30% were affected. The incidence remained unchanged after this.

Shurtleff et al. (1976) found that their patients were equally divided into three groups – curves ranging from 30° to 39°, curves ranging from 40° to 59°, and curves greater than 59°.

Management

The appropriate form of management of scoliosis in myelomeningocele will depend on careful evaluation of the patient's general and local condition. Furthermore, the need for intervention will be dictated by the degree of the deformity, the progression of the deformity and the effect that the deformity might have on any particular child. A certain deformity in one child may be affected to a greater or lesser extent than another child with the same deformity. Careful neurological assessment of shunt function is required. A change in neurological picture may demand further such investigation prior to intervening surgically. The advent of the MRI scan has assisted greatly by providing a means of examining the morphology of the brain, the ventricular size, and the base of the brain at the level of the foramen magnum and the spinal cord. Previously, syringomyelia or diastematomyelia that was not evident on plain radiographs and where neurological signs were not obvious may have gone undetected. Other relevant features of the assessment of the child with scoliosis is to note carefully their ambulatory status, their seating requirements and seating balance and any evidence of pressure breakdown. It is important to note the sensory level in these children and that useful muscle power might be in jeopardy in reconstructing a spinal deformity surgically. Preoperative full length AP and lateral radiographs of the spine with the patient in the upright and supine position are obtained. If there is any significant flexion deformity of the hips then a supine view is obtained with the hips flexed at least 45° and abducted 30° (Moe et al., 1978). Bending films that are very useful in idiopathic scoliosis are usually not of major benefit in spina bifida patients. However, CT scans may provide useful information, particularly with congenital anomalies of the spine, and also are of importance for assessment of dimensions of the pedicles for fixation by pedicle screws.

The decision to undertake major spinal surgery in children with myelomeningocele must only be undertaken after appropriate discussion with the family of the child, the neurosurgeon and physician co-ordinator of the spina bifida clinic. It is important to remember that these major operations can be life threatening in small children with deficiencies in multiple organ systems. The longevity of the child if surgery is not undertaken must be considered in the decision-making process.

Aims of scoliosis management

The aim of orthopaedic management in myelomeningocele is to maintain stable posture for both standing and sitting. Stable posture implies that the pelvis should be level and the trunk should sit vertically on this level pelvis without the need for hand support. Subsidiary aims of management are the maintenance of reasonable length of the trunk, the removal of convexities which may be the site of pressure sores, the preservation of good respiratory function and a satisfactory cosmetic appearance.

Prophylaxis

The study of hydrosyringomyelia, outlined above, indicates an important area for prophylaxis. It is suggested that the curve can be halted, or even reversed, by adequate shunting procedures.

Another important area is that of early diagnosis of scoliosis. Frequently, orthopaedic surgeons become so obsessed with leg deformity that they do not look at the back. Every child over the age of 5 years should have, as a routine, 12-monthly radiographs of the spine.

Fixed deformities of the hips should be vigorously treated in order to prevent intrapelvic causes leading to pelvic obliquity. Such obliquity might aggravate a developing scoliosis and increase its harmful effects.

Non-operative management (see also Chapter 6)

Non-operative treatment for scoliosis in myelomeningocele has a very limited place. There is difficulty in fitting a brace to a child who has anaesthetic skin, is often overweight, who has an ileal conduit and requires considerable leg bracing. Plaster casts are appropriate merely as postoperative immobilization and not as a definitive form of treatment.

There is a place for bracing in children with rapidly progressing scoliosis (with curves in excess of 30°) who are considered too young for surgery. If such a child can be fitted with a Milwaukee brace and still be mobile in their lower limb braces then a period of conservative management is of advantage. If such a child is subjected to early surgery then there is stunting of growth, and a likelihood of the internal fixation being difficult to apply to the small and porotic bones.

The object of brace management is to limit progression of the curve and encourage the spine to stiffen in a position which is as straight as possible. Exercises to the spine are therefore not indicated. If a brace programme is in trouble because the child tolerates the brace poorly or is developing pressure sores,

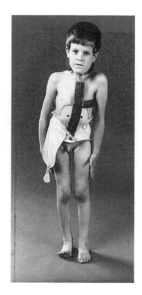

Figure 12.22 Photograph of a spina bifida patient with scoliosis that was controlled with a Milwaukee brace.

then this method of management should be discontinued. Brace management should not be continued for too long, merely until the child is large enough for surgery. Congenital deformities will not respond to bracing.

Hall and Bobechko (1973) reports successful use of the Boston brace in myelomeningocele. Drennan (1976) reports experience with an anterior opening brace with swivel supports. These supports fit into brackets on the wheelchair in such a way that a suspension effect is obtained.

The Milwaukee brace is the most effective orthosis. We have used it successfully in myelomeningocele (*Figure 12.22*). Moe *et al.* (1978) also reports its successful use. The pelvic girdle may require modification to allow for an ileal conduit. The lateral holding pad should be large and softly lined. The skin under the pelvic girdle and the lateral pad should be inspected twice daily. Moe and his colleagues suggest that the child can sometimes sleep without the brace as the curve is of a collapsing type and not likely to increase at night.

Indications for surgery

Increasing deformity in the ambulant child
In some children with low-level lesions in whom ambulation is possible, an increasingly severe scoliotic deformity can threaten ambulation because of increasing trunk imbalance. There is a significant risk that the child will become non-ambulant if a fusion of the spine to the sacrum is necessary and this must be made

clear to the family before surgery. Therefore, in some children fusion short of the lumbosacral level may be indicated even at the risk of having to return later to complete the fusion to the sacrum once the child has ceased ambulation.

Increasing deformity with associated pelvic obliquity in the non-ambulant child

In these children progressive lumbar scoliosis and increasing pelvic obliquity will lead to a progressive imbalance in seating and lead to soft tissue ulceration over the greater tuberosity or ischium on the lower side. In these children therefore it is necessary to set a goal of having trunk balance over a level pelvis.

Pain

Pain is an uncommon indication for surgery to the spine in spina bifida children; however, not all children are insensate over the level of the deformity of the spine.

Cosmesis

While this may be a significant factor in performing surgery in idiopathic scoliosis, in the spina bifida child ambulation and sitting balance are much higher on the priority list.

Operative management

Until about 1980 instrumentation available consisted of the Dwyer apparatus anteriorly and Harrington instrumentation posteriorly (Harrington, 1962; Dwyer *et al.*, 1969). Since that time there have been numerous advances in the instrumentation systems that are available and in general terms these are all directed to enabling segmental or near-segmental level instrumentation of spinal deformity. The Dwyer system has been supplanted by systems that incorporate the use of screws and rods. The Zielke apparatus evolved from the Dwyer system and utilizes a threaded rod and screws for segmental correction of the spine (Zielke *et al.*, 1976). More recently solid rod systems have been employed.

Two important developments in posterior spinal instrumentation systems have occurred since the writing of the previous edition of this text, the first being the Luque rod system which utilizes fixation to the spine with sublaminar wires around a smooth rod (Luque, 1982). The next landmark change was the development of the Cotrel–Dubousset system, which allowed for multiple levels of fixation of the spine using either hooks or pedicle screws (Cotrel and Dubousset, 1984). In spina bifida patients numerous surgeons have developed other techniques to pass wires through the pedicles or through the neural foraminae over the bifid

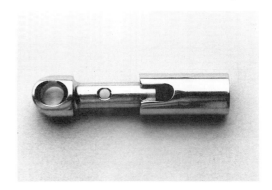

Figure 12.23 Photograph of an implant that provides a connection between the vertical rod, commonly Luque in style, with a transverse sacral bar.

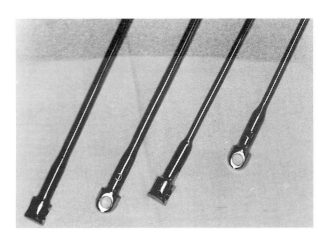

Figure 12.24 Modified rods that connect directly to a sacral bar.

area. Varying forms of fixation to the pelvis have been developed with the distal end of the Luque rods being passed either into the tables of the iliac wings or fashioned into an inverted hook to sit on the alar of the sacrum.

In our institution, we have also developed an implant that allows fixation of a Luque rod system to a sacral bar with sublaminar wiring over the proximal segment (*Figures 12.23, 12.24*).

A study of our spina bifida patients undergoing surgery for scoliosis in the decade from 1974 to 1983 (Mazur *et al.*, 1986a) revealed that an anterior fusion was an essential part in the surgical plan of these patients. It has also highlighted the problems in fixation with the early spinal systems. Furthermore, it showed that although there is a significant incidence of infection in children undergoing spinal surgery in myelomeningocele, the infection developed only following the posterior approach to the spine and did not develop in any child with the anterior procedure.

Further lessons were learned from evaluation of

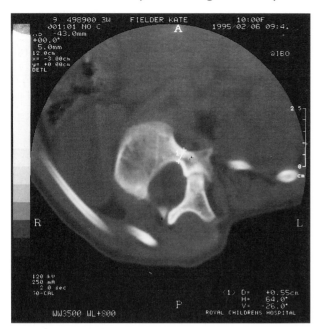

Figure 12.25 CT scan performed to measure the diameter of the pedicles that might be used for implantation of pedicle screws.

the implants used. It was evident that Harrington hook fixation in both the proximal and distal ends of the spine was less stable than desirable. A review of our patients indicates that in a proximal portion of the spine, segmental fixation with multiple hook systems or sublaminar wires is necessary. Two individual Luque rods were found to be less stable than one unitary Luque rod. Fixation distally to the pelvis was best using the sacral bar with a custom made implant that connected the bar to the Luque rod.

Pedicle screws can be utilized in the lumbar spine in these patients where the pedicle size permits (*Figure 12.25*). The pedicle screws can provide segmental fixation for improved stability of the construct, which allows earlier mobilization. Furthermore, in cases where the apex of the lumbar curve is higher and where the lumbosacral portion of the spine is not deformed the pedicle screws may allow stable fixation and correction of the deformity without fusion to the pelvis. These systems can be combined with either hook systems or sublaminar wires proximally.

Age of intervention

The most satisfactory age for correction and fusion for scoliosis is over the age of 10 years in girls and 12 years in boys (Moe *et al.*, 1978). However, an increasing deformity with soft tissue problems may demand earlier intervention. While a fusion at a younger age may produce a somewhat shorter trunk height, it should be recognized that for children in

wheelchairs slightly reduced height is not necessarily a disadvantage.

Choice of technique
Congenital scoliosis. Congenital curves in general and in spina bifida patients are likely to be more rigid and to progress with growth. Intervention therefore should be directed at preventing progression of these deformities and, where appropriate, correction of secondary curves that have developed as a consequence of the primary congenital deformity. The congenital deformities often require intervention at an earlier age than paralytic curves. These curves, however, are often in ambulant patients and hence it is preferable to attempt to prevent progression of these deformities by an anterior approach to the spine with a short fusion and a cessation of growth from the congenital anomaly. Correction of the deformity is usually of less importance in congenital anomalies or can be attained with an anterior instrumentation system and avoid a posterior approach with the risk for neural injury.

Paralytic scoliosis
Ambulant child. In the ambulant child it is desirable to avoid fusion to the pelvis. Where anterior instrumentation alone is possible we recommend the use of the Zielke procedure or one of the screw solid rod systems (*Figure 12.26a–d*). If anterior instrumentation alone is inadequate then, because of either the deformity or associated osteoporosis, posterior instrumentation might be required. In this setting pedicle screws can be used in the lumbar spine; however, the size of the pedicles must be ascertained prior to surgery, and often only a 5-mm diameter screw can be implanted (*Figure 12.25*).

Non-ambulant patients. *(a) Where the deformity does not extend to the lumbosacral junction.* In these patients if a satisfactory correction can be obtained by dissection of the discs anteriorly, with or without instrumentation, then it may be desirable to halt the fusion in the mid-lumbar spine and leave one or more lumbar discs unfused. If some mobility can be maintained in the lower lumbar spine then a modest degree of pelvic obliquity can be accepted and the seating balance supplemented by an appropriately shaped cushion.

(b) Where the curve involves the sacrum. In these children there is usually severe pelvic obliquity and it is not possible to avoid fusion to the sacrum. The instrumentation is used to correct the deformity. The curve is often very severe and an anterior approach followed by halo-femoral traction is utilized as the primary procedure. After 2 weeks of traction the posterior surgery with fixation to the pelvis is obtained by passing a sacral bar through the iliac wings and the body of the sacrum

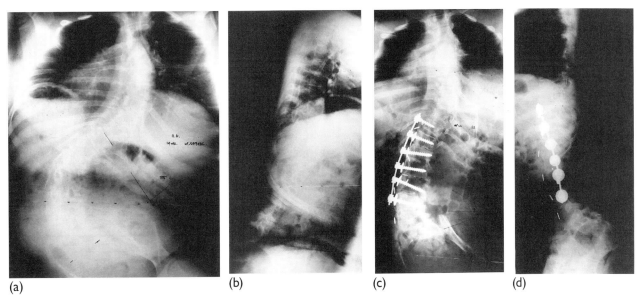

(a)   (b)   (c)   (d)

Figure 12.26(a–d)   Pre- and postoperative radiographs of the spine of a 14-year-old boy who had a severe spinal deformity instrumented with a Zielke construction. Although there has been a big improvement in the scoliosis and the lordosis, further correction would require instrumentation to the pelvis. The gain in correction must be weighed against the loss of mobility and added stress transmitted to the ischia.

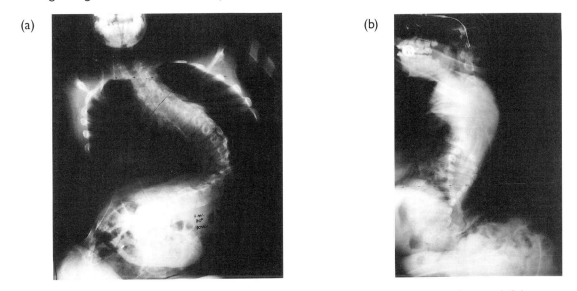

(a)   (b)

Figure 12.27(a,b)   Preoperative AP and lateral radiographs of a 10-year-old girl with spina bifida, severe pelvic obliquity and respiratory compromise. Note the extreme lordosis in addition to the severe scoliosis. She underwent an anterior release and fusion followed by halo-femoral traction and then posterior spinal fusion to the sacrum.

and fixing this to a modified Luque rod (*Figures 12.27, 12.28*). Alternatively, the Galveston technique can be utilized where the pelvis is adequate.

The anterior approach to the scoliotic spine. The technique of the Dwyer procedure is well described in the literature and need not be reiterated. Here we would merely indicate modifications that have significantly reduced operative time.

(a) Incision.   The incision is made over the rib one above the highest vertebral body to be included in the fusion with the patient positioned on the side with the convexity of the curve uppermost. This incision instead of passing across the abdomen, however, is directed towards the iliac crest on the affected side. This allows adequate exposure of the spine and also exposure of the iliac crest for bone graft harvesting.

(a)

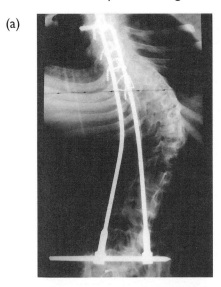

(b)

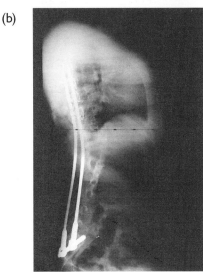

Figure 12.28(a,b) Postoperative AP and lateral radiographs showing the fixation to the pelvis via the sacral bar with sublaminar wires in the thoracic spine. Note that the very extensive bifid spine allowed fixation under only a small number of laminae. Stable fixation was obtained and maintained.

(b) **Division of the diaphragm.** In many descriptions marking sutures are placed in the diaphragm for re-attachment at the time of the closure. We found this to be unnecessary and the diaphragm can be divided using the diathermy and then repaired without problem at the time of closure.

(c) **Ligation of the segmental vessels.** In many instances the segmental vessels can be isolated and divided with diathermy rather than the use of sutures or vacular clips.

(d) **Disc excision.** There are numerous methods of removing the intervertebral discs. We have found the use of a sharp chisel to separate the cartilaginous endplate from the bone of the vertebra allows removal of most of the intervertebral disc in one piece rather than removal piece meal with a nibbler.

(e) **Bone grafting.** We have found that where anterior systems are utilized it is necessary to use a solid bone graft in the intervertebral space to resist kyphosis production. For this reason the blocks of iliac crest are utilized rather than the segmented excised rib.

(f) **Closure and drainage.** If one inspects the lung at the completion of the procedure and there is no air leak visible from an inadvertent injury, then the chest can be closed over a simple Redivac or equivalent drainage system. This obviates the need for an underwater sealed bottle or proprietary drainage system. The standard Redivac drain should be readily available in all operating theatres and is a far less costly device.

Technique for the implantation of the sacral bar. With the patient positioned prone on an appropriate frame or pillows a mid-line incision is made and subcutaneous tissue and muscle layers are dissected off the bony posterior elements of the spine. It is usually easier to start in the intact thoracic spine and work distally and once the bifid area is reached it is possible then to follow the margins of the upturned laminae and transverse processes distally and avoid perforation of the dura. This dissection proceeds distally until the alar of the sacrum is exposed on both sides. To insert the sacral bar, a stab wound is made in the buttock through which the sacral bar will be drilled into the lateral aspect of the ilium passing through both tables of the ilium and into the ipsilateral alar of the sacrum. If the surgeon is not experienced in this technique they may wish to use a K-wire initially to obtain a satisfactory position of the sacral bar.

Once the tip of the sacral bar is seen passing into the superior aspect of the alar of the sacrum it is then drilled through the body of the sacrum passing anterior to the neural canal and posterior to the abdominal contents. The bar then exits along the line of the opposite alar, the exit passing through both tables of the pelvis on the opposite side of the patient (*Figures 12.29, 12.30*).

During the passage of the sacral bar the fixation device is passed over the rod as it enters the alar and a second device is fixed to the rod as it emerges from the body of the sacrum on the opposite side. Then the Luque rods attached to these devices are fixed to the thoracic spine and where possible to the intervening lumbar spine (*Figures 12.31–12.33*).

Technique for pedicle screw fixation. The exposure of the

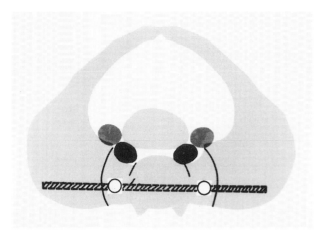

Figure 12.29 Diagramatic representation of the desired passage of the sacral bar through the body of the sacrum, posterior to the great vessels and anterior to the spinal canal.

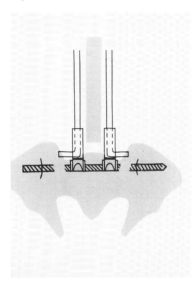

Figure 12.30 Illustration of the connection between the sacral bar and the vertical rods.

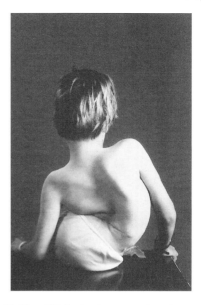

Figure 12.31 Clinical photograph of a spina bifida boy with a severe scoloitic deformity.

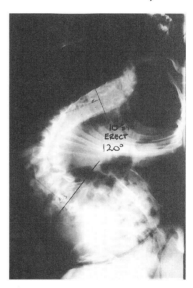

Figure 12.32 AP radiograph of the spine of the boy in *Figure 12.31*.

spine through the mid-line incision is carried out in a standard manner. The levels at which pedicle screw fixation is desired are exposed subperiosteally including both the inner and outer aspects of the pedicles at those levels. Numerous devices have been made for preparation of the whole insertion of pedicle screws into the pedicles; however, the author favours a small curette. The advantage of a small curette is that the blunt end should follow the softer canal of the pedicle and lessen the likelihood of penetration of the cortex as it is recognized that these children are often osteoporotic. Once satisfactory holes have been made in the pedicles of the adjacent vertebrae, pedicle screws are inserted so that prior to implantation of the rods there are four pedicle screws *in situ*. The rods to be fixed to the thoracic spine are then implanted into these pedicle screws and linked by a transverse fixation device. It is necessary to construct a four-screw unit to enable load sharing between the four pedicle screws as the intrinsic strength of the posterior elements of the bifid spine is far less than that of a normal spine. The rods are then brought to the intact thoracic vertebrae and attached with either hooks or sublaminar wires (*Figure 12.34a–c*).

Postoperative care

The initial postoperative period demands close observation to look for shunt malfunction and sepsis. The

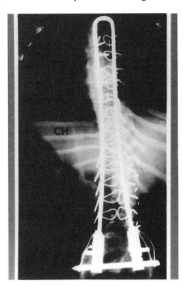

Figure 12.33 Postoperative PA radiograph of the boy in *Figure 12.31* after an anterior release and fusion halo-femoral traction for 2 weeks followed by posterior fusion with a sacral bar and modified Luque rod with sublaminar wires.

patients are maintained on minimal fluid loads to lessen the shunt demands. The patients are often small and the surgical procedures long and demanding and thus blood losses must be carefully monitored so replacements are adequate. Prophylactic antibiotics are routinely employed. The patients are nursed flat in bed initially with log-rolling, taking care to look for pres-

sure areas in insensate parts of the body. The degree of stability of the spinal implant construction will dictate the mobility allowed. Most patients are fitted with a polypropylene brace, with front and back shells and shoulder straps that provides support but can be removed for bathing and skin care. Caution should be exercised with regard to sitting and wheelchair use until fusion is assured.

Complications

Risk of sudden death
In many of the series published there are patients who died unexpectedly in the postoperative period (Winston *et al.*, 1977). This may be due to insufficiency of the CSF shunt under the increased stresses of a major surgical and physiological insult. Intracerebral haemorrhage has also caused sudden death; however, this may also be due to shunt insuffuciency.

Hardware failure
Hook pullout, hook–rod dissociation and rod fracture are a significant concern in all methods of instrumentation. This arises from a combination of poor bone stock and dysplastic bone that is extensively stripped during the surgical approach. Delay in fusion is common. An anterior approach affords an increased area for fusion and also increases the flexibility of the spine which reduces the load in implants during correction of deformity.

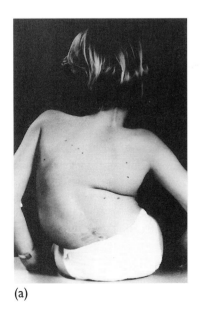

(a)

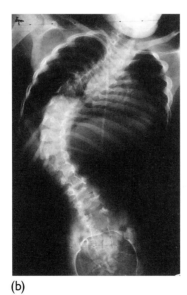

(b)

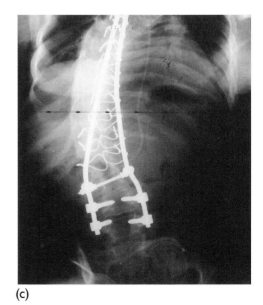

(c)

Figure 12.34(a–c)   Clinical photograph, pre- and postoperative radiographs of a spina bifida boy aged 10 years at the time of surgery. He underwent both an anterior and posterior spinal fusion utilizing the pedicle screw technique as described.

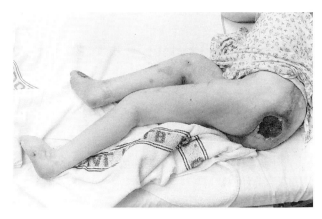

Figure 12.35 Clinical photograph of a teenage girl who had a fusion to the sacrum following a kyphectomy. She developed an acute kyphosis as her sacroiliac joints became unstable and this led to deformity and pressure on the posterior aspect of the sacrum and skin breakdown.

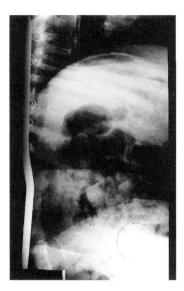

Figure 12.37 Lateral radiograph of the same girl in sitting. Note the displacement of the femoral heads in relation to the sacrum (i.e. the end of the rod). This indicates gross motion through the sacroiliac joints.

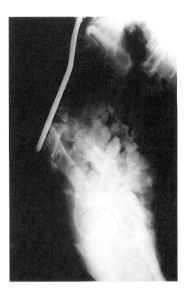

Figure 12.36 Lateral radiograph of the lumbosacral spine of the girl lying prone showing the relationship of the femoral heads to the sacrum.

Progression of deformity

This may occur with hardware failure but may also arise in the presence of a solid fusion with deformity progressing at the next unfused level either proximally or distally (*Figures 12.35–12.37*).

Infection

Intraoperative and postoperative antibiotic administration is routine in these children. Any focus of contamination or infection must be sought out in the preoperative work-up. During surgery tissues must be treated with great care to avoid necrosis and dead spaces must be eliminated.

Cerebrospinal fluid drainage

All children with spina bifida will have scarring of the dura and any surgical exposure of the vertebrae may result in the dura being opened. This is intentional in correcting the 'kyphotics'. The dural opening should be repaired where possible. Patches of muscle or fascia can be employed. If there is persistent CSF leakage that cannot be surgically addressed a long drain tube from the surgical site is passed subcutaneously to exit some distance from the wound. The drain is then gradually shortened in the postoperative period. On occasions a CSF fistula will require formal exploration and repair.

Chapter 13

Anaesthesia

Kester Brown

A remarkable feature of anaesthesia for patients with spina bifida is the scant reference to the subject in the literature. This account is an update of the chapter in the second edition of this work by W H J Cole who had extensive experience in the anaesthetic management of these patients.

It is necessary to include all the factors that together make up good anaesthesia practice. General anaesthesia is usually the preferred method. Certain points are important – careful handling of induction and recovery so that emotional disturbances are minimized, conservation of superficial veins, selecting a time for operation when the child is in an optimal state of general health, and adequate volume replacement including blood when significant blood loss occurs.

General Health

The child's general health is frequently not as good as that of a normal child of the same age. Because of the reduced activity of the child there is commonly reduced pulmonary function. Up to the age of 3 years there is generally reduced weight for age; over the age of 4 years, obesity is common.

Mental State and Effect of Previous Anaesthetics

About one-third of these children have intellectual impairment with or without emotional disturbances. Intellectual disability and emotional problems increase the difficulties of those who have the responsibility of providing medical care; complications may have a greater adverse effect in the intellectually impaired child.

Most of these children have had surgery early in life. In some, an effect of this has been to create an emotional disturbance manifested by a fear of anaesthetics, operations and operating theatres. It has been shown that orthopaedic operations hold more fear than do any other procedures for spina bifida children. Apprehension and fear can be reduced by adequate premedication and the presence of a parent at the induction of anaesthesia can provide reassurance to the child and help to the anaesthetist in handling these patients.

Venous Access

Venous access in the legs is less distressing to the child if sensation is diminished. The veins are often very small and fragile and some may have been damaged by previous intravenous therapy. An external jugular vein or other central venous access may be necessary. As few veins as possible should be transgressed and continuous infusions should be guarded carefully.

Neurological Defects

Although there is diminution of sensation in the lower extremities this is not usually of such a degree that one can employ unusually light depths of anaesthesia or omit anaesthetic procedures completely. One would expect that there would be some reduction of autonomic control of blood vessels in the legs, so that increased vigilance should be exercised in relation to blood loss.

Oral Health

Varying degrees of dental caries, and gingival infection are common. Such conditions constitute an additional danger to the patient and to the anaesthetist.

Preanaesthetic Assessment and Preparation for Anaesthesia

Since children suffering from spina bifida are less able than normal children to overcome complications it is advisable that the child be as fit as possible at the time of operation and be free of any infections. It is important to remember that more than two-thirds of children with spina bifida are normal intellectually. Impairment is usually associated with hydrocephalus.

Anaesthetic Procedures

Because of the neurological disorder it is desirable to employ general anaesthesia for all operations. Experience suggests that drug responses in these patients do not differ from those in normal children and that sensitization to anaesthetic agents is rare or non-existent in these patients.

If venous access is obtained anaesthesia can be induced with a suitable dose of intravenous anaesthetic agent. Some children fear the needle and ask to breathe an inhalation anaesthetic; non-irritating inhalational anaesthetic agents enable rapid and seemingly pleasant induction particularly with sevoflurane.

A less commonly used alternative is to give an intramuscular injection of ketamine ($4 \, mg \, kg^{-1}$ of body weight) to produce unconsciousness.

Anaesthesia is maintained by administering nitrous oxide plus an inhalational supplement. A satisfactory method is with the patient breathing spontaneously with a face or laryngeal mask. This is applicable to all operative procedures in which the patient lies on the back and in which there is no major blood loss. In many instances the method is applicable with the patient turned to a lateral position.

Endotracheal anaesthesia is desirable when the patient lies in the prone position and may also be used in major procedures that are longer and are associated with significant blood loss.

Major hip surgery may involve major blood loss and require blood transfusion. It is indicated when blood loss exceeds 20% of blood volume, which is $70 \, ml \, kg^{-1}$, there are continuing losses, or when the blood pressure is not maintained with other fluids. If the patient is anaemic, preoperatively transfusion may begin earlier. As bleeding commonly continues during the early postoperative period the rate of drainage into the suction bottle should be observed frequently. Blood loss should be replaced if the patient is already being transfused or signs of hypovolaemia develop.

For operations designed to correct kyphosis and other procedures that involve blood losses which are large in relation to the blood volume of the patient, it is desirable to have an infusion set with a large-bore cannula and a transfusion pump so that replacement at a rapid rate can be achieved. Blood pressure must be monitored. During operation, blood loss can be estimated by pack weighing and observation of the amount of blood in the sucker bottle.

Blood Loss and Induced Hypotension in Scoliosis Surgery

Blood loss can be significant during scoliosis surgery although the total loss tends to decrease with experience, especially when the same anaesthetist is working with the same surgical team. Induced hypotension can substantially reduce operative blood loss (from over $40-50 \, ml \, kg^{-1}$ to less than $10 \, ml \, kg^{-1}$). This reduction in blood loss is accompanied by much shorter operating time because the surgeon has a clearer view of the operating field and does not have to spend time removing blood from the site.

Various drugs have been used to induce hypotension. The direct vascular smooth muscle dilator, sodium nitroprusside, has been used as an intravenous infusion providing easily controlled conditions due to its very short action. The blood pressure rises to normal within 5 minutes of stopping the infusion. The rate is controlled either with a pump or with a device such as the 'Dial a flow' which allows fine control of flow to maintain a systolic pressure of 60–70 mmHg. Usually 50 mg of sodium nitroprusside is diluted in 500 ml of fluid ($1 \, mg \, kg^{-1}$ in 100 ml in a burette makes it easy to know the dose given in smaller children). The rate of infusion should not exceed $3 \, mg \, kg^{-1}$ over a 4-hour period. If the desired pressure cannot be achieved with flows less than this, there is a danger of toxicity. This should not happen as other drugs with hypotensive actions are often used in combination with, or as an alternative to, sodium nitroprusside. Isoflurane, which lowers blood pressure by a peripheral action, is often used instead of halothane, which achieves hypotension mainly by myocardial depression. Esmolol, a very short-acting beta adrenergic blocker can also be used by infusion to slow heart rate and reduce myocardial contractility.

Blood pressure monitoring is important when

this technique is used. Continuous read out from an intra-arterial line is usually recommended but the technique may be used with frequent blood pressure measurements using a non-invasive monitor.

When patients are vasodilated it is important to give extra intravenous fluids to maintain an adequate blood volume.

LATEX ALLERGY AND ANAPHYLAXIS

These patients, particularly if they have had many operations, have often been exposed to latex in such things as urinary catheters and surgical gloves. They, therefore, have an increased likelihood of sensitization. Difficulty blowing up a balloon may be a clue to this. It is important for anaesthetists to recognise the signs of anaphylaxis – usually bronchospasm and/or hypotension – and to institute rapidly treatment with adrenaline and intravenous fluids, including colloids, so that fatalities are avoided.

Latex is present in many items used in the operating theatre and special precautions should be taken to ensure a latex-free environment if patients are known to be susceptible.

References and Further Reading

Abraham E, Verinder DGR & Sharrard WJW (1977) The treatment of flexion contracture of the knee in myelomeningocele. *Journal of Bone and Joint Surgery*, **59(B)**, 433.

Abraham E, Lubicky JP, Songer MN & Millar EA (1996) Supramalleolar osteotomy for ankle valgus in myelomeningocele. *Journal of Pediatric Orthopaedics*, **16**, 774.

Adams RD, Denny-Brown D & Pearson CM (1962) *Diseases of Muscle*, 2nd edn., p. 310. New York: Hoeber.

Allen BLJ & Ferguson RL (1979). The operative treatment of myelomeningocoele spinal deformity. *Orthopedic Clinics of North America*, **10**, 845.

Alliaume A (1950) Fracture des os longs dans les myelomeningoceles. *Archives francaises de pediatrie*, **7**, 294.

Alman BA, Bhandari M & Wright JG (1996) Function of dislocated hips in children with lower level spina bifida. *Journal of Bone and Joint Surgery*, **78(B)**, 294.

Anderson EM (1973) Cognitive deficits in children with spina bifida and hydrocephalus: a review of the literature. *British Journal of Educational Psychology*, **43**, 257.

Anderson E (1976) Impairment of motor (manual) skill in children with spina bifida, myelomeningocele and hydrocephalus. *British Journal of Occupational Therapy*, **39(4)**, 91.

Anderson EM & Spain B (1977) *The Child with Spina Bifida*. London: Methuen.

Anschuetz R, Freehafer A, Shaffer J & Dixon M (1984) Severe fracture complications in myelodysplasia. *Journal of Pediatric Orthopaedics*, **4**, 22.

Appleton PL, Minchom PE, Ellis NC, Elliott CE, Boll V & Jones P (1994) The self concept of young people with spina bifida: A population based study. *Developmental Medicine and Child Neurology*, **36(3)**, 198.

Aronson DD & Middleton DL (1991) Extra-articular subtalar arthrodesis with cancellous bone graft and internal fixation for children with myelomeningocele. *Developmental Medicine and Child Neurology*, **33(3)**: 232.

Aronson DD, Kahn RH, Canady A, Bollinger RO & Towbin R (1991) Instability of the cervical spine after decompression in patients who have Arnold–Chiari malformation. *Journal of Bone and Joint Surgery*, **73A**, 898.

Arregui J, Cannon B, Murray J & O'Leary JJ (1965) Long term evaluation of ischiectomy in the treatment of pressure ulcers. *Plastic and Reconstructive Surgery*, **36(6)**, 583.

ASAMI Group (1991) *Operative Principles of Ilizarov* (ed. by Bianchi Maiocchi A & Aronson J). Milan: Williams & Wilkins.

Asher M & Olson J (1983) Factors affecting the ambulatory status of patients with spina bifida cystica. *Journal of Bone and Joint Surgery*, **65(A)**, 350.

Atar D, Grant AD & Lehman WB (1990) New approach to limb deformities in neuromuscular patients. *Bulletin of the Hospital for Joint Diseases Orthopaedic Institute*, **50(2)**, 99.

Bailey BN (1967) *Bedsores*. London: Arnold.

Baker RH & Sharrard WJW (1973) Correction of lordoscoliosis in spina bifida by multiple spinal osteotomy and fusion with Dwyer fixation: a preliminary report. *Developmental Medicine and Child Neurology*, Suppl., **29**, 12.

Banta JV & Hamada JS (1976) Natural history of kyphotic deformity on myelomeningocoele. *Journal of Bone and Joint Surgery*, **58(A)**, 279.

Banta JV, Sutherland DH & Wyatt M (1981) Anterior tibial transfer to the os calcis with Achilles tenodesis for calcaneal deformity in myelomeningocele. *Journal of Pediatric Orthopaedics*, **1**, 125.

Banta JV, Lin R, Peterson M & Daganais T (1990) The team approach in the care of the child with myelomeningocele. *Journal of Prosthetics and Orthotics*, **2**, 263.

Banta JV, Bonnani C & Prebluda J (1993) Latex anaphylaxis during spinal surgery in children with myelomeningocele. *Developmental Medicine and Child Neurology*, **35(6)**, 543.

Barakat LP & Linney JA (1992) Children with physical handicaps and their mothers: The interrelation of social support in maternal adjustment and child adjustment. *Journal of Pediatric Psychology*, **17(6)**, 725.

Barden GA, Meyer LC & Stelling FH (1975) Myelodysplastics: fate of those followed for twenty years or more. *Journal of Bone and Joint Surgery*, **57(A)**, 643.

Barr JS (1950) Poliomyelitic hip deformity and the erector spinae transplant. *Journal of the American Medical Association*, **144**, 813.

Barson AJ (1970) Spina bifida: the significance of the level and extent of the defect to the morphogenesis. *Developmental Medicine and Child Neurology*, **12(2)**, 129.

Bax MCO, Smyth DPL & Thomas AP (1988) Health care of physically handicapped adults. *British Medical Journal*, **296**, 1153.

Bazih J & Gross RH (1981) Hip surgery in the lumbar level myelomenongocele patient. *Journal of Pediatric Orthopaedics*, **1**, 405.

Beal S (1967) The occurrence of spina bifida cystica in South Australia. *Medical Journal of Australia*, **2(13)**, 597.

Beckman J (1987) The Louisiana State University Reciprocating Gait Orthoses. *Physiotherapy*, **73**, 386.

Beeker TW & Scheers MM (1986) The hip joint in spina bifida accompanied by myelomeningocele: A review of cases in a spina bifida team. *Neuro Orthopaedics*, **2**, 87.

Bensman A, Long D, Merrill D, Horrobin M, Easton J & Lai C (1971) Myelomeningocele birth defect.

Habilitation of the child. *Minnesota Medicine*, **54(8)**, 599.

Benton IJ, Salvati EA & Root L (1975) Reconstructive surgery in the myelomeningocele hip. *Clinical Orthopaedics and Related Research*, **110**, 261.

Bernstein ML, Esseltine D, Azouz EM & Forbes P (1989) Deep venous thrombosis complicating myelomeningocele: report of three cases. *Pediatrics*, **84(5)**, 856.

Birch R (1976) Surgery of the knee in children with spina bifida. *Developmental Medicine and Child Neurology*, Suppl. 37, **18(6)**, 111.

Bliss DG & Menelaus MB (1986) The results of transfer of tibialis anterior to the heel in patients who have a myelomeningocele. *Journal of Bone and Joint Surgery*, **68(B)**, 1258.

Blum RW (1983) The adolescent with spina bifida. *Clinical Paediatrics (Adolescent Medicine)*, **22(5)**, 331.

Blum RW, Resnick ND, Nelson R & St Germaine A (1991) Family and peer issues among adolescents with spina bifida and cerebral palsy. *Pediatrics*, **88**, 2.

Boothman R (1975) Some observations on the management of the child with a spina bifida. *British Medical Journal*, **1(5950)**, 145.

Brinker MR, Rosenfeld SR, Feiwell E, Granger SP, Mitchell DC & Rice JC (1994) Myelomeningocele at the sacral level: Long-term outcome in adults. *Journal of Bone and Joint Surgery*, **76(A)**, 1293.

Brocklehurst G (1976) Spina bifida for the clinician. *Clinics in Developmental Medicine*, No. 57. London: Heinemann.

Broome HL & Basmajian JV (1971) Survival of iliopsoas muscle after Sharrard procedure. An electromyographic study. *American Journal of Physical Medicine*, **50(6)**, 301.

Broughton NS, Wright J & Menelaus MB (1993a) Range of knee motion in normal neonates. *Journal of Pediatric Orthopaedics*, **13**, 263.

Broughton NS, Menelaus MB, Cole WG & Shurtleff DB (1993b) The natural history of hip deformity in myelomeningocele. *Journal of Bone and Joint Surgery*, **75(B)**, 760.

Broughton NS, Graham G & Menelaus MB (1994) The high incidence of foot deformity in patients with high level spina bifida. *Journal of Bone and Joint Surgery*, **76(B)**, 548.

Brown A (1965) Paralytic lesions: orthopaedic procedures. In *Symposium on Spina Bifida, London, 1965. Proceedings*. London: National Fund for Research into Poliomyelitis and other Crippling Diseases. (Action for the Crippled Child Monograph.)

Buisson JS & Hamblen DL (1972) Electromyographic assessment of the transplanted iliopsoas muscle in spina bifida cystica. *Developmental Medicine and Child Neurology*, Suppl. 27, 29.

Burkus JK, Moore DW & Raycroft JF (1983) Valgus deformity of the ankle in meylodysplastic patients. *Journal of Bone and Joint Surgery* **65(A)**, 1157.

Burney DW & Hasma WR (1963) Spina bifida with

myelomeningocele. *Clinical Orthopaedics and Related Research*, **30**, 167.

Butler P & Major R (1987) The parawalker – a rational approach to the provision of reciprocal ambulation for paraplegic patients. *Physiotherapy*, **73(8)**, 393.

Cameron AH (1956) The spinal cord lesion in spina bifida cystica. *Lancet*, **2**, 171.

Canale ST, Hammond NL, Cotler JM & Snedden HE (1975) Pelvic displacement osteotomy for chronic hip dislocation in myelodysplasia. *Journal of Bone and Joint Surgery*, **57(A)**, 177.

Capelli M, McGrath PJ, Daniels T, Manion I & Shillenger J (1994) Marital quality of parents of children with spina bifida: A case comparison study. *Journal of Developmental and Behavioural Paediatrics*, **15(5)**, 320.

Carlioz H, de la Caffiniere JY & Queneau P (1971) 22 psoas transplantations by Sharrard's method. *Revue de Chirurgie Orthopedique et Reparatrice de L'appareil Moteur*, **57**, Suppl. 1, 187.

Carr TL (1956) The orthopaedic aspects of one hundred cases of spina bifida. *Postgraduate Medical Journal*, **32**, 201.

Carroll NC (1987) Assessment and management of the lower extremity in myelodysplasia. *Orthopedic Clinics of North America*, **18**, 709.

Carroll NC & Sharrard, WJ (1972) Long-term follow-up of posterior iliopsoas transplantation for paralytic dislocation of the hip. *Journal of Bone and Joint Surgery*, **54(A)**, 551.

Carstens C, Schmidt E, Fromm B & Schiltenwolf M (1992) Results of surgical therapy of knee flexion contractions in patients with myelomeningocele. *Zeitschrift fur Orthopadie und Ihre Grenzgebiete*, **130**, 207.

Carter CO (1969) Spina bifida and anencephaly: a problem in genetic–environmental interaction. *Journal of Biological Sciences*, **1**, 71.

Carter CO 1976) Genetics of common simple malformations. *British Medical Bulletin*, **32**, 21.

Carter CO & Evans K (1973a) Children of adult survivors with spina bifida cystica. *Lancet*, **2**, 924.

Carter CO & Evans K (1973b) Spina bifida and anencephalus in Greater London. *Journal of Medical Genetics*, **10**, 209.

Carter CO & Fraser Roberts JA (1967) The risk of recurrence after two children with central nervous system malformation. *Lancet*, **1**, 306.

Carter CO, Evans KA & Till K (1976) Spinal dysraphism: a genetic relation to neural tube malformation. *Journal of Medical Genetics*, **13**, 343.

Cecotto C (1968) Myelo-vertebral malformations. *Policlinico Sezione Pratica*, **76(19)**, 615.

Chakour K (1971) Deformities of the lower extremities and prosthetic devices in children with myelodysplasia. *Archiv fur Orthopadische und Unfall-Chirurgie*, **70(2)**, 101.

Charney E, Melchionni J & Smith D (1991) Community ambulation by children with myelomeningocele and high-level paralysis. *Journal of Pediatric Orthopaedics*, **11**, 579.

Cherny WB, Boop FA *et al.* (1995) Bloodless kyphectomy for correction of neonatal kyphoscoliosis.

Chiari (1974) Medial displacement osteotomy of the pelvis. *Clinical Orthopaedics and Related Research*, **98**, 55.

Cholmeley JA (1953) Elmslie's operation for the calcaneus foot. *Journal of Bone and Joint Surgery*, **35(B)**, 46.

Chuinard EG & Peterson RE (1963) Distraction–compression bone-graft arthrodesis of the ankle: a method especially applicable in children. *Journal of Bone and Joint Surgery*, **45(A)**, 481.

Cochran JH Jr, Edstrom LE & Dibbell DG (1981) Usefulness of the innervated tensor fascia lata flap in paraplegic patients. *Annals of Plastic Surgery*, **7(4)**, 286.

Coleman JJ & Jurkiewicz MJ (1984) Methods of providing sensation to anaesthetic areas. *Annals of Plastic Surgery*, **12(2)**, 177.

Collman RD & Stoller A (1962) Epidemiology of congenital anomalies of the central nervous system with special reference to patterns in the state of Victoria, Australia. *Journal of Mental Deficiency Research*, **6**, 22.

Colonna PC (1936) An arthroplastic operation for congenital dislocation of the hip: a two stage procedure. *Surgery, Gynaecology and Obstetrics*, **63**, 777.

Corry IS, Duffy CM, Cosgrove AP & Graham HK (1996) Measurement of oxygen consumption in disabled children by the cosmed K2 portable telemetry system. *Developmental Medicine and Child Neurology*, **38**, 585.

Cotrel Y & Dubousset J (1984) Nouvelle technique d'osteosynthese rachidienne segmentaire par voie posterieure. *Rev. Arch. Ortoped*, **70**, 489.

Cotta H, Parsch K & Schulitz KP (1971) The treatment of lumbar kyphosis in spina bifida cystica. *Zeitschrift fuer Orthopadie und ihre Grenzgebiete*, **108(4)**, 567.

Crandall RC, Birkebak RC & Winter RB (1989) The role of hip location and dislocation in the functional status of the myelodysplastic patient. A review of 100 patients. *Orthopedics*, **12**, 675.

Cruess RL & Turner NS (1970) Paralysis of hip abductor muscles in spina bifida. Results of treatment by the Mustard procedure. *Journal of Bone and Joint Surgery*, **52(A)**, 1364.

Curtis BH (1973) The hip in the myelomeningocele child. *Clinical Orthopaedics and Related Research*, **90**, 11.

Czeizel A & Dudas I (1992) Prevention of first occurrence of neural tube defects by periconceptional vitamin supplementation. *New England Journal of Medicine*, **327**, 1832.

Daniel RK & Faibisoff B (1982) Muscle coverage of pressure points – the role of myocutaneous flaps. *Annals of Plastic Surgery*, **8(6)**, 446.

Daniel RK, Terzis JK & Cunningham DM (1976) Sensory skin flaps for coverage of pressure sores in paraplegic patients. *Plastic and Reconstructive Surgery*, **58(3)**, 317.

Daniel RK, Kerrigan CL & Gard DA (1978) The great potential of the intercostal flap for torso reconstruction. *Plastic and Reconstructive Surgery*, **61(5)**, 653.

Davidson H (1994) The Isocentric Reciprocating Gait Orthosis. *Association of Prosthetists and Orthotists Newsletter*, **1**.

Davidson RG & Sheffield LJ (1978) Hazards of prenatal detection of neural tube defects by screening material serum for alpha fetoprotein. *Canadian Medical Association Journal*, **118**, 1186.

Davis JB (1977) The salop skate. *Physiotherapy*, **63(4)**, 115.

de Carvalho Neto J, Dias LS & Gabrieli AP (1996) Congenital talipes equinovarus in spina bifida: Treatment and results. *Journal of Pediatric Orthopaedics*, **16**, 782.

De Sousa L & Carroll N (1976) Ambulation of the braced myelomeningocele patient. *Journal of Bone and Joint Surgery*, **58(B)**, 1112.

De Vries E (1928) Spina bifida occulta and myelodysplasia with unilateral clubfoot beginning in adult life. *American Journal of the Medical Sciences*, **175**, 365.

Dias LS (1982) Surgical management of knee contractures in myelomeningocele. *Journal of Pediatric Orthopaedics*, **2**, 127.

Dias LS (1983) Hip. In *Myelomeningocele: Orthopaedic Treatment* (ed. by Schafer MF & Dias LS), p. 105. Baltimore: Williams & Wilkins.

Dias LS (1985) Valgus deformity of the ankle joint: pathogenesis of fibular shortening *Journal of Pediatric Orthopaedics*, **5(2)**, 176.

Dibell DG (1974) Use of a long island flap to bring sensation to the sacral area in young paraplegics. *Plastic and Reconstructive Surgery*, **54(2)**, 220.

Dibell DG, McCraw JB & Edstrom LE (1979) Providing useful and protective sensibility to the sitting area in patients with meningomyelocele. *Plastic and Reconstructive Surgery*, **64(6)**, 796.

Diokno AC, Kass E & Lapides J (1976) A new approach to myelodysplasia. *Journal of Urology*, **116**, 771.

Donaldson WF (1972) Hip problems in the child with myelomeningocele. *American Academy of Orthopaedic Surgeons Symposium on Myelomeningocele*, p. 176. St Louis: CV Mosby.

Donaldson WF (1974) Neural spinal dysraphism. In *Spinal Deformity in Neurological and Muscular Disorders*, p. 140. St. Louis: CV Mosby.

Doran PA & Guthkelch AN (1961) Studies in spina bifida cystica. *Journal of Neurology Neurosurgery and Psychiatry*, **24**, 331.

Doran PA & Guthkelch AN (1963) Studies on spina bifida. IV. The frequency and extent of the paralysis. *Journal of Neurology Neurosurgery and Psychiatry*, **26**, 545.

Dorner S (1975) The relationship of physical handicap to stress in families with an adolescent with spina bifida. *Developmental Medicine and Child Neurology*, **17**, 765.

Dorner S (1976) Adolescents with spina bifida: How they

see their situation. *Archives of Disorders of Childhood*, **51**, 539.

Dorner S (1977) Sexual interest and activity in adolescents with spina bifida. *Journal of Child Psychology and Psychiatry*, **18**, 229.

Drennan JC (1976) Orthotic management of the myelomeningocele spine. *Developmental Medicine and Child Neurology*, **18**, Suppl. 37, 97.

Drennan JC & Sharrard WJ (1971) The pathological anatomy of convex pes valgus. *Journal of Bone and Joint Surgery*, **53(B)**, 455.

Duckworth T & Smith TW (1974) The treatment of paralytic convex pes valgus. *Journal of Bone and Joint Surgery*, **56(B)**, 305.

Duffy CM, Hill AE, Cosgrove AP, Corry IS & Graham HK (1996a) Energy consumption in children with spina bifida and cerebral palsy: A comparative study. *Developmental Neurology and Child Neurology*, **38**, 238.

Duffy CM, Hill AE, Cosgrove AP, Corry IS, Mollan RAB & Graham HK (1996b) Three dimensional gait analysis in spina bifida. *Journal of Pediatric Orthopaedics*, **16**, 786.

Duffy CM, Hill AE, Cosgrove AP, Corry IS & Graham HK (1996c) The influence of abductor weakness on gait in spina bifida. *Gait and Posture*, **4**, 34.

Duffy CM, Hill AE & Graham HK (1997) The influence of flexed knee gait on the energy cost of walking in children. *Developmental Medicine and Child Neurology*, **39**, 239.

Duncan JW, Lovell WW, Bailey SC & Ransom D (1976) Surgical treatment of kyphosis in myelomeningocele. *Journal of Bone and Joint Surgery*, **58(A)**, 155.

Dunne KB, Gingher N, Olsen LM & Shurtleff DB (1986) A survey of the medical and functional status of members of the adult network of the Spina Bifida Association of America. Washington DC: Spina Bifida Association of America.

Dunne KB, Bishop J, Wright S & Menelaus MB (1992) Are adults with spina bifida receiving adequate medical and rehabilitation care? *Developmental Medicine and Child Neurology*, **34(9)** Suppl. 66.

Dunne KB, Arata M, Grover S & Bryan AD (1996) Pregnancy in women with spina bifida – antenatal complications. *Developmental Medicine and Child Neurology*, **38(8)**, Suppl. 74, 7.

Dupré PH & Walker G (1972) Knee problems associated with spina bifida. *Developmental Medicine and Child Neurology*, Suppl. 27, 152.

Dwyer AF (1968) Screw and cable correction of scoliosis. (Abstract). In British Medical Association/Australian Medical Association Joint Annual Meeting and Third Australian Medical Congress. *Medical Journal of Australia*, **2**, Suppl. 39.

Dwyer AF, Newton NC & Sherwood AA (1969) An anterior approach to scoliosis. A preliminary report. *Clinical Orthopaedics and Related Research*, **62**, 192.

Dwyer FC (1959) Osteotomy of the calcaneum for pescavus. *Journal of Bone and Joint Surgery*, **41(B)**, 80.

Dziakas P (1968) On the sternal muscle in abnormalities with craniorachischisis. (German) *Anatomischer Anzeiger*, **122(2)**, 156.

Eckstein HB & Vora RM (1972) Spinal osteotomy for severe kyphosis in children with myelomeningocele. *Journal of Bone and Joint Surgery*, **54(B)**, 328.

Edvardsen P (1972) Physeo-epiphyseal injuries of lower extremities in myelomeningocele. *Acta orthopedica scandinavica*, **43(6)**, 550.

Eggers GWN (1952) Transplantation of hamstring tendons to femoral condyles in order to improve hip extension and to decrease knee flexion in cerebral spastic paralysis. *Journal of Bone and Joint Surgery*, **34(A)**, 827.

Ekus L & McHugh LA (1987) A new look at the RGO protocol. *Clinical Prosthetics and Orthotics*, **11(2)**, 79.

Emery JL (1974) Deformity of the aqueduct of sylvius in children with hydrocephalus and myelomeningocele. *Developmental Medicine and Child Neurology*, **16**, 40.

Evans D (1961) Relapsed club foot. *Journal of Bone and Joint Surgery*, **43(B)**, 722.

Evans K, Hickman V & Carter CO (1974) Handicap and social status of adults with spina bifida cysticia. *British Journal of Preventive and Social Medicine*, **28**, 85.

Eyring EJ, Wanken JJ & Sayers MP (1972) Spine osteotomy for kyphosis in myelomeningocele. *Clinical Orthopaedics and Related Research*, **88**, 24.

Feiwell E, Sakai D & Blatt T (1978) The effect of hip reduction on function in patients with myelomeningocele. *Journal of Bone and Joint Surgery*, **60(A)**, 169.

Feller A & Sternberg H (1929) Die Wirbelkorperspalt und ihre formale Genese. *Virchows Archiv*, **272**, 613.

Field B (1977) Surveillance of malformations in Sydney in 1976. *Medical Journal of Australia*, **2**, 797.

Fillauer Incorporated (1993) *Reciprocating Gait Orthosis Including the Horizontal Cable System*. A pictorial description and application manual. PO Box 5189 Chattanooga, Tennessee.

Filler AG, Britton JA, Uttley D & Marsh HT (1995) Adult post repair myelomeningocele and tethered cord syndrome: good surgical outcome after abrupt neurological decline. *British Journal of Neurosurgery*, **9(5)**, 659.

Fitzpatrick WF (1974) Sexual function in the paraplegic patient. *Archives of Physical Medicine and Rehabilitation*, **55**, 221.

Flandry F, Burke S, Roberts J *et al.* (1986) Functional ambulation in myelodysplasia: The effect of orthotic selection on physical and physiologic performance. *Journal of Pediatric Orthopaedics*, **6(6)**, 661.

Forrest D (1974) Spina bifida, practical and ethical considerations in its treatment. *Modern Medicine*, **17**, 108.

Fraser FC (1974) Genetic counselling. *American Journal of Human Genetics*, **26**, 636.

Fraser RK & Hoffman EB (1991) Calcaneus deformity in the ambulant patient with myelomeningocele. *Journal of Bone and Joint Surgery*, **73(B)**, 994.

Fraser RK & Menelaus MB (1993) The management of

tibial torsion in patients with spina bifida. *Journal of Bone and Joint Surgery*, **75(B)**, 495.

Fraser RK, Bourke HM, Broughton NS & Menelaus MB (1995) Unilateral dislocation of the hip in spina bifida. A long-term follow-up. *Journal of Bone and Joint Surgery*, **77(B)**, 615.

Frawley PA, Broughton NS & Menelaus MB (1996) Anterior release for fixed flexion deformity of the hip in spina bifida. *Journal of Bone and Joint Surgery*, **78(B)**, 299.

Frawley P, Broughton NS & Menelaus MB (1998) The incidence of foot deformities in low level spina bifida patients. *Journal of Pediatric Orthopaedics* (in press).

Freehafer AA, Vessely JC & Mack RP (1972) Iliopsoas muscle transfer in the treatment of myelomeningocele patients with paralytic hip deformities. *Journal of Bone and Joint Surgery*, **54(A)**, 1715.

Freeman JM (1974) *Practical Management of Meningomyelocele*. Baltimore: University Park Press.

Fuchs A (1909) Uber den Klinischen Nachweis kongenitaler Defektbildungen in den unteren Ruckenmarksabschnitten ('Myelodysplasie'). *Wiener medizinische Wochenschrift*, **(59)**, 2141, 2261.

Furman L & Mortimer JC (1994) Menarche and menstrual function in patients with myelomeningocele. *Developmental Medicine and Child Neurology*, **36(10)**, 910.

Gage JR (1991) Gait analysis in cerebral palsy. *Clinics in Developmental Medicine*, No. **121**. London: MacKeith Press.

Gallien R, Morin F & Marquis F (1989) Subtalar arthrodesis in children. *Journal of Pediatric Orthopaedics*, **9(1)**, 59.

Gardner WJ (1968) Myelocele: rupture of the neural tube? *Clinical Neurology and Neurosurgery*, **15**, 57–59.

Georgiadis GM & Aronson DD (1990) Posterior transfer of the anterior tibial tendon in children who have a myelomeningocele. *Journal of Bone and Joint Surgery*, **72(3)**, 392.

Ger R & Levine SA (1976) The management of decubitus ulcers by muscle transposition. *Plastic and Reconstructive Surgery*, **58(4)**, 419.

Gilbert JN, Jones KL, Rorke LB, Chernoff GF & James HE (1986) Central nervous system anomalies associated with meningomyelocele, hydrocephalus and the Arnold–Chiari malformation: re-appraisal of theories regarding the pathogenesis of posterior neural tube closure defects. *Neurosurgery*, **18**, 559.

Gillespie RB & Wedge JH (1974) The problems of scoliosis in paraplegic children. *Journal of Bone and Joint Surgery*, **56(A)**, 1767.

Goessens H & Parsch K (1971) Surgical treatment of knee and foot deformities in spina bifida. *Acta orthopaedica belgica*, **37(3)**, 216.

Goldsmith S (1967) *Designing for the Disabled*. McGraw-Hill.

Goldstein F & Kepes JJ (1966) The role of traction in the development of the Arnold–Chiari malformation. An experimental study. *Journal of Neuropathology and Experimental Neurology*, **25**, 654.

Golski A & Menelaus MB (1976) The treatment of intoed gait in spina bifida patients by lateral transfer of the medial hamstrings. *Australian and New Zealand Journal of Surgery*, **46(2)**, 157.

Gordon YB, Kitau MJ, Letchworth AT, Grudzinfkas JH, Usherwood M McD & Chard T (1978) Fetal wastage as a result of an alpha-fetoprotein screening program. *Lancet*, **1(8066)**, 677.

Gressang J (1974) Perceptual processes of children with myelomeningocele and hydrocephalus. *American Journal of Occupational Therapy*, **28(4)**, 226.

Grice DS (1952) An extra-articular arthrodesis of the subastragalar joint for the correction of paralytic flat feet in children. *Journal of Bone and Joint Surgery*, **37(A)**, 246.

Grice DS (1955) Further experience with extra-articular arthrodesis of the subtalar joint. *Journal of Bone and Joint Surgery*, **37**, 246.

Griffith ER, Tonks MA & Timms RJ (1973) Sexual function in spinal cord injured patients; a review. *Archives of Physical Medicine and Rehabilitation*, **54**, 539.

Grimm R (1976) Hand function and tactile perception in a sample of children with myelomeningocele. *American Journal of Occupational Therapy*, **30(4)**, 234.

Gucker T, III (1964) The role of orthopaedic surgery in the long-term management of the child with spina bifida. *Archives of Physical Medicine and Rehabilitation*, **45**, 82.

Gugenheim JJ, Gerson LP, Sadler C & Tullos HS (1982) Pathologic morphology of the acetabulum in paralytic and congenital hip instability. *Journal of Pediatric Orthopaedics*, **2**, 397.

Guthkelch AN (1964) Studies of spina bifida cystica (part V): anomalous reflexes in congenital spinal palsy. *Developmental Medicine and Child Neurology*, **6**, 264.

Guttman L (1955) Problem of treatment of pressure sores in spinal paraplegics. *British Journal of Plastic Surgery*, **8**, 196.

Guttman L (1973) *Spinal Cord Injuries*. London: Blackwell.

Guttman L (1976) *Spinal Cord Injuries – Comprehensive Management and Research*, 2nd edn. Oxford: Blackwell.

Hagberg B (1972) The sequelae of spontaneously arrested infantile hydrocephalus. *Developmental Medicine and Child Neurology*, **4**, 583.

Hall JE (1964) Congenital scoliosis treated by Harrington instrumentation and spinal fusion. *Journal of Bone and Joint Surgery*, **46(B)**, 784.

Hall JE (1972) The anterior approach to spinal deformities. *Orthopedic Clinics of North America*, **3**, 81.

Hall JE & Bobechko WP (1973) Advances in the management of spinal deformities in myelodysplasia. *Clinical Neurology and Neurosurgery*, **20**, 164.

Hall JE & Poitras B (1977) The management of kyphosis in patients with myelomeningocele. *Clinical Orthopaedics and Related Research*, **128**, 33.

Hall PV, Campbell RL & Kalsbeck JE (1975)

Meningomyelocele and progressive hydromyelia. *Journal of Neurosurgery*, **43**, 457.

Hall PV, Lindseth RE, Campbell RL & Kalsbeck JE (1976) Myelodysplasia and developmental scoliosis: a manifestation of syringomyelia. *Spine*, **1**, 48.

Hallock H (1942) Surgical stabilisation of dislocated paralytic hips: an end-result study. *Surgery, Gynaecology and Obstetrics*, **75**, 721.

Hallock H (1950) Arthrodesis of the hip for instability and pain in poliomyelitis. *Journal of Bone and Joint Surgery*, **32(A)**, 904.

Hamsa WR & Burney DW (1963) Open correction of recurrent talipes equinovarus: a study of end results. *Clinical Orthopaedics and Related Research*, **26**, 104.

Handelsman JE (1971) Orthopaedic aspects of spina bifida cystica. *South African Journal of Surgery*, **9(4)**, 183.

Harrington PR (1962) Treatment of scoliosis. *Journal of Bone and Joint Surgery*, **44(A)**, 591.

Hauben DJ, Smith AR, Sonneveld GJ & Van der Meulen JC (1983) The use of the vastus lateralis musculocutaneous flap for the repair of trochanteric pressure sores. *Annals of Plastic Surgery*, **10(5)**, 359.

Hay MC & Walker G (1973) Plantar pressures in healthy children and in children with myelomeningocele. *Journal of Bone and Joint Surgery*, **55(B)**, 828.

Hayden PW, Davenport LH & Campbell MM (1979) Adolescents with myelodysplasia: Impact of physical disability on emotional maturation. *Pediatrics*, **64**, 53.

Hayes JT & Gross HP (1963) Orthopedic implications of myelodysplasia. *Journal of the American Medical Association*, **184**, 762.

Hayes JT, Gross HP & Dow S (1964) Surgery for paralytic defects secondary to myelomeningocele and myelodysplasia. *Journal of Bone and Joint Surgery*, **46(A)**, 1577.

Henderson A & Pehoski C (1995) *Hand Function in the Child: Foundations for Remediation*. St Louis, Missouri: Mosby-Year Book.

Heydemann JS & Gillespie R (1987) Management of meningocele kyphosis in the older child by kyphectomy and segmental spinal instrumentation. *Spine*, **12**, 37.

Hight B, Redelman K & Hall PV (1976) Myelodysplasia: A progressive paraplegia and scoliosis. *Journal of Neurosurgical Nursing*, **8(1)**, 28.

Hobbs MST, Carney A, Field B, Simpson D & Kerr C (1974) Incidence of anencephalus and spina bifida and variation risks according to parental birthplaces in three Australian states. (Abstract). *British Journal of Preventive and Social Medicine*, **28**, 67.

Hodges D (1972) Handicapped adventure. *Social Work Today*, **3(10)**, 7.

Hoffer MM, Feiwell E, Perry J & Bonnett G (1973) Functional ambulation in patients with myelomeningocele. *Journal of Bone and Joint Surgery*, **55(A)**, 137.

Hogshead HP & Ponsetti IV (1964) Fascia lata transfer to erector spinae for the treatment of flexion-abduction contractures of the hip in patients with poliomyelitis

and meningomyelocele: evaluation of results. *Journal of Bone and Joint Surgery*, **46(A)**, 1389.

Holgate L (1970) *Physiotherapy for Spina Bifida. Early Treatment*. Surrey, UK: Jupiter Press.

Holgate L (1990) *Checklist and Guidelines for Employment and Training*. London: Association for Spina Bifida and Hydrocephalus.

Hollingsworth RP (1975) An X-ray study of valgus ankles in spina bifida children with valgus flat foot deformity. *Proceedings of the Royal Society of Medicine*, **68(8)**, 481.

Holmes LB, Driscoll SG & Atkins L (1976) Etiologic heterogenecity of neural-tube defects. *New England Journal of Medicine*, **294**, 365.

Holt R (1996) Surgical management of spinal deformity in spina bifida. Singapore Orthopaedic Association Annual Scientific Meeting, Singapore.

Holzman RS (1997) Clinical management of latex-allergic children. *Anesthesia & Analgesia*, **85(3)**, 529.

Hoppenfeld S (1967) Congenital kyphosis in myelomeningocele. *Journal of Bone and Joint Surgery*, **49(B)**, 276.

Hostler (1977) The right to life. *Journal of Medical Ethics*, **3**, 143.

Howe GW, Feinstein C, Reiss D, Molock S & Burger K (1993) Adolescent adjustment to chronic physical disorders: 1. Comparing neurological and non-neurological conditions. *Journal of Child Psychology and Psychiatry and Allied Disciplines*, **34(7)**, 1153.

Huff C & Ramsey P (1978) Myelodysplasia: The influence of the quadriceps and hip abductor muscles on ambulatory function and stability of the hip. *Journal of Bone and Joint Surgery*, **60(A)**, 432.

Hull W, Moe JH & Winter RB (1974) Spinal deformity in myelomeningocele: natural history, evaluation and treatment. *Journal of Bone and Joint Surgery*, **56(A)**, 1767.

Hunt G (1992) Open spina bifida: Cambridge Cohort in their 20s. *European Journal of Paediatric Surgery*, **2**, 39.

Hunt GM & Holmes AE (1976) Factors relating to intelligence in treated cases of spina bifida cystica. *American Journal of Diseases of Children*, **130**, 823.

Hunt GM & Poulton A (1995) Open spina bifida: A complete cohort reviewed 25 years after closure. *Developmental Medicine and Child Neurologia*, **37**, 19.

Hunt GM, Walpole L, Gleave J & Gairdner D (1973) Predictive factors in open myelomeningocele with special reference to sensory level. *British Medical Journal*, **4**, 197.

Hurwitz DJ, Swartz WM & Mathes SJ (1981) The gluteal thigh flap: a reliable, sensate flap for the closure of buttock and perineal wounds. *Plastic and Reconstructive Surgery*, **68(4)**, 521.

Ilizarov GA (1992) *Transosseous Osteosynthesis*. Berlin: Springer.

Ito J, Grant JA & McLone DG (1995) Outcome for an unselectively treated cohort of children with myelomeningocele. *European Journal of Pediatric Surgery*, **5**, Suppl., 51.

Jackson RW (1966) Correction of spinal curvature in

paraplegics by the method of Harrington fusion. *Medical Services Journal of Canada*, **22**, 486.

James CC & Lassman LP (1962) Spinal dysraphism. The diagnosis and treatment of progressive lesions in spina bifida occulta. *Journal of Bone and Joint Surgery*, **44(B)**, 828.

James CC & Lassman LP (1964) Diastematomyelia: a critical survey of 24 cases submitted to laminectomy. *Archives of Disease in Childhood*, **39**, 125.

James JI (1975) The management of infants with scoliosis. *Journal of Bone and Joint Surgery*, **57(B)**, 422.

Janda JP, Skinner SR & Barto PS (1984) Posterior transfer of tibialis anterior in low-level myelodysplasia. *Developmental Medicine and Child Neurology*, **26(1)**, 100.

Jefferson RJ & Whittle MW (1990) Performance of three walking orthoses for the paralysed: a case study using gait analysis. *Prosthetics and Orthotics International*, **14**, 103.

Johnson JTH & Robinson RA (1968) Anterior strut grafts for severe kyphosis: results of three cases with a preceding progressive paraplegia. *Clinical Orthopaedics*, **56**, 25.

Johnson LM (1995) To investigate and establish a regime for the management of perineal pressure care in children with spina bifida. Melbourne: Royal Childrens Hospital.

Jones CCM & Lassman LP (1972) *Spinal Dysraphism*. London: Butterworth.

Jones GB (1954) Paralytic dislocation of the hip. *Journal of Bone and Joint Surgery*, **36(B)**, 375.

Jones T (1891) Spina bifida occulta: no paralytic symptoms until 17 years of age – spine trephined to relieve pressure on the cauda equina: recovery. *British Medical Journal*, **1**, 173.

Jrujic H & Frecaparisi T (1982) Distal hamstring release in knee flexion deformity. *International Orthopaedics*, **6**, 103.

Katsen M, Handelsman JE, Costas S & Shneier N (1973) Experience in a spinal defects clinic. *South African Medical Journal*, **47(40)**, 1912.

Kaufmann J (1975) Orthopedic aspects in the care of children with spina bifida. *Paediatrie und Grenzgebiete*, **14(2)**, 115.

Kendall H, Kendall F & Wadsworth G (1971) *Muscle Testing and Function*, 2nd edn. Baltimore: Williams & Wilkins.

Kiburz JA (1994) The sections and concerns of the school age siblings of children with myelmeningocele. *Issues in Comprehensive Paediatric Nursing*, **17(4)**, 223.

Kielke K (1978) *Skoliose und Kyphose*. Stuttgart: Hippokrates.

Kilfoyle RM, Foley JJ & Norton PL (1965) Spine and pelvic deformity in childhood and adolescent paraplegia. *Journal of Bone and Joint Surgery*, **47(A)**, 659.

King JC, Currie DM & Wright E (1994) Bowel training in spina bifida. Importance of education, patient compliance, age, and anal reflexes. *Archives of Physical Medicine and Rehabilitation*, **75(3)**, 243.

King JD & Hall JE (1970) *Hyperlordosis Following Lumboperitoneal Shunts*. Toronto: Scoliosis Research Society.

Kinsman SL & Doehring MC (1996) The cost of preventable conditions in adults with spina bifida. *European Journal of Pediatrics*, **6**, Suppl. 17.

Kirtly C (1992a) A medially-mounted orthotic hip-joint for paraplegic walking systems. Preliminary Report on the 'Walkabout' Device. Polymedic PO Box 5022, Gold Coast Mail Centre, Queensland, Australia.

Kirtly C (1992b) Principles and practice of paraplegic locomotion: Experience with the Walkabout walking system. *Australian Orthotic and Prosthetics Magazine*, **7(2)**, 4.

Klein RW (1964) An experimental prosthesis for lower extremity omelia. *Medical Journal of Australia*, **1(13)**, 476.

Knutson L & Clark D (1991) Orthotic devices for ambulation in children with cerebral palsy and myelomeningocele. *Physical Therapy*, **71(12)**, 947.

Kronenberger WG & Thompson RJ Jr (1992a) Psychosocial adaptation of mothers of children with spina bifida: Association with dimensions of social relationships. *Journal of Paediatric Psychology*, **17(1)**, 1.

Kronenberger WG & Thompson RJ Jr (1992b) Medical stress, appraised stress, and the psychological adjustment of mothers of children with myelomeningocele. *Journal of Developmental and Behavioural Paediatrics*, **13(6)**, 405.

Krupp S, Kuhn W & Zaech GA (1983) The use of innervated flaps for the closure of ischial pressure sores. *Paraplegia*, **21(2)**, 119.

Kumer S, Cowell R & Townsend P (1984) Physeal, metaphyseal, and diaphyseal injuries of the lower extremities in children with myelomeningocele. *Journal of Pediatric Orthopaedics*, **4(1)**, 25.

Kupka J, Rey OT, Geddes N & Carroll NC (1978) Developmental landmarks in spina bifida. *Orthopedic Clinics of North America*, **9(1)**, 97.

Lapides J, Diokno AC & Silver SJ (1972) Clean intermittent self catheterisation in the treatment of urinary tract disease. *Journal of Urology*, **107**, 458.

Laurence KM (1970) Vertebral abnormalities in first degree relatives of cases of spina bifida and of anencephaly. *Archives of Diseases of Childhood*, **45(240)**, 274.

Laurence KM (1977) Impact of antenatal diagnosis for central nervous system malformation in high-risk pregnancies and pregnancy screening in a high-risk community *Zeitschrift fur Kinderchirurgie und Grenzgebiete*, **22(4)**, 383.

Laurence KM & Beresford A (1975) Continence, friends, marriage and children in 51 adults with spina bifida. *Developental Medicine and Child Neurology*, **17**, Suppl. 35, 123.

Laurence KM & David PA (1964) A sociogenetic survey of the major central nervous system malformations in South Wales. *Journal of the College of General Practitioners Research Newsletters*, **8**, Suppl. 2, 46.

Laurence KM & Tew BJ (1971) The natural history of

spina bifida cystica and cranium bifidum cysticum: Major central nervous system malformations in South Wales. *Archives of Disorders of Childhood*, **46(245)**, 127.

Laurence KM, Bligh AS & Evans KT (1968a) Vertebral and other abnormalities in parents and sibs of cases of spina bifida cystica and of anencephaly. *Developmental Medicine and Child Neurology*, Suppl. **16**, 107.

Laurence KM, Carter CO & David PA (1968b) Major central nervous system malformations in South Wales. *British Journal of Preventive and Social Medicine*, **22**, 146 & **22**, 212.

Lemire RJ (1975) *Normal and Abnormal Development of the Human Nervous System*. Hagerstown: Harper & Rowe.

Levitt RL, Canale ST & Gartland JJ (1974) Surgical correction of foot deformity in the older patient with myelomeningocele. *Orthopedic Clinics of North America*, **5(1)**, 19.

Lewis E (1976) The management of stillbirth. *Lancet*, **2**, 619.

Liandres AZ (Experiences in the rehabilitation of children with paralytic spina bifida). (Russian) *Ortopedia Travmatologia i Protezirovanie*, **29(10)**, 31.

Lie HR, Borjeson MC, Lagerkvist V, Rasmussen F, Hagelsteen JH & Lagergren J (1994) Children with myelomeningocele: The impact of disability on family dynamics and social conditions. A Nordic study. *Developmental Medicine and Child Neurology*, **36(11)**, 1000.

Lindberg C, Brown JC & Bonnett CA (1975) The surgical treatment of spine deformity in myelodysplasia. Presented to Scoliosis Research Society, Louisville.

Lindseth RE (1976) Treatment of the lower extremity in children paralysed with myelomeningocele. *A.A.O.S. Instructional Course Lectures*, **25**, 76.

Lindseth RE & Glancy J (1974) Polypropylene lower-extremity braces for paraplegia due to myelomeningocele. *Journal of Bone and Joint Surgery*, **56(A)**, 556.

Lintner SA & Lindseth RE (1994) Kyphotic deformity in patients who have a myelomeningocele. Operative treatment and long-term follow-up. *Journal of Bone and Joint Surgery*, **76(9)**, 1301.

Little DM, Gleeson MJ, Hickey DP, Donovan MG & Murphy DM (1994) Renal transplantation in patients with spina bifida. *Urology* **44(3)**, 1319.

Loder RT, Shapiro P, Towbin R & Aronson DD (1991) Aortic anatomy in children with myelomeningocele and congenital lumbar kyphosis. *Journal of Pediatric Orthopaedics*, **11**, 31.

Lopponen T, Saukkonen AL, Serlo W, Lanning P & Knimp N (1995) Slow pubertal linear growth but early pubertal growth spurt in patients with shunted hydrocephalus. *Pediatrics*, **95(6)**, 917.

Lorber J (1971) Results of treatment of myelomeningocele. *Developmental Medicine and Child Neurology*, **13** 279.

Lourenco A, Dias L, Thomas SES & Sarwark J (1992) *Gait Analysis in Myelomeningocele: A Comparative Study of Children Walking With and Without Support.* Proceedings from the Seventh Annual East Coast Clinical Gait Laboratories Conference, Richmond.

Lovell LM (1973) Playgroup for multiply handicapped children. *Physiotherapy*, **59(8)**, 251.

Lowe GP & Menelaus MB (1978) The surgical management of kyphosis in older children with myelomeningocele. *Journal of Bone and Joint Surgery*, **60(B)**, 40.

Luque ER (1982) Segmental spinal instrumentation for correction of scoliosis. *Clinical Orthopaedics and Related Research*, **163**, 192.

Mackenzie NG & Emery JL (1971) Deformities of the cervical cord in children with neurospinal dysraphism. *Developmental Medicine and Child Neurology*, **25**, 58.

Mackinnon SE, Delton AL, Patterson GA & Gruss JS (1985) Medial antebrachial cutaneous – lateral femoral cutaneous neurotization to provide sensation to pressure-bearing areas in the paraplegic patient. *Annals of Plastic Surgery*, **14(6)**, 541.

McAndrew I (1976) *Children with a Handicap and their Families*. Melbourne: Ability Press.

McAndrew I (1977) *Adolescents and Young People with Spina Bifida*. Melbourne: Ability Press.

McAndrew I (1979) Adolescents and young people with spina bifida. *Developmental Medicine and Child Neurology*, **21**, 616.

McCall R & Schmidt T (1986) Clinical experience with the Reciprocal Gait Orthosis in myelodysplasia. *Journal of Pediatric Orthopaedics*, **6(2)**, 157.

McCall R, Douglas R & Rightor N (1983) Surgical treatment in patients with myelodysplasia before using the L.S.U. reciprocation-gait system. *Orthopedics*, **6(7)**, 843.

McCraw JB, Dibbell DG & Carraway JH (1977) Clinical definition of independent myocutaneous vascular territories. *Plastic and Reconstructive Surgery*, **60(3)**, 341.

McDonald C, Jaffe K & Shurtleff D (1986a) Assessment of muscle strength in children with meningomyelocele: accuracy and stability of measurements over time. *Archives of Physical Medicine and Rehabilitation*, **67**, 855.

McDonald C, Jaffe K, Mosca V & Shurtleff D (1986b) Ambulatory outcome of children with myelomeningocele: Effect of lower-extremity muscle strength. *Developmental Medicine and Child Neurology*, **33**, 482.

McDonald C, Jaffe K, Shurtleff D & Menelaus M (1986c) Modifications to the traditional description of neurosegmental innervation in myelomengingocele. *Developmental Medicine and Child Neurology*, **33**, 473.

McKay DW, Jackman KV, Nason SS & Eng GE (1976) McKay stabilisation in myelomeningocele. *Developmental Medicine and Child Neurology*, Suppl. **37(18)**, 6.

McKeown T & Record RG (1951) Seasonal incidence of congenital malformations of the central nervous system. *Lancet*, **1**, 192.

McKibbin B (1973) The use of splintage in the

management of paralytic dislocation of the hip in spina bifida cystica. *Journal of Bone and Joint Surgery*, **55(B)**, 163.

McKibbin B & Porter RW (1967) The incidence of vitamin-C deficiency in meningomyelocele. *Developmental Medicine and Child Neurology*, **9**, 338.

McKibbin B, Roseland PA & Duckwith T (1968) Abnormalities in vitamin C metabolism in spina bifida. *Developmental Medicine and Child Neurology*, Suppl. **15**, 55.

McLone DG (1989) Spina bifida today: problems adults face. *Seminars in Neurology*, **9(3)**, 169.

McLone DG (1992) Continuing concepts in management of children with spina bifida. *Pediatric Neurosurgery*, **18(5–6)**, 254.

McLone DG, Herman JM, Gabrieli AP & Dias L (1990–1991) Tethered cord as a cause of scoliosis in children with myelomeningocele. *Pediatric Neurosurgery*, **16(1)**, 8.

McMaster WC & Silber I (1975) An urological complication of Dwyer instrumentation. *Journal of Bone and Joint Surgery*, **57(A)**, 710.

Malhotra D, Puri R & Owen R (1984) Valgus deformity of the ankle in children with spina bifida aperta. *Journal of Bone and Joint Surgery*, **66**, 381.

Mannor DA, Weinstein SL & Dietz FR (1996) Long-term follow up of chiari pelvic osteotomy in mylenomeningocele. *Journal of Pediatric Orthopaedics*, **16**, 769.

Marshall PD, Broughton NS, Menelaus MB & Graham HK (1996) Surgical release of knee flexion contractures in myelomeningocele. *Journal of Bone and Joint Surgery*, **78(B)**, 912.

Martin MC (1964) Physiotherapy in relation to myelomeningocele. *Physiotherapy, London*, **50**, 50.

Martin MC (1967) Spina bifida. *Physiotherapy, London*, **53**, 299.

Martin P (1975) Marital breakdown in families of patients with spina bifida cystica. *Developmental Medicine and Child Neurology*, **17**, 757.

Matson DD (1969) *Neurosurgery of Infancy and Childhood*, 2nd edn. Springfield, Illinois: Thomas.

Mazur J & Menelaus M (1991) Neurologic status of spina bifida patients and the orthopedic surgeon. *Clinical Orthopaedics and Related Research*, **264**, 54.

Mazur J, Menelaus MB, Dickens DRV & Doig WG (1986a) Efficacy of surgical management for scoliosis in myelomeningocoele: Correction of deformity and alteration of functional status. *Journal of Pediatric Orthopaedics*, **6**, 568.

Mazur J, Stillwell A & Menelaus M (1986b) The significance of spasticity in lower and upper limbs in myelomeningocele. *Journal of Bone and Joint Surgery*, **68(B)**, 213.

Mazur JM, Shurtleff DB, Menelaus MB & Colliver J (1989) Orthopaedic management of high-level spina bifida: early walking compared with early use of a wheelchair. *Journal of Bone and Joint Surgery*, **71(A)**, 56.

Mebust WK, Foret JD & Volk WL (1969) Fifteen years experience with urinary diversion in myelomeningocele patients. *Journal of Urology*, **101**, 177.

Melzak J (1969) Paraplegia among children. *Lancet*, **2(610)**, 45.

Menelaus MB (1967) Orthopaedic management in meningomyelocele. In *Proceedings of the Fifth International Congress of the World Federation of Physical Therapy, Melbourne, 1967*, p. 41. Melbourne: Australian Physiotherapy Association.

Menelaus MB (1969) Dislocation and deformity of the hip in children with spina bifida cystica. *Journal of Bone and Joint Surgery*, **51(B)**, 238.

Menelaus MB (1971) Talectomy for equinovarus deformity in arthrogryposis and spina bifida. *Journal of Bone and Joint Surgery*, **53(B)**, 468.

Menelaus MB (1976a) The hip in myelomeningocele – management directed towards a minimum number of operations and a minimum period of immobilisation. *Journal of Bone and Joint Surgery*, **58(B)**, 448.

Menelaus MB (1976b) Orthopaedic management of children with myelomeningocele: a plea for realistic goals. *Developmental Medicine and Child Neurology*, Suppl. 37, **18(6)**, 3.

Menelaus MB (1980) *The Orthopaedic Management of Spina Bifida Cystics*, 2nd edn. Edinburgh: Churchill Livingstone.

Micheli LJ & Hall JE (1974) The management of spine deformities in the myelomeningocele patient. *Medical Annals of the District of Columbia*, **43(1)**, 21.

Milhorat TH (1972) *Hydrocephalus and the Cerebrospinal Fluid*. Baltimore: Williams & Wilkins.

Miller E & Sethi L (1971a) The effect of hydrocephalus on perception. *Developmental Medicine and Child Neurology*, Suppl. **25**, 77.

Miller E & Sethi L (1971b) Tactile matching in children with hydrocephalus. *Neuropadiatrie*, **3**, 191.

Milunsky A & Alpert E (1976) Prenatal diagnosis of neural tube defects 1 and 11. *Journal of Obstetric Gynecologic and Neonatal Nursing*, **48**, 1.

Minchom PE, Ellis NC, Appleton PL *et al.* (1995) Impact of functional severity on self concept of young people with spina bifida. *Archives of Disease in Childhood*, **73(1)**, 48.

Minns RA, Sobkowiak CA, Skardoutsou A, Dick K, Elton RA, Brown JK & Forfar JO (1977) Upper limb function in spina bifida. *Zeitschrift fur Kinderchirurgie und Grenzgebiete*, **22(4)**, 493.

Mita K, Akataki K, Itoh K, Ono Y, Ishida N & Oki T (1993) Assessment of obesity of children with spina bifida. *Developmental Medicine and Child Neurology*, **35(4)**, 305.

Moe JH, Winter RB, Bradford DS & Longstein JE (1978) *Scoliosis and Other Spinal Deformities*. Philadelphia: Saunders.

Morgan DJ, Blackburn M & Bax M (1995) Adults with spina bifida and/or hydrocephalus. *Postgraduate Medical Journal*, **71(831)**, 17.

MRC Vitamin Study Research Group (1991) Prevention of neural tube defects: Results of the Medical Research Council Vitamin Study. *Lancet*, **338**, 131.

Murphy EA & Chase GA (1975) *Principles of Genetic Counselling.* Chicago: Year Book Medical Publications.

Mustard WT (1952) Iliopsoas transfer for weakness of the hip abductors. *Journal of Bone and Joint Surgery,* **34(A)**, 647.

Mustard WT (1959) A follow-up study of iliopsoas transfer for hip instability. *Journal of Bone and Joint Surgery,* **41(B)**, 289.

Nahai F, Silverton JS, Hill HL & Vasconez LO (1978) The tensor fascia lata musculocutaneous flap. *Annals of Plastic Surgery,* **1(4)**, 372.

Naik DR & Emery JL (1968) The position of the spinal cord segments related to the vertebral bodies in children with meningomyelocele and hydrocephalus. *Developmental Medicine and Child Neurology,* Suppl. **16**, 62.

Neto J, Dias L, Gabrielli AP (1996) Congenital talipes equinovarus in spina bifida: treatment and results. *Journal of Pediatric Orthopaedics,* **16**, 782.

Nicol RO & Menelaus MB (1983) Correction of combined tibial torsion and valgus deformity of the foot. *Journal of Bone and Joint Surgery,* **65(B)**, 641.

Nola GJ & Vistnes LM (1980) Differential response of skin and muscle in the experimental production of pressure sores. *Plastic and Reconstructive Surgery,* **66(5)**, 728.

Norton PL & Foley JJ (1959) Paraplegia in children. *Journal of Bone and Joint Surgery,* **41(A)**, 1291.

Ober FR (1927) An operation for the relief of paralysis of the gluteus maximum muscle. *Journal of the American Medical Association,* **88**, 1063.

O'Brien JP (1974) The surgical management of paralytic scoliosis. *Journal of Bone and Joint Surgery,* **56(B)**, 566.

Ogilvie C & Sharrard WJ (1986) Hemitransplantation of the tendo calcaneus in children with spinal neurological disorders. *Journal of Bone and Joint Surgery,* **68(B)**, 767.

Olney BW & Menelaus MB (1988) Triple arthrodesis in spina bifida patients – a longterm followup. *Journal of Bone and Joint Surgery,* **70(B)**, 234.

Padget DH (1970) Neuroschisis and human embryonic maldevelopment. *Journal of Neuropathology and Experimental Neurology,* **29**, 192.

Park TS, Hoffman HJ, Hendrich EB & Humphreys RB (1983) Experience with surgical decompression of the Arnold–Chiari malformation in young infants with myelomeningocele. *Neurosurgery,* **13**, 147.

Park WM & Watt I (1975) The preoperative artographic assessment of children with spina bifida cystica and severe kyphosis. *Journal of Bone and Joint Surgery,* **57(B)**, 112.

Parker B & Walker G (1975) Posterior psoas transfer and hip instability in lumbar myelomeningocele. *Journal of Bone and Joint Surgery,* **57(B)**, 53.

Parry SW & Mathes SJ (1982) Bilateral gluteus maximus myocutaneous advancement flaps: sacral coverage for ambulatory patients. *Annals of Plastic Surgery,* **8(6)**, 443.

Parsch K (1973) Grice extra-articular arthrodesis (results, extensions in the range of indication). (German) *Zeitschrift fuer Orthopadie und ihre Grensgebiete,* **109(3)**, 458.

Parsch K & Goessens H (1971) Surgical treatment of spinal column and hip deformities in spina bifida. *Acta orthopaedica belgica,* **37(3)**, 230.

Parsch K & Manner G (1976) Prevention and treatment of knee problems in children with spina bifida. *Developmental Medicine and Child Neurology,* Suppl. 37, **18(6)**, 114.

Parsch K & Schulitz KP (1971) Early orthopedic therapy of the child with cystic spina bifida. (German) *Zeitschrift fuer Orthopadie und ihre Grensgebiete,* **109(3)**, 458.

Parsch K, Rosska K & Goessens H (1970) Does hip dislocation in meningomyelocele require a special treatment? Apropos of 30 transplantations of the psoas by Sharrard's technic. *Revue de Chirurgie Orthopedique et Reparatrice de L'appareil Moteur,* **56(7)**, 683.

Patrick GM, Mohany JF & Disney AP (1994) The prognosis for end stage renal failure in spinal cord injury and spina bifida – Australia and New Zealand, 1970–1991. *Australian and New Zealand Journal of Medicine,* **24(1)**, 36.

Patten BM (1952) Overgrowth of the neural tube in young human embryos. *Anatomical Record,* **113**, 381.

Peach B (1965) Arnold–Chiari malformation. *Archives of Neurology,* **12**, 613.

Pemberton PA (1965) Pericapsular osteotomy of the ilium for treatment of congenital subluxation and dislocation of the hip. *Journal of Bone and Joint Surgery,* **47(A)**, 65.

Pena CE, Miller F, Budzilovich GN & Feigin I (1968) Arthrogryposis multiplex congenita: report of two cases of a radicular type with familial incidence. *Neurology, Minneapolis,* **18**, 926.

Perry J (1992) *Gait Analysis: Normal and Pathological Function.* Thorofare: Slack, NJ, USA.

Phillips DL, Field RE, Broughton NS & Menelaus MB (1995). Reciprocating orthoses for children with myelomeningocele: a comparison of two types. *Journal of Bone and Joint Surgery,* **77(B)**, 110.

Phillips DP & Lindseth RE (1992) Ambulation after transfer of adductors, external oblique and tensor fascia lata in myelomeningocele. *Journal of Pediatric Orthopaedics,* **12**, 712.

Pollack IF, Kinnunen D & Leland Albright A (1996) The effect of early craniocervical decompression on functional outcome in neonates and young infants with myelodysplasia and symptomatic chiari 11 malformations: Results from a prospective series. *Neurosurgery,* **38**, 703.

Poulton M (1975) Walking aid for young paraplegics. *Physiotherapy,* **61(9)**, 275.

Pouw R (1977) Assessment of pre-school abilities based on spina bifida children. *British Journal of Occupational Therapy,* **40(3)**, 61.

Ralis Z & Duckworth T (1973) Morphology of vertical talus. *Journal of Bone and Joint Surgery,* **55**, 428.

Ramirez OM, Ramasastry SS, Granick MS, Pang D & Futrell JW (1987) A new surgical approach to closure of large lumbosacral meningomyelocele defects. *Plastic and Reconstructive Surgery*, **80(6)**, 799.

Record RG & McKeown T (1949) Congenital malformations of the central nervous system: a survey of 930 cases. *British Journal of Preventive and Social Medicine*, **3**, 183.

Richards IDG, Roberts CJ & Lloyd S (1972) Area differences in prevalence of neural tube malformations in South Wales. *British Journal of Preventive and Social Medicine*, **26**, 89.

Rickwood AM, Grundy DJ & Thomas DG (1984) Danger of inadequate urological supervision of patients with congenital neuropathic bladder. *British Medical Journal (Clinical Research Edition)*, **288(6431)**, 1677.

Riley M & Halliday J (1996) Congenital malformations in Victoria 1983–1994. Department Human Services, Melbourne, Australia. ISBN 07306 54072.

Ritter MA & Wilson PD (1968) Colonna capsular arthroplasty. A long-term follow up of forty hips. *Journal of Bone and Joint Surgery*, **50(A)**, 1305.

Robin GC (1972) Scoliosis of spina bifida and infantile paraplegia. *Israel Journal of Medical Sciences*, **8(11)**, 1823.

Robin GC (1973) Scoliosis and neurological disease. *Israel Journal of Medical Sciences*, **9(5)**, 578.

Romness MJ & Menelaus MB (1995) Triple arthrodesis: a technique for the underformed or valgus foot. *Orthopaedics and Traumatology*, **2**, 114.

Rose GK & Henshaw JT (1972) A swivel walker for paraplegics: medical and technical considerations. *Biomedical Engineering*, **7(9-2)**, 420.

Rose G, Stallard J, Sankarankutty M (1981) Clinical evaluation of spina bifida patients using Hip Guidance Orthosis. *Developmental Medicine and Child Neurology*, **23**, 30.

Rosen DS (1994) Transition from paediatric to adult-oriented health care for the adolescent with chronic illness or disability. *Adolescent Medicine: State of the Art Reviews*, **5(2)**, 241.

Rosenstein B, Greene W, Herrington R & Blum A (1987) Bone density in myelomeningocele: The effects of ambulatory status and other factors. *Developmental Medicine and Child Neurology*, **29**, 486.

Rossak K, Parsch K & Schulitz KP (1970) Treatment of hip joint luxation in myelomeningocele. *Archiv fur Orthopadische und Unfall-Chirurgie*, **67(3)**, 199.

Rotenstern D, Adams M & Reigel DH (1995) Adult stature and anthropomorphic measurements of patients with myelomeningocele. *European Journal of Paediatrics*, **154(5)**, 398.

Rowley-Kelly FL & Reigel DH (1993) *Teaching the Student with Spina Bifida*. Baltimore: Paul H Brookes.

Rudeberg A, Donati F & Kaiser G (1995) Psychosocial aspects in the treatment of children with myelomeningocele: An assessment after a decade. *European Journal of Paediatrics*, **154(9)**, Suppl. 4, S85.

Rueda J & Carroll NC (1972) Hip instability in patients with myelomeningocele. *Journal of Bone and Joint Surgery*, **54(B)**, 422.

Ryan DR, Ploski C & Emans JB (1991) Myelodysplasia – the musculoskeletal problem: Habilation from infancy to adulthood. *Physical Therapy*, **71**, 935.

Salter RB (1961) Innominate osteotomy in the treatment of congenital dislocation and subluxation of the hip. *Journal of Bone and Joint Surgery*, **43(B)**, 518.

Samuelsson L & Eklof O (1988) Scoliosis in myelomeningocele. *Acta orthopedica scandinavica*, **59**, 122.

Samuelsson L & Skoog M (1988) Ambulation in patients with myelomeningocele: A multivariate statistical analysis. *Journal of Pediatric Orthopaedics*, **8**, 569.

Sand PL, Taylor N, Hill M, Kosky N & Rawlings M (1974) Hand function in children with myelomeningocele. *American Journal of Occupational Therapy*, **28**, 87.

Sandhu PS, Broughton NS & Menelaus MB (1995) Tenotomy of the ligamentum patellae in spina bifida: Management of limited flexion range at the knee. *Journal of Bone and Joint Surgery*, **77(B)**, 832.

Sandler AD, Worley G, Leroy EC, Stanley FD & Kalman S (1996) Sexual function and erection capability among young men with spina bifida. *Developmental Medicine and Child Neurology*, **38**, 823.

Satin-Smith MS, Katz LL, Thornton P, Gruccio D & Moshang T Jr (1996) Arm span as measurement of response to growth hormone (GH) treatment in a group of children with myelomeningocele and GH deficiency. *Journal of Clinical Endocrinology and Metabolism*, **81(4)**, 1654.

Schafer MF & Dias LAS (1983) *Myelomeningocele. Orthopaedic Treatment*. Baltimore: Williams & Wilkins.

Scheier HJ (1969) On the use of the instruments by P Harrington for the correction and internal fixation of scoliosis. (German) *Zeitschrift fuer Orthopadie und ihre Grenzgebiete*, **106(2)**, 253.

Schopler S & Menelaus M. Significance of the strength of the quadriceps muscles in children with myelomeningocele. *Journal of Pediatric Orthopaedics*, **7**, 507.

Segal LS, Mann DC, Feiwell E & Hoffer MM (1989) Equinovarus deformity in arthrogryposis and myelogeningocele: evaluation of primary talectomy. *Foot and Ankle*, **10(1)**, 12.

Sellers MJ & Nevin NC (1984) Periconceptional vitamin supplementation and the prevention of neural tube defects in SE England and West Ireland. *Journal of Medical Genetics*, **21**, 325.

Shaer CN, Slater JE, Mostello LA & Tosi LL (1992) Rubber specific IGE in children with spina bifida: Identification and management. *European Journal of Paediatrics*, Suppl. 1, 36.

Shanahan MD, Douglas DL, Sharrard WJ, Duckworth T & Betts R (1985) The long-term results of the surgical management of paralytic pes cavus by soft tissue release and tendon transfer. *Zeitschrift fur Kinderchirurgie*, **40(1)**, 37.

Sharrard WJW (1959) Congenital paralytic dislocation of

the hip in children with myelomeningocele. *Journal of Bone and Joint Surgery*, **41(B)**, 622.

Sharrard WJW (1962) The mechanism of paralytic deformity in spina bifida. *Developmental Medicine and Child Neurology*, **4**, 310.

Sharrard WJW (1964a) Spina bifida. *Physiotherapy, London*, **50**, 44.

Sharrard WJW (1964b) The segmental innervation of the lower limb muscles in man. *Annals of the Royal College of Surgeons*, **35**, 106.

Sharrard WJW (1964c) Posterior iliopsoas transplantation in the treatment of paralytic dislocation of the hip. *Journal of Bone and Joint Surgery*, **46(B)**, 426.

Sharrard WJW (1967a) Paralytic deformity in the lower limb. *Journal of Bone and Joint Surgery*, **49(B)**, 731.

Sharrard WJW (1967b) Modern trends in the treatment of spina bifida: methods of assessment and their relation to treatment by early closure. *Proceedings of the Royal Society of Medicine*, **60**, 767.

Sharrard WJW (1968) Spinal osteotomy for congenital kyphosis in myelomeningocele. *Journal of Bone and Joint Surgery*, **50(B)**, 466.

Sharrard WJW (1973) The orthopaedic surgery of spina bifida. *Clinical Orthopaedics and Related Research*, **92**, 195.

Sharrard WJW (1975) The orthopaedic management of spina bifida. *Acta orthopedica scandinavica*, **46(3)**, 356.

Sharrard WJW & Drennan JC (1972) Osteotomy – excision of the spine for lumbar kyphosis in older children with myelomeningocele. *Journal of Bone and Joint Surgery*, **54(B)**, 50.

Sharrard WJW & Grosfield I (1968) The management of deformity and paralysis of the foot in myelomeningocele. *Journal of Bone and Joint Surgery*, **50(B)**, 456.

Sharrard WJW & Smith TW (1976) Tenodesis of flexor hallucis longus for paralytic clawing of the hallux in childhood. *Journal of Bone and Joint Surgery*, **58(B)**, 224.

Sharrard WJW & Webb J (1974) Supra-malleolar wedge osteotomy of the tibia in children with myelomeningocele. *Journal of Bone and Joint Surgery*, **56(B)**, 458.

Sharrard WJW, Zachary RB & Lorber J (1967) The long-term evaluation of a trial of immediate and delayed closure of spina bifida cystica. *Clinical Orthopaedics and Related Research*, **50**, 197.

Shepherd R (1975) The prevention of generalized developmental delay in the spina bifida child. Lecture from the 1st National Spina Bifida Congress, Sydney, Australia.

Sherk HH & Ames MD (1975) Talectomy in the treatment of the myelomeningocele patient. *Clinical Orthopaedics and Related Research*, **110**, 218.

Shively RE, Schafer ME & Kernahan DA. (1980) The spread of sensibility into previously anaesthetic skin following intercostal flap transfer in a paraplegic. *Annals of Plastic Surgery*, **5(5)**, 396.

Shurtleff DB (ed.) (1986) *Myelodysplasias and Extrophies:*

Significance, Prevention and Treatment. Orlando: Grune & Stratton.

Shurtleff DB & Dunne KB (1986) Adults and adolescents with meningomyelocele. In *Myelodysplasias and Extrophies: Significance, Prevention and Treatment*. (ed. by Shurtleff DB), p. 433. Florida: Grune & Stratton.

Shurtleff DB & Lemire RJ (1995) Epidemiology, etiologic factors, and prenatal diagnosis of open spinal dysraphism. *Neurosurgery Clinics of North America*, **6(2)**, 183.

Shurtleff DB, Goiney R, Gordon LH & Livermore N (1976) Myelodysplasia: the natural history of kyphosis and scoliosis. A preliminary report. *Developmental Medicine and Child Neurology*, Suppl. 37, **18(6)**, 126.

Shurtleff D, Menelaus M, Staheli L *et al.* (1986) Natural history of flexion deformity of the hip in myelodysplasia. *Journal of Pediatric Orthopaedics*, **6**, 666.

Simmons EH (1968) Observations on the technique and indications for wedge resection of the spine. *Journal of Bone and Joint Surgery*, **50(A)**, 847.

Simpson D (1976) Congenital malformations of the nervous system. *Medical Journal of Australia*, **1**, 700.

Slater JE (1989) Rubber anaphylaxis. *New England Journal of Medicine*, **320**, 1126.

Smith ED (1965) *Spina Bifida and the Total Care of Spinal Myelomeningocele*. Springfield, Illinois: Thomas.

Smith ET, Pevey JK & Shindler TO (1963) The erector spinae transplant – a misnomer. *Clinical Orthopaedics and Related Research*, **30**, 144.

Smith GK (1966) Total care in spina bifida cystica. In *Industrial Society and Rehabilitation – problems and solutions: Proceedings of the 10th World Congress of the International Society for Rehabilitation of the Disabled, Wiesbaden, 1966*, p. 75. Heidelberg: ISRD.

Smith GK (1976) Spina bifida. In *Clinical Paediatric Surgery*, 2nd edn, p. 100. London: Blackwell.

Smith GK & Smith ED (1973) Selection for treatment in spina bifida cystica. *British Medical Journal*, **4**, 189.

Smithells RW & Chin ER (1965) Spina bifida in Liverpool. *Developmental Medicine and Child Neurology*, **7**, 258.

Society for Research into Hydrocephalus and Spina Bifida (1965) Proceedings of a symposium on spina bifida. National Fund for Research in Poliomyelitis and Other Crippling diseases, London. Supplements to *Developmental Medicine and Child Neurology*, Nos. 11 (1966), 13 (1967), 15 (1968), 16 (1968), 20 (1969), 22 (1970), 25 (1971), 27 (1972), 29 (1973), 32 (1974), 35 (1975).

Somerville EW (1959) Paralytic dislocation of the hip. *Journal of Bone and Joint Surgery*, **41(B)**, 279.

Sousa J, Telzrow R, Holm R, McCartin R & Shurtleff D (1983) Developmental guidelines for children with myelodysplasia. *Physical Therapy*, **63(1)**, 21.

Spain B (1974) Verbal and performance ability in pre-school children with spina bifida. *Developmental Medicine and Child Neurology*, **16**, 773.

Spears FS, Littlewood KE & Liu DW (1995) Anaesthesia

for the patient with allergy to latex. *Anaesthesia and Intensive Care*, **23(5)**, 623.

Specht EE (1975) Congenital paralytic vertical talus. An anatomical study. *Journal of Bone and Joint Surgery*, **57(A)**, 842.

Spielrein RE (1963) An engineering approach to ambulation without the use of external power sources, of severely handicapped individuals. *Journal of the Australian Institute of Engineers*, **35**, 321.

Sriram K, Bobechko WP & Hall JE (1972) Surgical management of spinal deformities in spina bifida. *Journal of Bone and Joint Surgery*, **54(B)**, 666.

Stark GD (1971) Neonatal assessment of the child with a myelomeningocele. *Archives of Diseases of Childhood*, **46(248)**, 539.

Stark GD (1975) Myelomeningocele: the changing approach to treatment. In *Recent Advances in Paediatric Surgery*, No. 3, p. 73. London: Churchill Livingstone.

Stark GD (1977) *Spina Bifida: Problems and Management*. London: Blackwell.

Stark GD & Baker GC (1967) The neurological involvement of the lower limbs in myelomeningocele. *Developmental Medicine and Child Neurology*, **9**, 732.

Stark GD & Drummond M (1971) The spinal cord lesion in myelomeningocele. *Developmental Medicine and Child Neurology*, Suppl. 25, **13(6)**, 1.

Stark GD & Drummond M (1973) Results of selective early operation in myelomeningocele. *Archives of Diseases of Childhood*, **48**, 676.

Steele HH (1973) Triple osteotomy of the innominate bone. *Journal of Bone and Joint Surgery*, **55(A)**, 343.

Steele HH & Adams DJ (1972) Hyperlordosis caused by the lumboperitoneal shunt procedure for hydrocephalus. *Journal of Bone and Joint Surgery*, **54(A)**, 1537.

Stern MB, Grant SS & Isaacson AS (1967) Bilateral distal tibial and fibular epiphyseal separation associated with spina bifida: a case report. *Clinical Orthopaedics and Related Research*, **50**, 191.

Stevens PM & Toomey E (1988) Fibular–Achilles tenodesis for paralytic ankle valgus. *Journal of Paediatric Orthopaedics*, **8**, 169.

Stillwell A (1979) The physiotherapist's role in the treatment of spina bifida. *Australian Journal of Physiotherapy*, **Dec**, 91.

Stillwell A & Menelaus M (1983) Walking ability in mature patients with spina bifida. *Journal of Pediatric Orthopaedics*, **3**, 184.

Stone AR (1995) Neurologic evaluation and urologic management of spinal dysraphism. *Neurosurgery Clinics of North America*, **6(2)**, 269.

Supan TJ & Hovorka CF (1995) A review of ankle–foot orthosis adjustments/replacements in young cerebral palsy and spina bifida patients. *Journal of Prosthetics and Orthotics*, **7**, 15.

Sutherland AD (1977) The management of spinal deformity in patients with myelomeningocele. *Records of the Adelaide Children's Hospital, Australia*, **1**, 492.

Sutherland D (1988) *The Development of Mature Walking. Clinics in Developmental Medicine* No. **104/105**. Oxford: MacKeith Press.

Swank M & Dias L (1992) Myelomeningocele: a review of the orthopaedic aspects of 206 patients treated from birth with no selection criteria. *Developmental Medicine and Child Neurology*, **34**, 1047.

Symposium on Spina Bifida, London, 1965. *Proceedings*. London: National Fund for Research into Poliomyelitis and other Crippling Diseases. (Action for the Crippled Child Monograph.)

Taillard W, Compere J, Vasey H & Berney J (1969) Orthopedics of spina bifida. (French) *Annales de Chirurgie Infantile*, **10(1)**, 87.

Talbot HS (1955) The sexual function in paraplegia. *Journal of Urology*, **73(1)**, 91.

Tamaki N, Shirataki K, Kojima N, Shouse Y & Matsumoto S (1988) Tethered cord syndrome of delayed onset following repair of myelomeningocele. *Journal of Neurosurgery*, **69**, 393.

Tappit-Emas E (1983) Physical therapy intervention. In *Myelomeningocele: Orthopedic Treatment* (ed. by Schafer M & Dias L), p. 6. Baltimore: Williams & Wilkins.

Tappit-Emas E (1994) Spina bifida. In *Paediatric Physical Therapy*, 2nd edn. (ed. by Tecklin JS), p. 135. Philadelphia: Lippincott.

Taylor LJ (1986) Excision of the proximal end of the femur for hip stiffness in myelomeningocele. *Journal of Bone and Joint Surgery*, **68(B)**, 75.

Tew B & Laurence KM (1984) The relationship between intelligence and academic achievements in spina bifida adolescents. *Z Kinderchir*, **39**, Suppl. 2, 122.

Thomas LI, Thompson TC & Straub LR (1950) Transplantation of the external oblique muscle for abductor paralysis. *Journal of Bone and Joint Surgery*, **32(A)**, 207.

Thompson MS, Cavin E & Phippen WG (1964) Fractures of the femora associated with spina bifida. *Military Medicine*, **129**, 841.

Till K (1969) Congenital malformations of the lower back in childhood. *Proceedings of the Royal Society of Medicine*, **62(7)**, 727.

Tomlinson P & Sugarman ID (1995) Complication with shunts in adults with spina bifida. *British Medical Journal*, **311(7000)**, 286.

Torode IP & Godette G (1995) A new method of fixation of myelomeningocoele kyphosis. *Journal of Pediatric Orthopaedics*, **15**, 202.

Torode IP, Gillespie R & Van Olm JMJ (1984) Surgical management of congenital kyphosis in myelomeningocele (Abstract). *Journal of Bone and Joint Surgery*, **66(B)**, 780.

Tosi LL, Slater JE, Shaer CN & Mostello LA (1993) The surgical implications of latex sensitivity in children with spina bifida. *European Journal of Paediatric Surgery*, **3**, Suppl. 1, 34.

Tuck WH (1974) The Stanmore cosmetic caliper. *Journal of Bone and Joint Surgery*, **56(B)**, 115.

Turner A (1986) Upper limb function of children with

myelomeningocele. *Developmental Medicine and Child Neurology*, **28**, 790.

Turner JW & Cooper RR (1971) Posterior transposition of tibialis anterior through the interosseous membrane. *Clinical Orthopaedics and Related Research*, **79**, 71.

Tzimas NA & Badell-Ribera A (1969) Orthopedic and habilitation management of patients with spina bifida and myelomeningocele. *Medical Clinics of North America*, **53(3)**, 502.

Vankoski SJ, Sarwark JF, Moore C & Dias L (1995) Characteristic pelvic, hip and knee kinematic patterns in children with lumbosacral myelomeningocele. *Gait and Posture*, **3(1)**, 51.

Variend S & Emery JL (1973) The weight of the cerebellum in children with myelomeningocele. *Developmental Medicine and Child Neurology*, Suppl. **29**, 77.

Variend S & Emery JL (1974) The pathology of the central lobes of the cerebellum in children with myelomeningocele. *Developmental Medicine and Child Neurology*, Suppl. **32**, 99.

Vogel L & Lubicky J (1995) Ambulation with parapodia and Reciprocation Gait Orthoses in pediatric spinal cord injury. *Developmental Medicine and Child Neurology*, **37**, 957.

Wald NJ & Cuckle H (1977) Maternal serum alpha fetoprotein measurement in antenatal screening for anencephaly and spina bifida in early pregnancy. Reports of a collaborative study of alpha fetoprotein in relation to neural tube defect. *Lancet*, **1**, 1323.

Walker G (1971) The early management of varus feet in myelomeningocele. *Journal of Bone and Joint Surgery*, **53(B)**, 462.

Walker G & Cheong-Leen P (1973) Surgical management of paralytic vertical talus in myelomeningocele. *Developmental Medicine and Child Neurology*, Suppl. 29, **15(6)**, 112.

Walker JH, Thomas M & Russell IT (1971) Spina bifida – the parents. *Developmental Medicine and Child Neurology*, **13**, 462.

Wallace SJ (1973) The effect of upper-limb function on mobility of children with myelomeningocele. *Developmental Medicine and Child Neurology*, Suppl. **29**, 84.

Watson-Jones R (1926) Spontaneous dislocations of the hip. *British Journal of Surgery*, **14**, 36.

Weisl H & Matthews JP (1973) Posterior ilio-psoas transfer in the management of the hip in spina bifida: a review of 34 operations. *Developmental Medicine and Child Neurology*, Suppl. **29**, 100.

Weisl H, Fairclough JA & Jones DG (1988) Stabilisation of the hip in myelomeningocele. Comparison of posterior iliopsoas transfer and varus-rotation osteotomy. *Journal of Bone and Joint Surgery*, **70(B)**, 29.

Welbourn H (1975) Spina bifida children attending ordinary schools. *British Medical Journal*, **1**, 142.

Westin GW (1975) Tendon transfers about the foot, ankle, and hip in the paralysed lower extremity. *Journal of Bone and Joint Surgery*, **47(A)**, 1430.

Westin GW & DiFiore RJ (1974) Tenodesis of the tendo Achillis to the fibula for paralytic calcaneus deformity. *Journal of Bone and Joint Surgery*, **56(A)**, 1541.

Williams JJ, Graham GP, Dunne KB & Menelaus MB (1993) Late knee problems in myelomeningocele. *Journal of Pediatric Orthopaedics*, **13**, 701.

Williams PF (1965) Surgical advances in the management of deformities of the spine and lower limbs in spina bifida. *Australian and New Zealand Journal of Surgery*, **34**, 250.

Williams PF (1976) Restoration of muscle balance of the foot by transfer of the tibialis posterior. *Journal of Bone and Joint Surgery*, **58(B)**, 217.

Williams PF & Menelaus MB (1977) Triple arthrodesis by inlay grafting – a method suitable for the underformed or valgus foot. *Journal of Bone and Joint Surgery*, **59(B)**, 333.

Willson MA (1965) Multidisciplinary problems of myelomeningocele and hydrocephalus. *Physical Therapy Review*, **45**, 1139.

Wiltse LL (1972) Valgus deformity of the ankle. *Journal of Bone and Joint Surgery*, **54(A)**, 595.

Winchester P, Carollo J, Parekh R, Lutz L & Aston J (1993) A comparison of paraplegic gait performance using two types of Reciprocating Gait Orthoses. *Prosthetics and Orthotics International*, **17**, 101.

Winston K, Hall J, Johnson D & Micheli L (1977) Acute elevation of intracranial pressure following transection of non-functional spinal cord. *Clinical Orthopaedics and Related Research*, **128**, 41.

Winter RB, Moe JW & Eilers VE (1968) Congenital scoliosis: a study of 234 patients treated and untreated. *Journal of Bone and Joint Surgery*, **50(A)**, 1.

Wolf L & McLaughlin J (1992) Early motor development in infants with meningomyelocele. *Pediatric Physical Therapy*, **12**.

Wolman C & Basco DE (1994) Factors influencing self esteem and self consciousness in adolescents with spina bifida. *Journal of Adolescent Health*, **15(7)**, 543.

Wright JG, Menelaus MB, Broughton NS & Shurtleff D (1991) Natural history of knee contractures in myelomeningocele. *Journal of Pediatric Orthopaedics*, **11**, 725.

Wright JG, Menelaus MB, Broughton NS & Shurtleff D (1992) Lower extremity alignment in children with spina bifida. *Journal of Pediatric Orthopaedics*, **12**, 232.

Wynne-Davies R (1975) Congenital vertebral anomalies: aetiology and relationship to spina bifida cystica. *Journal of Medical Genetics*, **12(3)**, 280.

Yamada S, Zinke DE & Sanders D (1981) Pathophysiology of tethered cord syndrome. *Journal of Neurosurgery*, **54**, 494.

Yngve DA & Lindseth RE (1982) Effectiveness of muscle transfer in myelomeningocele hips measured by radiographic indices. *Journal of Pediatric Orthopaedics*, **2**, 121.

Yngve DA, Douglas R & Roberts JM (1984) The Reciprocating Gait Orthosis in myelomeningocele. *Journal of Pediatric Orthopaedics*, **4**, 304.

Younoszai MK (1992) Stooling problems in patients with

myelomeningocele (review). *Southern Medical Journal*, **85(7)**, 718.

Yount CC (1926) The role of the tensor fasciae femoris in certain deformities of the lower extremities. *Journal of Bone and Joint Surgery*, **8**, 171.

Zielke K (1978) *Skoliose und Kyphose*. Stuttgart: Hippokrates.

Zielke K, Stunkat R & Beaujean F (1976) Ventrale derotations – spondylese. *Archives Orthopedica Unfallchirurgica*, **85**, 257.

Ziller R (1974) Neuropathic osteolysis following arthrodesis of the ankle joint in myelodysplasia. *Beitrage zur Orthopadic und Traumatologie*, **21(7)**, 401.

Zimmerman MH, Smith CF & Oppenheim WL (1982) Supracondylar femoral extension osteotomies in the treatment of fixed flexion deformity of the knee. *Clinical Orthopaedics and Related Research*, **171**, 87.

Ziviani JM (1987) *The Performance of Handwriting in Children with Spina Bifida*. Fred & Eleanor Schowell Special Education Research Centre. Department of Education, University of Queensland, St Lucia, Queensland.

Index

6753852

3 1378 00675 3852

RY MATERIALS MUST BE RETURNED TO:
..RGE LIBRARY